T0256204

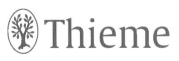

Imaging of Traumatic Brain Injury

Yoshimi Anzai, MD, MPH
Professor of Radiology
Director of Neuroradiology
Director of Head and Neck Imaging
Co-Director of the Radiology Health Service Research Section
Department of Radiology
University of Washington
Seattle, Washington

Kathleen R. Fink, MD
Assistant Professor of Neuroradiology
Department of Radiology
Harborview Medical Center
University of Washington
Seattle, Washington

Thieme
New York • Stuttgart • Delhi • Rio de Janiero

Thieme Medical Publishers, Inc.
333 Seventh Ave.
New York, NY 10001

Executive Editor: William Lamsback
Managing Editor: J. Owen Zurhellen IV
Assistant Managing Editor: Heather Allen
Senior Vice President, Editorial and Electronic Product Development:
    Cornelia Schulze
Production Editor: Sean Woznicki
International Production Director: Andreas Schabert
International Marketing Director: Fiona Henderson
Director of Sales, North America: Mike Roseman
International Sales Director: Louisa Turrell
Vice President, Finance and Accounts: Sarah Vanderbilt
President: Brian D. Scanlan
Printer: Asia Pacific Offset, Inc.

Library of Congress Cataloging-in-Publication Data

Imaging of traumatic brain injury / [edited by] Yoshimi Anzai,
Kathleen R Fink.
       p. ; cm.
   Includes bibliographic references
     ISBN 978-1-60406-728-6 (hardback) – ISBN 978-1-60406-729-3
(eISBN)
   I. Anzai, Yoshimi, editor. II. Fink, Kathleen R., editor.
   [DNLM: 1. Brain Injuries–diagnosis. 2. Brain Injuries–physiopa-
thology. 3. Neuroimaging–methods. 4. Prognosis. WL 354]
   RC387.5
   617.4'81044–dc23
                                  2014014207

Copyright © 2015 by Thieme Medical Publishers, Inc.

Thieme Publishers New York
333 Seventh Avenue, New York, NY 10001 USA
+1 800 782 3488, customerservice@thieme.com

Thieme Publishers Stuttgart
Rüdigerstrasse 14, 70469 Stuttgart, Germany
+49 [0]711 8931 421, customerservice@thieme.de

Thieme Publishers Delhi
A-12, Second Floor, Sector-2, Noida-201301
Uttar Pradesh, India
+91 120 45 566 00, customerservice@thieme.in

Thieme Publishers Rio, Thieme Publicações Ltda.
Argentina Building 16th floor, Ala A, 228 Praia do Botafogo
Rio de Janeiro 22250-040 Brazil
+55 21 3736-3631

Printed in China   5 4 3 2 1

ISBN 978-1-60406-728-6

Also available as an e-book:
eISBN 978-1-60406-729-3

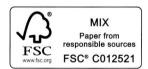

To all physicians and nurses serving for trauma patients at Harborview Medical Center, Seattle, Washington.

To my husband Satoshi and our daughter Erika for their love and support, and to my mother Kotoko Anzai who always believes in me.

Yoshimi Anzai

To my husband James, for his unwavering love and support, and to my beloved daughters Lucille and Michelle.

Kathleen R. Fink

Contents

Foreword

Traumatic brain injury is a leading cause of death and disability in the United States. The mortality and morbidity associated with traumatic brain injury have declined. Improved patient outcomes have resulted from improvements in emergency department diagnosis which leads to effective emergent treatment. CT is usually the initial imaging study performed on a patient with traumatic brain injury. Medical imaging helps to define the acute injury and, if necessary, to guide acute surgical intervention. It has also contributed to our understanding of the nature and pathophysiology of these injuries.

Overall, the use of CT in the emergency department increased more than threefold between 1996 and 2007; however when adjustments are made for variables such as severity of injury there may be little change in the utilization rate of cranial CT. Increased CT usage has likely resulted from the increased 24 hour availability of CT in emergency departments. Along with the increased use of emergent CT, has come a greater emphasis on accurate and rapid imaging interpretation. The role of the radiologist has become much more central to the health care delivery team. Radiologists who may not be specialty trained in emergency imaging or in neuroimaging are being increasingly called upon to provide a high level of contemporaneous imaging interpretation. The need to provide coordinated imaging assessment to the emergency department patient has never been greater. This book is an important and timely contribution to the field.

It is noteworthy that Dr. Anzai and Dr. Fink have compiled the latest information on traumatic brain injury in comprehensive volume. Both these neuroradiologists are well known for their many important contributions to the imaging literature. They have also included contributions from authors who have extensive experience in the imaging of traumatic brain injury.

The authors and their collaborators do not confine themselves to the imaging aspects of traumatic brain injury.

Epidemiology and decision rules are discussed in separate chapters. The special considerations of pediatric head trauma are explored. Outside the brain, but vital to the comprehensive care of the brain injured patient, are chapters detailing cerebrovascular injuries, skull base injuries, maxillofacial injuries, and orbital injuries. It is appropriate that the book concludes with a chapter about advanced imaging. Magnetic resonance techniques including diffusion tensor imaging, spectroscopy, susceptibility imaging, and functional imaging are illustrated. There are also brief discussions of magnetoencephalography and positron emission tomography. These advanced techniques have deepened our understanding of traumatic brain injury in selected patient cohorts. This chapter may serve as a preview to the next clinically relevant new imaging techniques to be applied to the care of traumatic brain injuries.

This book provides the radiologist with an important resource for the interpretation of images of the brain, face, and neck of the brain injured patient. To the clinician caring for the brain injured patient, it provides helpful guidelines for the ordering of imaging studies and insight into how the pathophysiology of injury is depicted by imaging. Those researchers studying traumatic brain injury will gain a better understanding of how the application of imaging guides therapy. To all the imagers, clinicians, and researchers interested in neurotrauma, I hope that you will enjoy having such a valuable resource.

Wayne S. Kubal, MD
President
American Society of Emergency Radiology
Professor of Medical Imaging
University of Arizona
Tucson, Arizona

Preface

Traumatic Brain Injury (TBI) is a leading cause of mortality and morbidity among youth in the United States. Patients with TBI are managed by a multidisciplinary group of medical professions, including Emergency Medicine, Trauma Surgery, Neurosurgery, Neurology, and Rehabilitation Medicine. Significant advancements in the management of TBI patients have been made in the last several years. Despite marked improvement of clinical care, however, many patients still live with disabilities and suffer the sequelae of TBI, which may significantly impact their quality of life.

Nearly all of the materials in this book came from Harborview Medical Center where we have the tremendous pleasure and privilege to work as neuroradiology faculty. Harborview Medicine Center is an essential entity of UW Medicine, and is the only Level I adult and pediatric trauma center in the state of Washington. Harborview also serves as a regional trauma center for Alaska, Idaho and Montana. Harborview Medical Center is a county hospital (owned by King County, Washington) and is governed by the University of Washington board of trustees. Annually, it provides over $200 million in charity care and serves as the one of the most prestigious institutions fighting against health disparity. This textbook draws upon our extensive experience at the Level I trauma center at Harborview Medical Center.

This textbook is designed to target a large audience, including radiology residents and fellows, as well as neuroradiologists in various clinical settings. It will also appeal to general radiologists that interpret imaging studies for trauma patients and other medical subspecialties, such as Emergency Medicine, Neurosurgery, and Neurology. This book was designed to provide an "image rich" textbook aligned with the recent emphasis on the case-based learning style. It is intended to cover a large population of TBI case materials beyond traumatic brain injury, including penetrating injury, pediatric TBI, extracranial injuries such as maxillofacial injury, orbital injury, and skull base injury. Written by experts in the field, this textbook contains over 250 high quality images with numerous pearls and summary boxes for easy and quick reference in the clinical setting.

Without question, imaging plays a significant role in the management of TBI patients. CT *still* serves as primary imaging study to triage TBI patients who need emergent surgery from those who can be safely observed in the acute trauma setting. Brain MR is well known to demonstrate more TBI lesions than CT. Brain MR imaging has been utilized increasingly in TBI patients as a problem solving tool as well as a means to predict outcome of patients with severe TBI. Some challenges remain, such as being able to accurately detect those patients with mild forms of TBI who are suffering from prolonged post-traumatic symptoms where CT or conventional brain MR reveals no abnormality. Advanced MR imaging and physiologic imaging tools are expected to play a larger role in the future to address this issue.

We hope readers find this book to be a valuable resource for the neuroimaging of the acutely injured patient, whether read cover to cover, or referenced when questions arise.

Acknowledgments

We would like to thank all of physicians at Harborview Medical Center who have demonstrated ongoing dedication and commitment to the care of traumatic brain injury patients, and their passion to improve diagnosis and management of TBI patients. We would also like to acknowledge all of the patients who are treated at HMC and in whose care we have had the privilege to participate.

Contributors

Jalal B. Andre, MD
Director of Neurological MRI
Harborview Medical Center
Assistant Professor of Neuroradiology
Department of Radiology
University of Washington
Seattle, Washington

Yoshimi Anzai, MD, MPH
Professor of Radiology
Director of Neuroradiology
Director of Head and Neck Imaging
Co-Director of the Radiology Health Service Research Section
Department of Radiology
University of Washington
Seattle, Washington

Jayson L. Benjert, DO
Assistant Professor of Neuroradiology
Department of Radiology
VA Puget Sound Health Care System
Seattle, Washington

Wendy A. Cohen, MD
Professor of Neuroradiology
Vice-Chair and Director, Radiology
Harborview Medical Center
Department of Radiology
Harborview Medical Center and University of Washington
Seattle, Washington

Roberta W. Dalley, MD
Associate Professor of Neuroradiology
Department of Radiology
University of Washington
Seattle, Washington

Kathleen R. Fink, MD
Assistant Professor of Neuroradiology
Department of Radiology
Harborview Medical Center and University of Washington
Seattle, Washington

Sarah J. Foster, MBBS
Department of Radiology
University of Washington
Seattle, Washington

Shivani Gupta, MD
Clinical Instructor
Faculty of Medicine
Department of Radiology
University of British Columbia
Vancouver, British Columbia

Nicholas D. Krause, MD
Partner Radiologist
Medical Imaging Northwest
Tacoma, Washington

Robert Linville, MD
Department of Radiology
University of Washington
Seattle, Washington

Carrie P. Marder, MD, PhD
Acting Instructor of Neuroradiology
Department of Radiology
University of Washington
Seattle, Washington

Mahmud Mossa-Basha, MD
Assistant Professor of Neuroradiology
Department of Radiology
University of Washington
Seattle, Washington

Jeffrey P. Otjen, MD
Assistant Professor of Pediatric Radiology
Department of Radiology
Seattle Children's Hospital and University of Washington
Seattle, Washington

Bahman S. Roudsari, MD, MPH, PhD
Department of Radiology
University of Washington
Seattle, Washington

Jonathan O. Swanson, MD
Assistant Professor of Pediatric Radiology
Department of Radiology
Seattle Children's Hospital and University of Washington
Seattle, Washington

1 Epidemiology of Traumatic Brain Injuries in the United States

Bahman S. Roudsari and Yoshimi Anzai

1.1 Overall Incidence

Traumatic brain injury (TBI) is one of the leading causes of injury-related mortality and morbidity worldwide.[1–3] In the United States, more than 1.7 million people sustain a TBI each year.[2] Of those, 1.4 million are treated and released from the emergency department (ED), more than 270,000 are hospitalized, and more than 53,000 die as a result of their injury.[1–3] In Europe, 235 per 100,000 individuals sustain TBI annually.[4] The World Health Organization estimates that by the year 2020, more than 10 million people will incur TBI annually worldwide.[5] Between 2002 and 2006, an average of 100 million ED visits and 37 million admissions were reported each year, of which 3 and 5% were TBI related, respectively. During the same period, 30% of injury-related deaths in the United States were attributable to TBIs.[5]

Although no recent studies have evaluated the incidence of TBIs, Faul and Langlois demonstrated an increasing trend in the incidence of TBI-related ED visits and hospital admissions in the United States from 2002 through 2006.[5,6] The incidence of TBI-related ED visits increased from 401 to 468 per 100,000, and the hospitalization rate increased from 86 to 94 per 100,000.[5,6]

1.1.1 Children

For the pediatric population, TBIs are of special importance because of their high incidence compared with other disabling diseases as well as their lifetime consequences.[7] In the United States, each year, more than 600,000 emergency department visits, 60,000 hospitalizations, and 6000 fatalities in patients aged 0 to 20 years are attributed to TBIs. [5,8,9] ► Fig. 1.1 summarizes the TBI-related ED visits, hospitalizations, and deaths from 2002 to 2006 according to age group based on the study performed by Faul and colleagues.[5]

1.1.2 Older Adults

Whereas recent studies suggest that the incidence of TBIs in children and young adults has decreased as a result of the implementation of injury-prevention programs, the opposite is true for older adults.[10] The aging of the population, the growing number of senior drivers, multidrug use by seniors, and the risk of drug-related falls are among the factors contributing to the increasing incidence of TBIs in the older adult population.[11,12] Besides being at higher risk for TBIs compared with younger patients, older adults are more susceptible to detrimental consequences of TBI, such as longer hospital stays, a higher rate of intensive care unit admissions, higher mortality rates, and poorer functional status at discharge after a moderate to severe TBI.[13–17]

1.1.3 War Veterans

It is well known that military personnel are susceptible to TBI, but since the September 11, 2001, attacks, the types of TBIs among soldiers have changed. A large number of U.S. soldiers in the Afghanistan and Iraq Wars have been exposed to new generations of explosives.[18] Because of advances in body-armor technology, faster evacuations from the scene of injury, and improvements in surgical care, the "at-scene" fatality rate has decreased, but the number of soldiers surviving disastrous TBIs while sustaining substantial disabilities has increased.[18–21] Because of the high frequency of TBIs in recent wars, they are considered the "signature injury of modern military operations." The Departments of Defense and Veterans Affairs have adopted special strategies to screen for TBIs, especially for veterans of the Afghanistan and Iraq Wars.[18,22]

1.2 Risk Factors

Among adults in the United States, alcohol is the most important modifiable risk factor for injuries, including TBIs.[23] The incidence of alcohol-related injuries has not decreased significantly in the past two decades, although alcohol-related driver fatalities remained relatively unchanged between 1999 and 2006, as reported by Roudsari et al.[23]

In recent years, the use of mobile devices has become an increasingly significant contributor to road-traffic crashes resulting in TBI.[24] A large study conducted in the United States and Europe revealed that among drivers 18 to 64 years of age, the prevalence of talking on a cell phone or using a mobile device for texting and e-mail while driving at least once in the past 30 days ranged from 21% in the United Kingdom to 69% in the

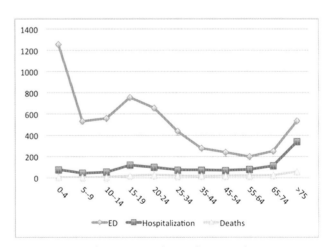

Fig. 1.1 Estimated average annual rates of traumatic brain injury–related emergency department (ED) visits, hospitalizations, and deaths by age group using the U.S. population in 2000 as the baseline for rate calculation, United States, 2002–2006. (Used with permission from Faul MXL, Wald MM, Coronado VG. Traumatic Brain Injury in the United States, Emergency Department Visits, Hospitalizations and Deaths 2002–2006. Atlanta, GA: Centers for Disease Control and Prevention, National Center for Injury Prevention and Control; 2010.)

United States. Distracted driving has become one of the most significant risk factors for TBI. Similarly, the use of mobile devices contributes to an increased incidence of pedestrian injuries.[25] When pedestrians use the Internet on a mobile device, their behaviors become significantly higher risk.

In the United States, the three major nonmodifiable risk factors for TBIs are age, sex, and race or ethnicity. Overall, children younger than 5 years are at the highest risk of TBI, followed by adolescents (i.e., 15 to 19 years) and adults 75 years and older.[5] Older adults (both men and women) are at higher risk for TBI-related mortality.[5] Similar to other types of injuries, men are at greater risk for TBI than women; in fact, about 60% of all TBIs are suffered by males.[5] ▶ Fig. 1.2 illustrates TBI-related ED visits

(▶ Fig. 1.2a), hospitalization (▶ Fig. 1.2b), and deaths (▶ Fig. 1.2c) based on age group and sex in the United States between 2002 and 2006.[5]

From 2002 through 2006, African Americans had the highest unadjusted ED visit and hospitalization rates compared with whites and American Indians, Alaska Natives, and Asians (▶ Fig. 1.3) but slightly lower TBI-related mortality rates (16.7 in 100,000) than whites (18.2 in 100,000). American Indians, Alaska Natives, and Asians had the lowest TBI-related mortality rates (10.1 in 100,000).[5]

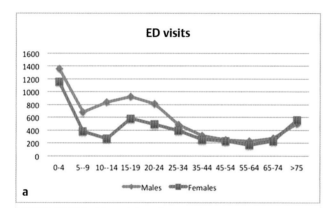
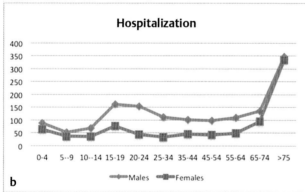
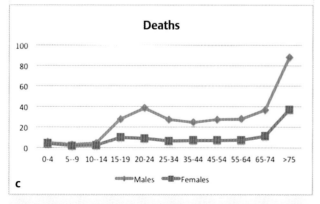

Fig. 1.2 Unadjusted emergency department (ED) visits (a), hospitalization (b), and mortality rates (c) per 100,000 for traumatic brain injuries in the United States, 2002–2006, categorized based on age group and sex using the U.S. population in 2000 as the baseline for the rate calculations.

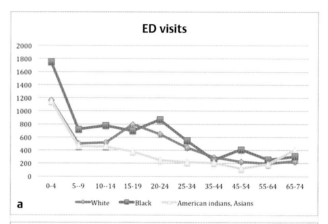
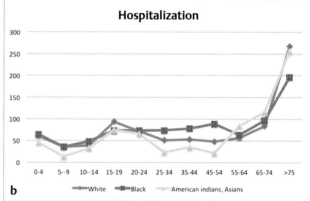
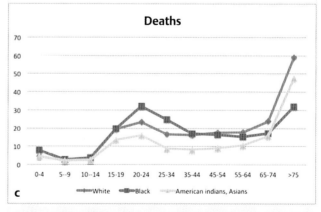

Fig. 1.3 Unadjusted emergency department (ED) visits (a), hospitalization (b), and mortality rates (c) for traumatic brain injury in the United States, 2002–2006, categorized based on age group and race or ethnicity using the U.S. population in 2000 as the baseline for the rate calculations.

1.3 Underlying Causes of Traumatic Brain Injury

The underlying cause of TBIs depends largely on the age group involved. For children and older adults, falls are the most common mechanism of TBI. For young and middle-aged adults, motor-vehicle or motorcycle collisions and assault are more prominent.[5] Concussion, or so-called mild TBI (mTBI), is the most common cause of TBI among young athletes. Concussion proves increasingly complex to deal with and may not be "mild" as the name implies.[26] This topic is discussed in detail in Chapter 12.

1.4 Short- and Long-Term Consequences of Traumatic Brain Injury

1.4.1 Mortality Rate

Most studies that have evaluated the effectiveness of preventive strategies for TBI have considered the mortality rate the main outcome of interest.[27] Mortality is easy to measure and has a minimal chance of misclassification; therefore, it is an appealing target for most injury-prevention programs. Studies conducted by the Centers for Disease Control and Prevention have demonstrated that between 1989 and 2007, the TBI-related mortality rate declined from 21.9 in 100,000 to 17.8 in 100,000.[2,28] However, not all age groups have experienced the same declining trend in mortality rates. Coronado and colleagues found that between 1997 and 2007, the mortality rate for TBIs decreased significantly among patients 0 to 44 years old but increased significantly among patients 75 and older.[2] Recent analyses have shown men to be three times more likely to die of TBI-related causes (28.8 in 100,000) than women (9.1 in 100,000).[2]

1.4.2 Children

Multiple studies have discussed the neuropsychological consequences of TBIs among children.[29-36] Previous studies suggested that reorganization of the brain after a TBI can minimize the short- and long-term consequences in a child's "flexible" brain. However, new findings indicate that childhood injury could have more detrimental consequences than previously expected, not only because of damage to the available brain tissue, but also because of disruption of developmental milestones, which could interrupt the process of acquiring new skills at a developmentally appropriate rate.[27,29,37-39] Pediatric neuropsychological impairments after a TBI can be categorized into two major categories: educational impairments and social or behavioral impairments.[35,40,41] Studies have estimated that up to one third of children might require support into their adolescence and adulthood because of social and educational impairments.[29]

A number of studies have demonstrated that the severity of injury is likely the most important factor in predicting future functional impairment.[31,37,42,43] The association between the severity of injury and functional impairments among mTBI patients remains open to debate. Although the vast majority of mTBI patients recover from injury, 15 to 20% suffer from reduced intellectual capabilities, attention disorder, memory impairment, linguistic problems, and academic failure in the postinjury years.[30,36,37,42,44,45] Fewer longitudinal studies have expanded our knowledge in regard to the long-term consequences of TBI on child development. Rivara and colleagues followed up on 729 pediatric patients with moderate to severe TBIs for 2 years.[27] They found that "the quality of life for children with moderate or severe TBI was lower at all follow-up times compared with baseline, but there was some improvement during the first 2 years after injury."[27]

Anderson and colleagues conducted one of the few long-term follow-up studies of TBI patients.[29] They found that after 10 years, the relationship between injury severity and cognitive impairment was most significant in the acute postinjury phase and much less evident 10 years later. Reports have conflicting conclusions about whether younger age at occurrence of the trauma is associated with poorer outcomes.[29,43,46]

1.4.3 Older Adults and Falls

Several studies have demonstrated higher mortality rates, longer hospital stays, and poorer functional outcomes in older adults compared with younger patients suffering from TBI.[14,47-50] Older patients also need more intense rehabilitation to recover their functional status and prevent permanent disability after injury.[50] Previous studies identified several risk factors for poor outcomes among older post-TBI patients, including but not limited to age,[14,47,50] male sex, minority status,[51] injury severity, comorbidities, and taking anticoagulation medication at the time of TBI.[49]

1.4.4 Other Long-Term Consequences

Quality of Life

Although objective measures such as length of hospital or intensive care unit stay and hospital expenses are easy to measure, they do not reflect the actual burden of TBIs on patients and their families. One factor often ignored in outcome studies is the quality of life after a TBI.[52-54] Pagulayan and colleagues evaluated the quality of life of TBI patients at 1 month, 3 years, and 5 years after TBI by using the Quality of Life (QoL) Questionnaire.[54] They concluded that although the physical components of QoL improved over time, the psychosocial domains remained lower than expected for TBI victims.[54]

In China, Hu et al followed up on 312 patients with moderate to severe TBI and used the Health-Related Quality of Life (HRQoL) Questionnaire to measure their quality of life compared with a control group of 381 patients without a history of TBI admitted at the same institution.[55] They found that despite rapid improvement in the HRQoL during the first 6 months after injury, TBI patients had significantly lower scores for all domains compared with their non-TBI counterparts. Severity of injury, female sex, and older age were among the main factors associated with poor quality of life in this study.[55]

Dementia

Although some studies have suggested an association between Alzheimer disease and TBI,[56,57] the mechanism for such an association is not well understood. In about 30% of TBI-

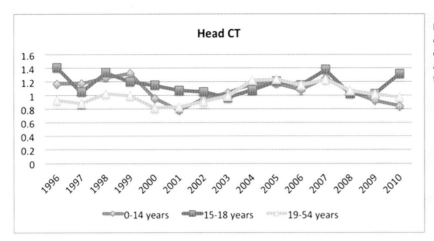

Fig. 1.4 Average number of computed tomograms (CT) of the head performed per patient during each hospitalization for each age category at Harborview Medical Center, Seattle, Washington, 1996–2010.

related fatalities, β-amyloid plaques, one of the pathological features of Alzheimer disease, were found.[57] It remains controversial whether TBI leads to Alzheimer disease. Not all dementia patients have a history of TBI, but survivors of TBI invariably develop dementia later in life. The combination of TBI and underlying brain changes associated with aging may facilitate development of cognitive disorders.[58,59] It has been suggested that maintaining or increasing cognitive reserve may help to prevent or delay the clinical manifestation of dementing disorders among TBI patients.

Depression and Other Psychiatric Disorders

Numerous studies report a higher prevalence of depression among TBI victims. The reported 1-year prevalence of depression varies from 12 to 50%.[60–62] Bombardier and colleagues reported that 53% of hospitalized trauma patients at a level I trauma center had major depressive disorder.[60] In addition, TBIs, both directly and indirectly through depression, have been associated with suicide.[63]

Costs

Unfortunately, despite the importance of high TBI-related morbidity and mortality rates, limited studies have focused on the financial burden of TBIs for patients, their families, and society as a whole.[2,64–67] Whereas mortality rates and the cost of hospital care are easy to examine, the indirect costs, including loss of productivity for patients and their families and short and long-term disabilities, are difficult to measure. It is estimated that in the United States three to five million individuals are suffering from long-term consequences of TBIs.[68–70]

To date, the study by Finkelstein and colleagues is the most comprehensive evaluation of the socioeconomic burden of TBIs; they estimated the annual cost of TBIs, including direct (medical and rehabilitation) and indirect (including loss of productivity) costs, to exceed $60 billion (in $U.S., year 2000).[65] However, these estimates do not include the growing number of war-related TBIs from the Iraq and Afghanistan Wars. In addition, their estimates do not include those who did not seek medical care. Sosin and colleagues have estimated that approximately one fourth of all TBI victims do not seek any medical care; as a result, the short- and long-term consequences of these injuries are not well understood.[71]

1.5 Use of Imaging in the Management of Traumatic Brain Injury

Computed tomography (CT) is the imaging modality of choice for the management of acute TBIs. Although several studies have criticized the escalating trend in the use of CT in the United States, information regarding its use for trauma patients is scarce. Using data from a level I trauma center in the United States, Roudsari et al demonstrated a slight increase in the use of head CTs between 1996 and 2006.[72] Using data from the only level I trauma center in Northwest United States, the same group of researchers observed little change in the use of head CTs between 1996 and 2010 after adjustment for confounding variables such as age, sex, mechanism and severity of injury, and length of stay in the hospital and intensive care unit stay (▶ Fig. 1.4).[73] Unfortunately, no multicenter study has been performed to evaluate variability in the use of imaging for trauma patients in the United States.

The association between repeat head CTs and outcome in patients with TBI has been the focus of debate. Thorson and colleagues reported that repeat head CT after mTBI and positive first head CT revealed progression of injury in 30% of patients before clinical deterioration of neurologic symptoms helped in the early identification of patients requiring craniotomy.[74] Another study comprising 1019 consecutive TBI patients at a level I trauma center reported that worsening findings on the scheduled repeat head CT for patients with an abnormal first CT more likely result in neurosurgical intervention compared with a stable scheduled second head CT.[59]

On the other hand, some investigators have reported that routine repeat head CT is not indicated for mTBI patients, even those whose initial head CT was positive for mTBI. Three factors independently predicted a worse repeat head CT: age 65 years or older, Glasgow Coma Scale score lower than 15, and multiple traumatic intracranial lesions noted on initial head CT.[75]

Magnetic resonance imaging (MRI) is not commonly used in the acute management of TBIs; however, MRI has critical value in the diagnosis and management of injuries that cannot be sufficiently evaluated by CT, such as diffuse axonal injuries. Unfortunately, no study has evaluated the evolving role of MRI in the setting of acute TBI. Extensive research is ongoing to detect imaging biomarkers for mTBI in terms of which patients remain symptomatic after mTBI and concussion. Many studies are currently based on the group comparison studies featuring diffusion tensor imaging, magnetic resonance perfusion, and resting-state functional imaging studies, but these topics are beyond the scope of this chapter and are discussed in detail in Chapter 12.

References

[1] Coronado VG, Thomas KE, Sattin RW, Johnson RL. The CDC traumatic brain injury surveillance system: characteristics of persons aged 65 years and older hospitalized with a TBI. J Head Trauma Rehabil 2005; 20: 215–228

[2] Coronado VG, Xu L, Basavaraju SV et al. Centers for Disease Control and Prevention (CDC). Surveillance for traumatic brain injury-related deaths—United States, 1997–2007. MMWR Surveill Summ 2011; 60: 1–32

[3] Corrigan JD, Harrison-Felix C, Bogner J, Dijkers M, Terrill MS, Whiteneck G. Systematic bias in traumatic brain injury outcome studies because of loss to follow-up. Arch Phys Med Rehabil 2003; 84: 153–160

[4] Tagliaferri F, Compagnone C, Korsic M, Servadei F, Kraus J. A systematic review of brain injury epidemiology in Europe. Acta Neurochir (Wien) 2006; 148: 255–268

[5] Faul MXL, Wald MM, Coronado VG. Traumatic Brain Injury in the United States, Emergency Department Visits, Hospitalizations and Deaths 2002–2006. Atlanta, GA: Centers for Disease Control and Prevention, National Center for Injury Prevention and Control; 2010

[6] Langlois JA, Rutland-Brown W, Wald MM. The epidemiology and impact of traumatic brain injury: a brief overview. J Head Trauma Rehabil 2006; 21: 375–378

[7] Stanley RM, Bonsu BK, Zhao W, Ehrlich PF, Rogers AJ, Xiang H. US estimates of hospitalized children with severe traumatic brain injury: implications for clinical trials. Pediatrics 2012; 129: e24–e30

[8] Centers for Disease Control and Prevention (CDC). Traumatic Brain Injury in the United States: Assessing Outcomes in Children. Atlanta, GA: CDC, National Center for Injury Prevention and Control; 2006

[9] Schneier AJ, Shields BJ, Hostetler SG, Xiang H, Smith GA. Incidence of pediatric traumatic brain injury and associated hospital resource utilization in the United States. Pediatrics 2006; 118: 483–492

[10] Ramanathan DM, McWilliams N, Schatz P, Hillary FG. Epidemiological shifts in elderly traumatic brain injury: 18-year trends in Pennsylvania. J Neurotrauma 2012; 29: 1371–1378

[11] Federal Highway Administration. Highway Statistics. Washington, DC: U.S. Department of Transportation; 1999

[12] Federal Highway Administration. Highway Statistics. Washington, DC: U.S. Department of Transportation; 2009

[13] Cagetti B, Cossu M, Pau A, Rivano C, Viale G. The outcome from acute subdural and epidural intracranial haematomas in very elderly patients. Br J Neurosurg 1992; 6: 227–231

[14] Hukkelhoven CW, Steyerberg EW, Rampen AJ et al. Patient age and outcome following severe traumatic brain injury: an analysis of 5600 patients. J Neurosurg 2003; 99: 666–673

[15] Mosenthal AC, Lavery RF, Addis M et al. Isolated traumatic brain injury: age is an independent predictor of mortality and early outcome. J Trauma 2002; 52: 907–911

[16] Pennings JL, Bachulis BL, Simons CT, Slazinski T. Survival after severe brain injury in the aged. Arch Surg 1993; 128: 787–793

[17] Susman M, DiRusso SM, Sullivan T et al. Traumatic brain injury in the elderly: increased mortality and worse functional outcome at discharge despite lower injury severity. J Trauma 2002; 53: 219–224

[18] Sayer NA. Traumatic brain injury and its neuropsychiatric sequelae in war veterans. Annu Rev Med 2012; 63: 405–419

[19] Sponheim SR, McGuire KA, Kang SS et al. Evidence of disrupted functional connectivity in the brain after combat-related blast injury. Neuroimage 2011; 54 s uppl 1: S21–S29

[20] Mac Donald CL, Johnson AM, Cooper D et al. Detection of blast-related traumatic brain injury in U.S. military personnel. N Engl J Med 2011; 364: 2091–2100

[21] Carlson KF, Kehle SM, Meis LA et al. Prevalence, assessment, and treatment of mild traumatic brain injury and posttraumatic stress disorder: a systematic review of the evidence. J Head Trauma Rehabil 2011; 26: 103–115

[22] DePalma RG, Burris DG, Champion HR, Hodgson MJ. Blast injuries. N Engl J Med 2005; 352: 1335–1342

[23] Roudsari B, Ramisetty-Mikler S, Rodriguez LA. Ethnicity, age, and trends in alcohol-related driver fatalities in the United States. Traffic Inj Prev 2009; 10: 410–414

[24] Centers for Disease Control and Prevention (CDC). Mobile device use while driving—United States and seven European countries, 2011. MMWR Morb Mortal Wkly Rep 2013; 62: 177–182

[25] Byington KW, Schwebel DC. Effects of mobile Internet use on college student pedestrian injury risk. Accid Anal Prev 2013; 51: 78–83

[26] Slobounov S, Gay M, Johnson B, Zhang K. Concussion in athletics: ongoing clinical and brain imaging research controversies. Brain Imaging Behav 2012; 6: 224–243

[27] Rivara FP, Koepsell TD, Wang J et al. Disability 3, 12, and 24 months after traumatic brain injury among children and adolescents. Pediatrics 2011; 128: e1129–e1138

[28] Centers for Disease Control and Prevention (CDC). Surveillance for Traumatic Brain Injury Deaths—United States, 1989–1998. Atlanta, GA: CDC; 2002

[29] Anderson V, Catroppa C, Godfrey C, Rosenfeld JV. Intellectual ability 10 years after traumatic brain injury in infancy and childhood: what predicts outcome? J Neurotrauma 2012; 29: 143–153

[30] Babikian T, Asarnow R. Neurocognitive outcomes and recovery after pediatric TBI: meta-analytic review of the literature. Neuropsychology 2009; 23: 283–296

[31] Ewing-Cobbs L, Barnes M, Fletcher JM, Levin HS, Swank PR, Song J. Modeling of longitudinal academic achievement scores after pediatric traumatic brain injury. Dev Neuropsychol. 2004; 25: 107–133

[32] Fay GC, Jaffe KM, Polissar NL, Liao S, Rivara JB, Martin KM. Outcome of pediatric traumatic brain injury at three years: a cohort study. Arch Phys Med Rehabil 1994; 75: 733–741

[33] Fay TB, Yeates KO, Wade SL, Drotar D, Stancin T, Taylor HG. Predicting longitudinal patterns of functional deficits in children with traumatic brain injury. Neuropsychology 2009; 23: 271–282

[34] Kirkwood MW, Yeates KO. Neurobehavioral outcomes of pediatric mild traumatic brain injury. In: Anderson V, Yeates KO, eds. Pediatric Traumatic Brain Injury: New Frontiers in Clinical and Translational Research. Cambridge UP: Cambridge, UK. 2010: 94–117

[35] Muscara F, Catroppa C, Eren S, Anderson V. The impact of injury severity on long-term social outcome following paediatric traumatic brain injury. Neuropsychol Rehabil 2009; 19: 541–561

[36] Yeates KO, Swift E, Taylor HG et al. Short- and long-term social outcomes following pediatric traumatic brain injury. J Int Neuropsychol Soc 2004; 10: 412–426

[37] Anderson V, Catroppa C, Morse S, Haritou F, Rosenfeld J. Functional plasticity or vulnerability after early brain injury? Pediatrics 2005; 116: 1374–1382

[38] Anderson V, Catroppa C, Morse S, Haritou F, Rosenfeld JV. Intellectual outcome from preschool traumatic brain injury: a 5-year prospective, longitudinal study. Pediatrics 2009; 124: e1064–e1071

[39] Giza CC, Prins ML. Is being plastic fantastic? Mechanisms of altered plasticity after developmental traumatic brain injury. Dev Neurosci 2006; 28: 364–379

[40] Fletcher JM, Levin HS, Lachar D et al. Behavioral outcomes after pediatric closed head injury: relationships with age, severity, and lesion size. J Child Neurol 1996; 11: 283–290

[41] Muscara F, Catroppa C, Anderson V. The impact of injury severity on executive function 7–10 years following pediatric traumatic brain injury. Dev Neuropsychol 2008; 33: 623–636

[42] Ewing-Cobbs L, Brookshire B, Scott MA, Fletcher JM. Children's narratives following traumatic brain injury: linguistic structure, cohesion, and thematic recall. Brain Lang 1998; 61: 395–419

[43] Ewing-Cobbs L, Fletcher JM, Levin HS, Francis DJ, Davidson K, Miner ME. Longitudinal neuropsychological outcome in infants and preschoolers with traumatic brain injury. J Int Neuropsychol Soc 1997; 3: 581–591

[44] Catroppa C, Anderson VA, Muscara F et al. Educational skills: long-term outcome and predictors following paediatric traumatic brain injury. Neuropsychol Rehabil 2009; 19: 716–732

[45] Yeates KO, Taylor HG, Rusin J et al. Longitudinal trajectories of postconcussive symptoms in children with mild traumatic brain injuries and their relationship to acute clinical status. Pediatrics 2009; 123: 735–743

[46] Anderson V, Moore C. Age at injury as a predictor of outcome following pediatric head injury: a longitudinal perspective. Child Neuropsychology 1995; 1: 187–202

[47] Bouras T, Stranjalis G, Korfias S, Andrianakis I, Pitaridis M, Sakas DE. Head injury mortality in a geriatric population: differentiating an "edge" age group with better potential for benefit than older poor-prognosis patients. J Neurotrauma 2007; 24: 1355–1361

[48] Fletcher AE, Khalid S, Mallonee S. The epidemiology of severe traumatic brain injury among persons 65 years of age and older in Oklahoma, 1992–2003. Brain Inj 2007; 21: 691–699

[49] Utomo WK, Gabbe BJ, Simpson PM, Cameron PA. Predictors of in-hospital mortality and 6-month functional outcomes in older adults after moderate to severe traumatic brain injury. Injury 2009; 40: 973–977

[50] LeBlanc J, de Guise E, Gosselin N, Feyz M. Comparison of functional outcome following acute care in young, middle-aged and elderly patients with traumatic brain injury. Brain Inj 2006; 20: 779–790

[51] Arango-Lasprilla JC, Rosenthal M, Deluca J et al. Traumatic brain injury and functional outcomes: does minority status matter? Brain Inj 2007; 21: 701–708

[52] Bullinger M, Azouvi P, Brooks N et al. TBI Consensus Group. Quality of life in patients with traumatic brain injury-basic issues, assessment and recommendations. Restor Neurol Neurosci 2002; 20: 111–124

[53] Dawson DR, Levine B, Schwartz M, et al. Quality of life following traumatic brain injury: a prospective study Brain Cogn 2000; 44: 35–39

[54] Pagulayan KF, Temkin NR, Machamer J, Dikmen SS. A longitudinal study of health-related quality of life after traumatic brain injury. Arch Phys Med Rehabil 2006; 87: 611–618

[55] Hu XB, Feng Z, Fan YC, Xiong ZY, Huang QW. Health-related quality-of-life after traumatic brain injury: a 2-year follow-up study in Wuhan, China. Brain Inj 2012; 26: 183–187

[56] Nemetz PN, Leibson C, Naessens JM et al. Traumatic brain injury and time to onset of Alzheimer's disease: a population-based study. Am J Epidemiol 1999; 149: 32–40

[57] Sivanandam TM, Thakur MK. Traumatic brain injury: a risk factor for Alzheimer's disease. Neurosci Biobehav Rev 2012; 36: 1376–1381

[58] Moretti L, Cristofori I, Weaver SM, Chau A, Portelli JN, Grafman J. Cognitive decline in older adults with a history of traumatic brain injury. Lancet Neurol 2012; 11: 1103–1112

[59] Moretti L, Cristofori I, Weaver SM, Chau A, Portelli JN, Grafman J. Cognitive decline in older adults with a history of traumatic brain injury. Lancet Neurol 2012; 11: 1103–1112

[60] Bombardier CH, Rimmele CT, Zintel H. The magnitude and correlates of alcohol and drug use before traumatic brain injury. Arch Phys Med Rehabil 2002; 83: 1765–1773

[61] Fann JR, Katon WJ, Uomoto JM, Esselman PC. Psychiatric disorders and functional disability in outpatients with traumatic brain injuries. Am J Psychiatry 1995; 152: 1493–1499

[62] Jorge RE, Robinson RG, Arndt SV, Starkstein SE, Forrester AW, Geisler F. Depression following traumatic brain injury: a 1 year longitudinal study. J Affect Disord 1993; 27: 233–243

[63] Teasdale TW, Engberg AW. Suicide after traumatic brain injury: a population study. J Neurol Neurosurg Psychiatry 2001; 71: 436–440

[64] Brewer-Smyth K, Burgess AW, Shults J. Physical and sexual abuse, salivary cortisol, and neurologic correlates of violent criminal behavior in female prison inmates. Biol Psychiatry 2004; 55: 21–31

[65] Finkelstein EA, Corso PS, Miller TR. The Incidence and Economic Burden of Injuries in the United States. New York, NY: Oxford University Press; 2006

[66] Kushel MB, Hahn JA, Evans JL, Bangsberg DR, Moss AR. Revolving doors: imprisonment among the homeless and marginally housed population. Am J Public Health 2005; 95: 1747–1752

[67] Silver JM, Yudofsky SC, Anderson KE. Aggressive disorders. In: Silver JM, McAllister TW, Yudofsky SC, eds. Textbook of Traumatic Brain Injury. Washington, DC: American Psychiatric Publishing. 2005: 259–277

[68] Centers for Disease Control and Prevention (CDC). Traumatic Brain Injury in the United States: A Report to Congress. Atlanta, GA: U.S. Department of Health and Human Services, CDC; 1999

[69] Selassie AW, Zaloshnja E, Langlois JA, Miller T, Jones P, Steiner C. Incidence of long-term disability following traumatic brain injury hospitalization, United States, 2003. J Head Trauma Rehabil 2008; 23: 123–131

[70] Zaloshnja E, Miller T, Langlois JA, Selassie AW. Prevalence of long-term disability from traumatic brain injury in the civilian population of the United States, 2005. J Head Trauma Rehabil 2008; 23: 394–400

[71] Sosin DM, Sniezek JE, Thurman DJ. Incidence of mild and moderate brain injury in the United States, 1991. Brain Inj 1996; 10: 47–54

[72] Roudsari B, Moore DS, Jarvik JG. Trend in the utilization of CT for adolescents admitted to an adult level I trauma center. J Am Coll Radiol 2010; 7: 796–801

[73] Roudsari BS, Psoter KJ, Vavilala MS, Mack CD, Jarvik JG. CT use in hospitalized pediatric trauma patients: 15-year trends in a level I pediatric and adult trauma center. Radiology 2013; 267: 479–486

[74] Thorson CM, Van Haren RM, Otero CA et al. Repeat head computed tomography after minimal brain injury identifies the need for craniotomy in the absence of neurologic change. J Trauma Acute Care Surg 2013; 74: 967–975

[75] Thomas BW, Mejia VA, Maxwell RA et al. Scheduled repeat CT scanning for traumatic brain injury remains important in assessing head injury progression. J Am Coll Surg 2010; 210: 824–832

2 Evidence-Based Imaging and Prediction Rules: Who Should Get Imaging for Mild Traumatic Brain Injury?

Mahmud Mossa-Basha

2.1 Introduction

It is estimated that more than 1.3 million people are treated for mild traumatic brain injury (mTBI) in emergency departments (EDs) in the United States each year.[1] Although most patients with mTBI can be sent home after a brief period of observation, a small proportion will show neurologic deterioration and may require hospitalization or, rarely, neurosurgical intervention. It has been reported that 10 to 15% of patients with mTBI whose Glasgow Coma Scale (GCS) scores of 15 will have acute abnormalities on noncontrast head computed tomography (CT), but only 1% of this group will have lesions that require intervention.[1-5] Between 5 and 15% of mTBI patients will have persistent disability 1 year after the initial injury, including persistent headaches, cognitive impairments, and difficulties with complex tasks.[6,7] Some patients with mTBI will not be able to return to routine activities and work for prolonged periods, taxing the U.S. economy an estimated 17 billion dollars yearly.[8] In patients with clinically important brain injury, CT imaging can provide an efficient and accurate diagnostic tool such that neurosurgical intervention can prevent adverse outcomes from intracranial hemorrhage, cerebral herniation, or hydrocephalus.

Overuse of CT in the evaluation of mTBI exposes the patient and the health care system to unnecessary costs, incurring $750 million in charges.[9] More than one million head CT scans are performed in the United States in the setting of mTBI, most secondary to falls or motor-vehicle accidents, and approximately 90 to 95% of these examinations are negative.[1,8-11] In recent years, there has been a fivefold increase in the use of head CT in the setting of mTBI, without an increase in the diagnosis of life-threatening conditions or the rates of hospital admissions.[12,13] A part of imaging overuse in the setting of mTBI is related to medical legal concerns, exemplified by the fact that states that have passed tort reform laws have the lowest ED CT imaging use rates for mTBI.

In addition to the health care costs, unnecessary head CT imposes ionizing radiation on the head, which is a serious concern, especially for pediatric trauma patients. Although the brain is not a radiosensitive organ and the radiation dose of a routine head CT is relatively low, approximately 2 millisieverts (similar to a chest radiograph), judicious use of CT scans is nevertheless essential. The cancer-related risk of ionizing radiation is age and gender specific, but it is estimated that there is one radiation-related cancer per 4360 to 14,680 head CT scans in adult patients, depending on age and sex.[14]

There is variability in the nomenclature used to describe mTBI, as well as the defining criteria and classification. Terms such as *minor TBI, mild TBI, concussion,* and *low-risk TBI* are used interchangeably. Most are classified as minimal or minor to mild; some define minimal injuries as having suffered no loss of consciousness or post-traumatic amnesia (LOC or PTA) and typically not requiring hospitalization. There are many definitions of mTBI, with minor variations, although most incorporate a history of LOC, amnesia, disorientation, or transient focal neurologic signs or seizure in the setting of blunt traumatic or acceleration/deceleration injury, with a GCS score of 13 to 15.[8,11,15,16] Some have advocated placement of patients with GCS scores of 13 into the "moderate" TBI group because of the significant number of injuries requiring neurosurgical intervention[17-19]; however, in most classification schemes, these patients are still included in the mTBI category. The New Orleans Criteria (NOC) defines mTBI as loss of consciousness after trauma in a neurologically intact patient with GCS score of 15.[2] Some have advocated inclusion of patients without LOC or PTA, considering that in this setting, if other risk factors for traumatic brain injury are present, intracranial abnormalities can be found at a similar rate to that in patients without LOC or PTA.[20]

The GCS was initially developed by Teasdale and Jeannette to reliably evaluate comatose patients with head injury and was meant to serve as a simple assessment tool by relatively inexperienced clinicians to serially and reliably evaluate comatose patients.[21-23] The scale was not developed to evaluate mTBI, although it has proven useful in moderate and severe TBI assessment and to guide the need for neurosurgical intervention. There is growing sentiment that TBI classifications based on GCS scores are limited, with grouping of heterogeneous trauma patient populations with very different prognoses into broad categories. One prospective study found that despite having GCS scores of 13 to 15, patients with intracranial injuries on imaging performed similarly to patients with moderate TBI on neuropsychological testing.[19] The Veterans Affairs and Department of Defense definition of mTBI includes normal structural imaging (i.e., head CT), thus classifying patients with imaging abnormality into moderate TBI. In the setting of mTBI, single-time-point GCS scores are of limited clinical value because they are not accurate for intracranial injury or prognosis. Rather, serial GCS score evaluation provides more prognostic information.[6]

2.2 Who Requires CT Imaging?

The difficulty facing clinicians is determining the apparently well-appearing, neurologically intact patients who may have underlying intracranial injury that will require neurosurgical intervention. A secondary and more elusive goal is to identify patients with risk for postconcussive symptoms. There is considerable heterogeneity in opinions regarding indications for ordering CT heads in the setting of mTBI. Some advocate ordering CT head examinations for all patients with mTBI, regardless of clinical presentation,[16,24,25] whereas others[26-29] advocate more judicious use of CT. CT ordering practices have varied significantly between institutions, as well as between clinicians from the same institution. The development of a clinical decision-making tool, using clinical history and physical examination, to identify blunt trauma patients with essentially no risk of intracranial injury on imaging has been a priority among ED physicians.[6,7,30] Such a tool would allow significant reductions in health care costs while also reducing patient exposure to radiation exposure. It is also important to ensure that any set of imaging decision rules is sensitive enough and has a high negative predictive value not to miss any cases of intracranial injury that would require neurosurgical intervention or lead to significant disability. It is important that any guidelines that are developed for CT ordering mTBI be easy to use for clinicians and easy to remember. It is also important that education of clinicians to the benefits of the rules be thorough and efficient, indicating the advantages of limiting overuse of CT in the ED, as well as the reliability and sensitivity of the implemented diagnostic algorithm for clinically significant intracranial injury. Typically, guidelines that are less complex and incorporate concrete definitions are easy to follow and have strong supporting evidence have higher rates of compliance.

Four clinical decision-making criteria have been developed to guide CT imaging in the setting of mTBI, aimed at including all cases of clinically significant intracranial imaging while also reducing unnecessary CT imaging. These include the Canadian CT Head Rules (CCHR), the New Orleans Imaging Criteria (NOC), the National Emergency X-Radiography Utilization Study II (NEXUS II), and the American College of Emergency Physicians (ACEP)/Centers for Disease Control and Prevention (CDC) Clinical Policy Recommendations.

2.2.1 Canadian CT Head Rules Criteria

The CCHR Criteria were developed from the initial evaluation of 3121 adult mTBI patients who had been treated in the ED of 10 major Canadian hospitals.[11] Inclusion criteria were age greater than 16, blunt head trauma resulting in witnessed LOC, the presence of amnesia or witnessed disorientation, initial ED GCS score of 13 or greater, and injury within 24 hours at the time of evaluation in the ED. Of the patients evaluated, 8% had clinically significant intracranial injury as determined by CT imaging (i.e., injuries that would require hospitalization and neurologic follow-up), and 1% required neurosurgical intervention. An additional 4% were also found to have clinically unimportant intracranial injuries, specifically focal subarachnoid hemorrhages or cerebral contusions measuring less than 5 mm in neurologically intact patients.

Based on this evaluation, a clinical decision rule was developed that included five high-risk factors for neurosurgical intervention:

- GCS lower than 15 at 2 hours after the initial injury
- Suspected open or depressed skull fracture
- Any sign of basal skull fracture
  - "Raccoon" eyes
  - Hemotympanum
  - Cerebrospinal fluid otorrhea/rhinorrhea
  - Battle's sign
- Vomiting at least twice
- Age 65 years or older

If any of these factors are present, there is a high likelihood of need for neurosurgical intervention. In addition, two medium-risk criteria were identified that portended clinically important intracranial injury without the need for neurosurgical intervention. These included dangerous mechanism of injury (e.g., pedestrian struck by a motor vehicle, a fall from greater than 3

feet or five stairs, being ejected from a motor vehicle) and amnesia after impact for longer than 30 minutes. The high-risk criteria had a sensitivity of 100%, identifying all 44 cases that required neurosurgical intervention, as well as a specificity of 68.7%. The CT imaging rate was 32%. When the high- and medium-risk criteria were considered, the sensitivity and specificity were 98.7% and 49.6%, respectively, with a CT imaging rate of 54%. Cranial CT imaging was considered mandatory in patients who fulfilled the high-risk criteria and was recommended in medium-risk patients. One important feature of the criteria is that they considered certain intracranial injuries as being not clinically important, specifically, a solitary contusion smaller than 5 mm, localized subarachnoid hemorrhage less than 1 mm thick, subdural hematoma measuring less than 4 mm, pneumocephalus, and closed depressed skull fracture not involving the inner table. Minor head injury is defined as witnessed LOC, definite amnesia, or witnessed disorientation in patients with a GCS score of 13 to 15.

Stiell et al[31] applied their CCHR prospectively at 12 different academic and community radiology practices in Canada and evaluated changes in ordering ED CT head imaging ordering before and after implementation of these rules. Six institutions were randomized into "intervention" sites, at which the CCHR were implemented, whereas six others served as "control" sites, in which there was no implementation or education of these rules. Between the two groups, in the evaluation of a total of 4531 patients, no cases were included in which clinically significant intracranial injuries were not imaged; however, the CT ordering rate increased at both the control and intervention sites between before and after implementation of the rules. At the intervention sites, the rate of use increased from 62.8 to 76.2% [a difference of 13.3% with 95% confidence interval (CI) of 9.7 to 17%), whereas the control sites showed an increase of 67.5 to 74.1% in use (a difference of 6.7%, with 95% CI of 2.6 to 10.8%).[31] This study again confirmed that the CCHRs have high sensitivity for clinically important intracranial injury, but implementation of these rules did not reduce, but rather increased, CT imaging use relative to control and baseline use. According to the authors, this result may have been secondary to inadequate education before rule implementation, an inability of the ED physicians to recall the rules, abnormally low use rates at the participating institutions before intervention, and a lack of compliance on the part of the ED physicians to implement the rules for a myriad of reasons.[31] Other reasons for this discrepancy could be the differences in health care systems between Canada and the United States and the lesser availability of CT scanners in Canada (only 30% of urgent care settings had CT scanners at the time) affecting utilization.[32] According to other trials, implementation of the CCHR can potentially decrease CT use in the ED by up to 37%.[5,33] U.S. health care savings estimates with appropriate implementation of this rule range from 120 to 400 million dollars annually.[33,34]

2.2.2 New Orleans Imaging Criteria

Haydel et al.[2] established and validated the NOC to clinically evaluate for the need of head CT examination in the setting of mTBI by initially prospectively evaluating the clinical information of 520 consecutive patients who visited the ED having mTBI and a GCS score of 15 and received CT imaging. The definition of mTBI was blunt head trauma with resultant LOC, normal findings on brief neurologic examination, and a GCS score of 15. Inclusion criteria were patients older than 3 years of age who went to the ED within 24 hours of injury. From this group, 56 patients had CT findings of acute intracranial injury, and each had one or more of the following clinical findings:

- Headache
- Vomiting
- Seizure
- Age over 60 years
- Drug or alcohol intoxication
- Short-term memory deficit
- Physical evidence of trauma above the clavicles

These clinical parameters represent the NOCriteria, and the presence of any of these indicates the need for CT imaging according to these criteria. In the second phase of their trial, 909 patients were prospectively evaluated using these guidelines. Fifty-seven cases of intracranial injury were found, for which the NOC showed 100% sensitivity. These criteria established CT imaging guidelines in the setting of mTBI but, more importantly, validated that if none of their seven clinical factors was present, they believed the patient would not have intracranial injury and could be safely sent home.

Whereas the NOC and the CCHR have indicated that age greater than 60 and 65 years, respectively, is a risk factor for intracranial injury, others have disputed this factor. Riccardi et al[35] retrospectively evaluated older patients (i.e., older than 65 years) with mTBI for the incidence of clinically significant intracranial injury, as well as the need for neurosurgical intervention. When evaluating a total of 2149 patients, all of whom received CT for mTBI, 2.18% had acute intracranial abnormalities, whereas only 0.14% required neurosurgical intervention. Patients between 65 and 79 years of age had acute abnormality on CT in 0.66% of cases, with a significant increase in patients older than 80 years, with a 3.33% rate of acute pathology. The rate of acute CT findings also increased in the setting of anticoagulation, most prominently in those treated with double antiplatelet agents. The group advocated that universal CT imaging of patients younger than 80 years in the setting of mTBI was not necessary but should be considered in mTBI patients receiving anticoagulation therapy.

2.2.3 NEXUS II Criteria

In the development of the NEXUS II criteria, 13,728 patients who underwent CT imaging in the setting of acute blunt head injury at 21 participating institutions were prospectively evaluated.[36] Of these patients, 917 had clinically important intracranial injury. Eight criteria were found that were independently and highly associated with intracranial abnormalities that required CT imaging:

- Evidence of significant skull fracture
- Scalp hematoma
- Neurologic deficit
- Altered level of alertness
- Abnormal behavior
- Coagulopathy
- Persistent vomiting
- Age 65 years or older

The presence of any of these criteria was 98.3% sensitive, correctly identifying 901 of the patients. This criteria system also identified 12.7% of the patients as very low risk based on the absence of any of the preceding listed risk factors. Specificity was 13.7%. Among patients with minor head injury, 330 patients were found to have intracranial abnormality, of which 314 were identified, for a sensitivity of 95.2%, negative predictive value of 99.1%, and specificity of 17.3%. Of the 16 patients missed (1.7% of intracranial injury cases) by the NEXUS II criteria, one required neurosurgical intervention, specifically intracranial pressure monitoring. Unlike the CCHR and NOC, NEXUS II and ACEP/CDC guidelines (discussed as follows) provide an evaluation tool for patients who had not suffered LOC or posttraumatic amnesia.

2.2.4 ACEP/CDC Guidelines

The ACEP/CDC produced a new set of guidelines for CT imaging in the setting of mTBI in adults in 2008 to update their prior guidelines from 2002.[6] The guidelines were based on published CT ordering rules in the setting of blunt trauma and a number of well-designed outcome trials. The primary change that was made from the 2002 guidelines was inclusion of patients with risk factors but without LOC or posttraumatic amnesia into the definition of mTBI, allowing for consideration of this patient population for CT imaging. This was changed because of interval studies that had been performed indicating that LOC and posttraumatic amnesia are not sufficient to identify all patients with acute intracranial injury.[3,20] Level A Recommendations of the guidelines indicate that for patients with LOC or posttraumatic amnesia, a noncontrast CT should be ordered if one or more of the following are present:

- Headache
- Vomiting
- Age older than 60 years
- Drug or alcohol intoxication
- Short-term memory deficits
- Physical evidence of trauma above the clavicle
- Post-traumatic seizure
- GCS score below 15
- Focal neurologic deficit
- Coagulopathy

Level B Recommendations of the guidelines indicate that for patients without LOC/PTA, a noncontrast head CT should be performed if one or more of the following are present:

- Focal neurologic deficit
- Vomiting
- Severe headache
- Age 65 years or older
- Physical signs of a basilar skull fracture
- GCS score lower than 15
- Coagulopathy
- Dangerous mechanism of injury[6] (e.g., ejection from a motor vehicle, pedestrian being struck, a fall from a height greater than 3 feet or five stairs)

For consideration of this policy, the following are the inclusion criteria: nonpenetrating trauma to the head, presentation to the ED within 24 hours of injury, GCS score of 14 or 15 at initial evaluation in the ED, and age older than 16 years.

2.3 Comparison of the mTBI CT Imaging Criteria

The CCHR and NOC have been extensively validated, both internally and externally.[1,2,5,31,33,37–39] Stiel et al[1] compared their CCHR with the NOC for head CT prospectively in nine EDs across Canada in a group of 1822 mTBI patients with GCS scores of 15. Both the CCHR and NOC were 100% sensitive in determining the need for head CT in patients who eventually required neurosurgical intervention, as well as in patients with clinically important intracranial injury; the investigators found that the CCHR criteria were more specific for both types of injuries. The CCHRs also resulted in fewer orders for CT imaging (52.1% vs. 88.0%). Prospective comparison of the CCHRs and the NOC in a cohort of 3181 patients in the Netherlands indicated that NOC were more sensitive than the CCHR for all intracranial injury and clinically important neurocranial trauma (97.7 and 99.4% vs. 83.4 and 87.2%), but both were able to detect all cases that required neurosurgical intervention.[5] The CCHR were able to reduce CT imaging by 37%, compared with 3% for the NOC. Melnick et al[33] showed that CCHR had the potential to decrease CT imaging in the setting of mTBI by 35% compared with 10% for the NOC. The NOC, however, had higher compliance by the ED physicians relative to the CCHR (90.5% vs. 64.7%). In a prospective observational cohort evaluation of 431 mTBI patients in a U.S. ED, Papa et al[38] found comparable sensitivity of the two guidelines (CCHR and NOC) for any intracranial injury, significant intracranial injury, and cases requiring neurosurgical intervention, but they found the CCHR to be more specific in all three outcomes relative to the NOC. Evaluation of the two rules in Tunisian ED between 2008 and 2011 found that compared with the NOC, the CCHR were more sensitive and specific for cases requiring neurosurgical intervention, as well as significant intracranial injury.[37]

A limitation of the CCHR is that it is relatively cumbersome and complex, making compliance by ED physicians more difficult. In addition, it requires monitoring the patient for 2 hours in the ED, increasing congestion within busy EDs. Some clinicians, including some of the ED physicians at the institutions that were used to validate the CCHR, have objected to the categorization of some intracranial injuries as being not significant and not considered in the criteria. The CCHRs prove to be the imaging guideline that consistently can reduce imaging use the most, indicated by its higher specificity compared head-to-head with the other guidelines. The NOC guidelines require that all patients with any sign of injury above the clavicle be imaged, including abrasions and lacerations. Although the NOC increased the sensitivity and negative predictive value and lowered the imaging threshold of the guideline, this requirement reduces the specificity and ability to limit imaging.

Both the NOC and CCHR must be applied within the limits of their inclusion criteria; specifically, to be considered, patients must have had LOC or PTA and must not have been receiving anticoagulants. It has been demonstrated that LOC and amnesia are not necessary for traumatic intracranial abnormality to be present.[3,34] Smits et al[34] compared mTBI patients who

presented with a risk factor for intracranial injury: 1708 with and 754 without LOC or amnesia; they found that there were comparable odds ratios for CT abnormalities between patients with known risk factors for intracranial injury with or without LOC or PTA. There was an equivalent need for neurosurgical intervention between the two groups as well. The group advocated that LOC and PTA be considered as risk factors for intracranial injury, but not as prerequisites for mTBI. The NEXUS II provides evaluation criteria that do not include LOC or amnesia as part of the definition of mTBI, and it thus allows for inclusion of these patients. The ACEP/CDC decided to modify their guidelines on imaging in the setting of mTBI in 2008 to include patients who had not suffered LOC or PTA as well.

As indicated, a number of guidelines dictate indications for CT imaging in the setting of blunt head injury, with extensive internal and external validation. Each set of rules has its strengths and weaknesses, and these must be considered when implementing these criteria. Based on these rules, however, it is clear that adult patients who have suffered acute blunt head trauma but did not experience LOC or PTA and do not have risk factors for intracranial injury do not require CT imaging in the ED.

2.4 Who Requires Magnetic Resonance Imaging?

No guidelines currently indicate that magnetic resonance imaging (MRI) should be performed in patients arriving in the ED with mTBI, as indicated and confirmed by the ACEP/CDC recommendations published in 2008.[40] Whereas conventional MRI is more sensitive than CT for small focal traumatic intracranial lesions, such as cerebral contusions, axonal shear injury, and extra-axial hematomas, at this point there is no consensus on the clinical relevance of these lesions and whether routine detection of these lesions will result in improved prognosis or reduced likelihood of long-term neuropsychological abnormalities or postconcussive symptoms.[41] Variable relationships have been indicated between focal traumatic lesions on MRI and long-term outcomes in the literature.[41–46] One study showed no difference in mTBI patients with or without MRI brain lesions on the Rivermead Postconcussion Symptoms questionnaire or in ability to return to work 6 months after the injury.[42] In two reports, Scheid et al[43,44] found no correlation burden of diffuse axonal hemorrhagic lesions and long-term functional outcomes or specific or global cognitive deficits. On the other hand, when evaluating 135 adult mTBI patients, using both CT and MRI, Yuh et al[46] found that 27 of 98 patients who had no acute abnormality on CT had intracranial injury on MRI, including hemorrhagic axonal injuries, brain contusions, and extra-axial hematomas. CT findings of subarachnoid hemorrhage and MRI findings of brain contusions of four or more hemorrhagic axonal shear injuries portended poorer outcomes on extended Glasgow outcome scale evaluation at 3 months post injury.[46] Diffusion tensor imaging and functional MRI techniques have also been explored in mTBI, and although these are very promising modalities, there currently is no clinical indication for their use in the setting of trauma or consensus on their applicability to outcomes for individual patients.

Conventional MRI is typically the modality of choice in evaluating patients with persistent symptoms in the subacute or chronic setting of mTBI. MRI is more likely to indicate the sequelae of prior injury than CT, although a negative conventional MRI does not preclude the presence of symptoms or abnormalities that are not detected.

References

[1] Stiell IG, Clement CM, Rowe BH et al. Comparison of the Canadian CT Head Rule and the New Orleans Criteria in patients with minor head injury. JAMA 2005; 294: 1511–1518

[2] Haydel MJ, Preston CA, Mills TJ, Luber S, Blaudeau E, DeBlieux PM. Indications for computed tomography in patients with minor head injury. N Engl J Med 2000; 343: 100–105

[3] Ibañez J, Arikan F, Pedraza S et al. Reliability of clinical guidelines in the detection of patients at risk following mild head injury: results of a prospective study. J Neurosurg 2004; 100: 825–834

[4] Mack LR, Chan SB, Silva JC, Hogan TM. The use of head computed tomography in elderly patients sustaining minor head trauma. J Emerg Med 2003; 24: 157–162

[5] Smits M, Dippel DW, de Haan GG et al. External validation of the Canadian CT Head Rule and the New Orleans Criteria for CT scanning in patients with minor head injury. JAMA 2005; 294: 1519–1525

[6] Jagoda AS, Bazarian JJ, Bruns JJ, Jr et al. American College of Emergency Physicians. Centers for Disease Control and Prevention. Clinical policy: neuroimaging and decisionmaking in adult mild traumatic brain injury in the acute setting. Ann Emerg Med 2008; 52: 714–748

[7] Rimel RW, Giordani B, Barth JT, Boll TJ, Jane JA. Disability caused by minor head injury. Neurosurgery 1981; 9: 221–228

[8] Gerberding JLBS, ed. Report to Congress on mild traumatic brain injury in the United States: steps to prevent a serious public health problem. In: Control NCfIPa. Atlanta, GA: Centers for Disease Control and Prevention; 2003

[9] Mower WR, Hoffman JR, Herbert M, Wolfson AB, Pollack CV, Jr, Zucker MI NEXUS II Investigators. National Emergency X-Radiography Utilization Study. Developing a clinical decision instrument to rule out intracranial injuries in patients with minor head trauma: methodology of the NEXUS II investigation. Ann Emerg Med 2002; 40: 505–514

[10] Rutland-Brown W, Langlois JA, Thomas KE, Xi YL. Incidence of traumatic brain injury in the United States, 2003. J Head Trauma Rehabil 2006; 21: 544–548

[11] Stiell IG, Wells GA, Vandemheen K et al. The Canadian CT Head Rule for patients with minor head injury. Lancet 2001; 357: 1391–1396

[12] McCaig LF. National Hospital Ambulatory Medical Care Survey: 1992 emergency department summary. Adv Data 1994: 1–12

[13] Pitts SR, Niska RW, Xu J, Burt CW. National Hospital Ambulatory Medical Care Survey: 2006 emergency department summary. Natl Health Stat Report 2008; 7: 1–38

[14] Smith-Bindman R, Lipson J, Marcus R et al. Radiation dose associated with common computed tomography examinations and the associated lifetime attributable risk of cancer. Arch Intern Med 2009; 169: 2078–2086

[15] Kay T, Adams R, Andersen T et al. Definition of mild traumatic brain injury. J Head Trauma Rehabil 1993; 8: 86–87

[16] Shackford SR, Wald SL, Ross SE et al. The clinical utility of computed tomographic scanning and neurologic examination in the management of patients with minor head injuries. J Trauma 1992; 33: 385–394

[17] Stein SC. Minor head injury: 13 is an unlucky number. J Trauma 2001; 50: 759–760

[18] Stein SC, Ross SE. The value of computed tomographic scans in patients with low-risk head injuries. Neurosurgery 1990; 26: 638–640

[19] Williams DH, Levin HS, Eisenberg HM. Mild head injury classification. Neurosurgery 1990; 27: 422–428

[20] Smits M, Hunink MG, Nederkoorn PJ et al. A history of loss of consciousness or post-traumatic amnesia in minor head injury: "conditio sine qua non" or one of the risk factors? J Neurol Neurosurg Psychiatry 2007; 78: 1359–1364

[21] Jennett B, Teasdale G, Galbraith S et al. Severe head injuries in three countries. J Neurol Neurosurg Psychiatry 1977; 40: 291–298

[22] Teasdale G, Jennett B. Assessment of coma and impaired consciousness: a practical scale. Lancet 1974; 2: 81–84

[23] Teasdale G, Jennett B. Assessment and prognosis of coma after head injury. Acta Neurochir (Wien) 1976; 34: 45–55

[24] Livingston DH, Loder PA, Koziol J, Hunt CD. The use of CT scanning to triage patients requiring admission following minimal head injury. J Trauma 1991; 31: 483–489

[25] Stein SC, Ross SE. Minor head injury: a proposed strategy for emergency management. Ann Emerg Med 1993; 22: 1193–1196

[26] Borczuk P. Predictors of intracranial injury in patients with mild head trauma. Ann Emerg Med 1995; 25: 731–736

[27] Gutman MB, Moulton RJ, Sullivan I, Hotz G, Tucker WS, Muller PJ. Risk factors predicting operable intracranial hematomas in head injury. J Neurosurg 1992; 77: 9–14

[28] Madden C, Witzkc DB, Arthur , Sanders B, Valente J, Fritz M. High-yield selection criteria for cranial computed tomography after acute trauma. Acad Emerg Med 1995; 2: 248–253

[29] Taheri PA, Karamanoukian H, Gibbons K, Waldman N, Doerr RJ, Hoover EL. Can patients with minor head injuries be safely discharged home? Arch Surg 1993; 128: 289–292

[30] Fabbri A, Servadei F, Marchesini G et al. Clinical performance of NICE recommendations versus NCWFNS proposal in patients with mild head injury. J Neurotrauma 2005; 22: 1419–1427

[31] Stiell IG, Clement CM, Grimshaw JM et al. A prospective cluster-randomized trial to implement the Canadian CT Head Rule in emergency departments. CMAJ 2010; 182: 1527–1532

[32] Haydel MJ. The Canadian CT head rule. Lancet 2001; 358: 1013–1014

[33] Melnick ER, Szlezak CM, Bentley SK, Dziura JD, Kotlyar S, Post LA. CT overuse for mild traumatic brain injury. Jt Comm J Qual Patient Saf 2012; 38: 483–489

[34] Smits M, Dippel DW, Nederkoorn PJ et al. Minor head injury: CT-based strategies for management—a cost-effectiveness analysis. Radiology 2010; 254: 532–540

[35] Riccardi A, Frumento F, Guiddo G et al. Minor head injury in the elderly at very low risk: a retrospective study of 6 years in an Emergency Department (ED). Am J Emerg Med 2013; 31: 37–41

[36] Mower WR, Hoffman JR, Herbert M, Wolfson AB, Pollack CV, Jr, Zucker MI NEXUS II Investigators. Developing a decision instrument to guide computed tomographic imaging of blunt head injury patients. J Trauma 2005; 59: 954–959

[37] Bouida W, Marghli S, Souissi S et al. Prediction value of the Canadian CT head rule and the New Orleans criteria for positive head CT scan and acute neurosurgical procedures in minor head trauma: a multicenter external validation study. Ann Emerg Med 2013; 61: 521–527

[38] Papa L, Stiell IG, Clement CM et al. Performance of the Canadian CT Head Rule and the New Orleans Criteria for predicting any traumatic intracranial injury on computed tomography in a United States Level I trauma center. Acad Emerg Med 2012; 19: 2–10

[39] Rosengren D, Rothwell S, Brown AF, Chu K. The application of North American CT scan criteria to an Australian population with minor head injury. Emerg Med Australas 2004; 16: 195–200

[40] Barbosa RR, Jawa R, Watters JM et al. Eastern Association for the Surgery of Trauma. Evaluation and management of mild traumatic brain injury: an Eastern Association for the Surgery of Trauma practice management guideline. J Trauma Acute Care Surg 2012; 73 Suppl 4: S307–S314

[41] Lee H, Wintermark M, Gean AD, Ghajar J, Manley GT, Mukherjee P. Focal lesions in acute mild traumatic brain injury and neurocognitive outcome: CT versus 3 T MRI. J Neurotrauma 2008; 25: 1049–1056

[42] Hughes DG, Jackson A, Mason DL, Berry E, Hollis S, Yates DW. Abnormalities on magnetic resonance imaging seen acutely following mild traumatic brain injury: correlation with neuropsychological tests and delayed recovery. Neuroradiology 2004; 46: 550–558

[43] Scheid R, Preul C, Gruber O, Wiggins C, von Cramon DY. Diffuse axonal injury associated with chronic traumatic brain injury: evidence from T2*-weighted gradient-echo imaging at 3 T. AJNR Am J Neuroradiol 2003; 24: 1049–1056

[44] Scheid R, Walther K, Guthke T, Preul C, von Cramon DY. Cognitive sequelae of diffuse axonal injury. Arch Neurol 2006; 63: 418–424

[45] Wilson JT, Wiedmann KD, Hadley DM, Condon B, Teasdale G, Brooks DN. Early and late magnetic resonance imaging and neuropsychological outcome after head injury. J Neurol Neurosurg Psychiatry 1988; 51: 391–396

[46] Yuh EL, Mukherjee P, Lingsma HF et al. TRACK-TBI Investigators. Magnetic resonance imaging improves 3-month outcome prediction in mild traumatic brain injury. Ann Neurol 2013; 73: 224–235

3 Neuroimaging of Traumatic Brain Injury

Yoshimi Anzai

3.1 Introduction

Traumatic brain injury (TBI) is a major public health and socioeconomic problem in the United States and throughout the world. The U.S. Centers for Disease Control and Prevention estimates that approximately 1.7 million Americans sustain a TBI annually, resulting in 1.3 million visits to the emergency department, 275,000 hospitalizations, and more than 50,000 deaths related to TBI annually.[1] Clearly, TBI is a leading cause of death among young adults in the United States. These numbers underestimate the actual magnitude of TBI because the statistics are unknown for those who do not seek medical care or who have no access to care. Moreover, long-term disability as a result of TBI is being increasingly recognized as a public health issue. It is estimated that at least 5.3 million Americans (up to 2% of the U.S. population) suffer from long-term or lifelong disability as a result of TBI.[2]

The common causes of TBI are falls, motor-vehicle crashes, bike accidents, sports-related injuries, assault and battery, and most recently blast injuries among soldiers returning from the Iraq and Afghanistan wars.[3] In Seattle, a city of motorcycle and bicycle enthusiasts, accidents are frequent and occasionally fatal among youth, despite mandatory bicycle-helmet-use laws in King County and Washington State.[4]

The vast majority of sports-related TBIs are so-called mild traumatic brain injury (mTBI), or concussion.[5] Concussion presents unique features of TBI in which emotional and behavioral psychological symptoms persist in some of the victims. Conventional imaging does not usually demonstrate abnormality, and advanced imaging has been tested with variable results. This topic is discussed in detail in Chapter 11 of this book.

Traditionally, The Glasgow Coma Scale (GCS) has classified TBI as mild (GCS 13–15), moderate (GCS 9–12), or severe (GCS 8 or lower). The GCS was developed in 1974 by Bryant Jennett, a neurosurgeon at the University of Glasgow.[6] The GCS is a simple, reproducible clinical assessment tool of the state of consciousness of a patient and has been used widely in first aid, emergency medical services, and intensive care unit settings for the last 16 years.[7,8] Three components of GCS score include eye response (4 points), verbal response (5 points), and motor response (6 points) (▶ Table 3.1). It is useful for estimating the prognosis for TBI patients; however, it does not provide mechanistic or pathophysiological information related to TBI. It is well known that clinical and imaging findings vary widely among patients classified for the same GCS score and that these patients often require different clinical management.[9] Moreover, the accuracy of the GCS score is often reduced by early sedation and intubation of TBI patients.[10]

One of the major downsides of GCS score is the limited utility of GCS for mTBI. GCS was not intended to address the level of injury or consciousness for patients with mTBI.

Table 3.1 Glasgow Coma Scale: coma score (E + M + V) = 3 to 15.

Eye opening (E)	
Spontaneously	4
To verbal stimuli	3
To pain	2
Never	I
Best motor response (M)	
Obeys commands	6
Localizes pain	5
Flexion withdrawal	4
Flexion abnormal	3
Extension abnormal	2
No response	1
Best verbal response (V)	
Orientated and converses	5
Disoriented and converses	4
Inappropriate words	3
Incomprehensible words	2
No response	1

Table 3.2 Extended Glasgow Outcome Scale (GOSE).

1	Death	D
2	Vegetative state	VS
3	Lower severe disability	SD -
4	Upper severe disability	SD +
5	Lower moderate disability	MD -
6	Upper moderate disability	MD +
7	Lower good recovery	GR -
8	Upper good recovery	GR +

Use of the structured interview is recommended to facilitate consistency in ratings.

The Glasgow Outcome Scale (GOS), on the other hand, focuses on how head injury affects the functional status of life. Each patient is assigned to one of five possible outcomes: death, persistent vegetative state, severe disability, moderate disability, and good recovery. Extended GOS further divides the outcomes into eight categories (▶ Table 3.2).[11]

3.2 Imaging Workups for Traumatic Brain Injury

In the acute traumatic phase, computed tomography (CT) scan remains the first line of diagnostic imaging to evaluate the severity of TBI and the extent of the injury, which helps in triaging patients who need surgical intervention from those who can safely be observed clinically.[12] Unconscious or obtunded patients who arrived in the emergency room need an immediate head CT to assess the presence of intracranial hemorrhage, cerebral edema, and/ or herniation. A large expanding hematoma or hematoma with active extravasation needs to be evacuated to control hemorrhage in a timely fashion. Normal head CT allows patients to be discharged from the ED unless clinical signs and symptoms suggest more serious injury.

The CT scan is also the best imaging modality to evaluate fractures in the skull or skull base. The location of such fractures potentially necessitates further imaging workup for vascular injury, such as traumatic dissection or venous thrombosis or occlusion. Chapter 7, Blunt Cerebrovascular Injury, covers this type of injury, and Chapter 9, Skull Base Trauma, covers the anatomy of the skull base and fractures therein. Chapter 10, Maxillofacial Trauma, and Chapter 11, Traumatic Orbital Injury, discuss these types of injuries in detail.

Little discussion has taken place as to which severe and moderate TBI patients require head CT at arrival: A question is, which patients with mTBI should receive head CT in the ED and which patients can safely avoid CT scan? A CT scan involves ionizing radiation. Even though brain is not a particularly radiosensitive organ, judicious use of head CT is essential, in particular, in the pediatric patient population. In addition, the cost associated with CT scan for minor head trauma should be weighed against the benefits of CT. Several prediction rules and guidelines have been developed and validated to address this question.[13–15] The prediction rules for head CT indication for mTBI are covered extensively in Chapter 22, Evidence-Based Imaging and Prediction Rules. It was reported that approximately 10 to 35% of head CT scans performed for minor head trauma in an urban level I trauma center did not meet the guidelines for an mTBI.[16]

Another common clinical question is whether or not to repeat head CT for patients with TBI. In an era of cost containment and judicious use of CT for radiation concern, this is a relevant question with conflicting evidence in literature. Meta-analysis of mTBI patients revealed that the routine follow-up head CT is not indicated unless patients present with clinical deterioration.[17] A prospective study enrolling all types of TBI patients addressing the impact of management by the repeat head CT between a "clinically indicated" group and "routine follow-up" without clinical deterioration showed that approximately 20% of patients who underwent repeat head CT for clinical deterioration resulted in changes in the case management; these changes were seen in more severely injured and younger patients. This study did not support the routine use of repeat head CT without clinical deterioration.[18] However, a recent study on repeat CT for 360 mTBI patients with abnormality on the initial head CT reported that approximately 30% of patients had injury progression even though clinical symptoms and signs remained stable in the first 8 hours.[19] Those patients had a higher injury severity score, intubation,

and higher mortality rates. The presence of a mass effect on the initial CT was independently associated with worsening CT findings.

Despite its higher sensitivity in detecting TBI lesions, magnetic resonance imaging (MRI) of the brain is not routinely used clinically for acute TBI, and its routine use is not supported in the literature,[20] in part because of relatively limited access to MRI and difficulty in monitoring patients with severe injury inside the scanner. Several studies reported that brain MRI showed more TBI lesions compared with the CT study at the time of the patient's arrival,[21] but the study also indicated that there was no significant impact on the management of patients with TBI in the acute trauma setting.[22] It has been reported that for about 30% of patients with mTBI with a negative head CT, brain MRI shows evidence of TBI. Most CT-negative, but MR-positive brain injuries are axonal injuries [diffuse axonal injury (DAI) and traumatic axonal injury (TAI)].

The workshop organized by the National Institute of Neurological Disorders and Stroke, with support from the Brain Injury Association of America, the Defense and Veterans Brain Injury Center, and the National Institute of Disability and Rehabilitation Research, outlined the problems related to the current TBI classification based on GCS and stated that "more widespread use of acute MRI will be important to provide additional detail necessary for accurate pathoanatomic classification, particularly of the TAI/DAI spectrum. Efforts should be coordinated to identify and eliminate barriers to the implementation of acute MRI for TBI clinical trials and to standardize and validate MRI grading system.[9]

Various magnetic resonance (MR) sequences have been investigated, including T2-weighted images, fluid-attenuated inversion recovery (FLAIR), gradient echo (GRE) images, susceptibility-weighted images (SWI), diffusion-weighted images (DWI), diffusion tensor images (DTI), and MR spectroscopy. A study of 56 mTBI patients revealed that SWI showed the largest number of lesions, followed by GRE images, FLAIR, and T2-weighted images.[23] Another study confirmed that SWI images revealed 30% more mTBI lesions compared with CT scans.[24]

Microhemorrhages, which are sometimes seen in TBI patients, may evolve over time. A study comparing 1.5 T and 3 T GRE images demonstrated 50% more lesions detected on 3 T compared with 1.5 T and a negative correlation between the number of lesions and the time interval from trauma in 1.5 T study but not in the 3 T study.[25]

3.3 Prediction of Clinical Outcomes

The degree of TBI can be better categorized based on the morphologic abnormality on CT scan. Attempts have been made to incorporate CT findings to predict the clinical outcomes of TBI patients. Maas et al developed the prognostic model based on 2269 moderate to severe TBI patients from multicenter clinical trials to predict the 6-month outcome using the information available at patient admission (i.e., the Marshall CT score). The model discriminated well in the development population [area under the receiver (AUR) operating characteristic curve (0.78–0.80)], as well as in the two external validity studies [area under the curve (AUC), 0.83–0.89] from Europe and North America.

Table 3.3 Rotterdam score of head CT: Predicting the probability of mortality in patients with TBI based on CT findings.

Prediction Value	Score
Basal Cisterns	
Normal	0
Compressed	1
Absent	2
Midline Shift	
No shift of shift < = 5 mm	0
Shift > 5 mm	1
Epidural mass lesion	
Present	0
Absent	1
Intraventricular blood or tSAH	
Absent	0
Present	1
Sun Score	+ 1

The scores range from 1 (mildest) to 6 (most severe). The actual mortality corresponding to the Rotterdam CT Score for the total score 1, 2, 3, 4, 5, and 6 is 0%, 6.8%, 16%, 26%, 53%, and 61%, respectively. Data from Maas AI, Hukkelhoven CW, Marshall LF, Steyerberg EW. Prediction of outcome in traumatic brain injury with computed tomographic characteristics: a comparison between the computed tomographic classification and combinations of computed tomographic predictors. Neurosurgery. 2005;57(6):1173–1182.

The CT findings used in the Marshall CT score include the presence or absence of a mass (hematoma) lesion, a midline shift of more than 5 mm, a compressed or absent cistern, and evacuated mass lesions. This evaluation was modified to develop the Rotterdam CT score,[26] which includes compression of the basilar cistern, midline shift greater than 5 mm, traumatic subarachnoid or intraventricular hemorrhage, and the presence of different types of mass lesions (▶ Table 3.3). Using this simple CT-based Rotterdam score, 6-month mortality was predicted (AUC 0.77) more accurately than using the Marshall score (AUR 0.67).[26]

A small study investigating the predictive values of CT, T2-weighted images, FLAIR, and SWI showed that the volume of T2 and FLAIR abnormality most consistently discriminates between good and poor outcomes groups as measured by Eye Opening (E)-GCS, whereas SWI was the most sensitive imaging study for showing parenchymal hemorrhage, although it failed to discriminate outcomes.[27] More recently, a multicenter study enrolling 135 mTBI patients demonstrated that 27% of mTBI patients with negative CTs had abnormality on MRI. This Transforming Research and Clinical Knowledge (TRACK) TBI study revealed that subarachnoid hemorrhage (SAH) is a predictor for poor outcomes after adjusting for demographics, clinical presentation, and socioeconomic status. More than one contusion on MR [odds ratio (OR) = 4.5] and more than four foci of hemorrhagic TAI (OR = 3.2) are independent predictors for a poor prognosis after adjusting for head CT, demographics, and clinical and socioeconomic factors.[28]

Extensive research using advanced MRI has been ongoing to address which mTBI patients suffer from neuropsychological deficits and need to refrain from activity to avoid a second impact injury. The current state of mTBI imaging research is discussed in detail in Chapter 12.

3.4 Imaging Findings of Primary Traumatic Brain Injury Lesions

In this chapter, the pathoanatomic description of TBI was made in accordance with the Head Injury Reporting and Data System (HIRADS) in collaboration with the American College of Radiology (ACR) Head Injury Institute. The HIRADS was created to standardize the terminology used to describe the CT or MR findings of traumatic brain injury and to gather data for investigation of natural history, effectiveness of intervention, and prediction of clinical outcomes across various institutions in the country.

The pathoanatomic classifications of TBI described in this chapter are as follows:
- Skull Fracture
- Epidural Hematoma (EDH)
- Subdural Hematoma (SDH)
- Subarachnoid Hemorrhage (SAH)
- Contusion
- Intracerebral hemorrhage
- Intraventricular hemorrhage
- Diffuse axonal injury (DAI) and Traumatic axonal injury (TAI)
- Brainstem injury
- Pituitary/hypothalamic injury
- Thalamus and Deep gray matter injury

3.4.1 Skull Fracture

A sign of skull fracture, such as scalp laceration or hematoma, is one of the indications for head CT. Skull radiography should not be performed because as it does not reveal any underlying brain injury. Limited sensitivity may lead to false assurance and is potentially dangerous. Lack of skull fracture does not exclude underling brain injury. One study showed that mTBI patients (GCS 14 or 15) of skull fractures had a fivefold higher risk of requiring neurosurgery compared with patients without skull fracture.[29]

Skull fracture is classified as either open or closed. Open fracture describes a fracture with an overlying skin defect, and may be frankly visible. The following are the types of skull fractures that commonly seen (▶ Fig. 3.1):
- Linear: A break from the outer to the inner table in a straight line or branching pattern without displacement of bone. Linear fracture itself has no significant clinical consequences unless it is associated with epidural hematoma (often associated with middle meningeal artery injury) or venous sinus injury or thrombosis (often transverse sinus).
- Depressed: Usually results from blunt head injury by an object (e.g., rock, hammer, baseball bat, or assault). Depressed fractures are often accompanied by severe TBI and a high risk of increasing intracranial pressure. Compound depressed fracture exposes the cranial content to extracranial space, bearing the risk of infection and contamination. Depressed

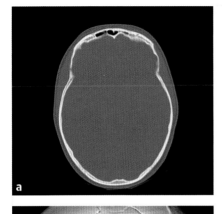

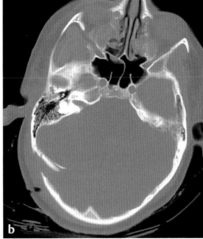

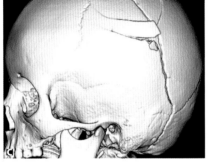

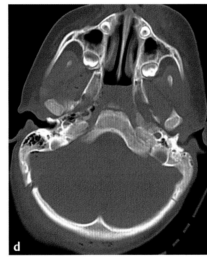

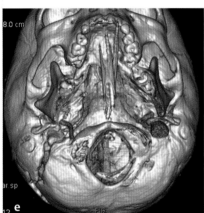

Fig. 3.1 Various skull fractures. (a) Linear fracture, (b) depressed fracture, (c) comminuted fracture, (d) diastatic fracture, (e) diastatic fracture involving the right occipitomastoid suture. Three-dimensional volumetric image provides an excellent overview of fracture configuration and alignment, which helps surgical planning.

skull fractures are usually treated surgically to remove pressure on the brain from fragmented bone pieces.
- Comminuted: Fracture into three or more pieces. Comminuted fractures are often associated with depressed fractures, where the pieces of fragments are displaced inward.
- Diastatic: Fractures involving one or more sutures, resulting in widening of fractured suture rather than break of bone. Diastatic fractures are common in infants and young children (i.e., younger than 3 years) because sutures are not yet fused. When seen in adults, diastatic fractures commonly occur in the lambdoid sutures. One of the complications for children with skull fracture is leptomeningeal cyst, which is a cerebrospinal fluid (CSF) collection caused by a dural tear, resulting in diastasis of suture and development of cyst in between. It is called a growing skull fracture (▶ Fig. 3.1b).
- Greenstick fractures: Incomplete fractures. Broken bones are not completely separated but rather bend or deform as if bending a greenstick. This is also more common in children.

The TBI lesions are classified into primary and secondary. Primary lesions refer to immediate parenchymal injury occuring at the time of injury. The primary injury includes EDH, SDH, SAH/intraventricular hemorrhage (IVH), TAI/DAI, contusions, and hematoma. Direct injury to the cerebral vasculature is also a type of primary lesion. Secondary lesions are potentially avoidable brain damages that occur at variable time after injury. The secondary injury include, but not limited to, cerebral swelling (edema), brain herniation, hydrocephalus, ischemia, infarction, CSF leak, and encephalomalacia. A brainstem injury can be a primary or secondary injury (discussed later).

3.4.2 Epidural Hematoma

An EDH is a collection of blood between the inner table of the skull and dura matter (▶ Fig. 3.2). In normal circumstances, no epidural space is present because of the firm attachment of the

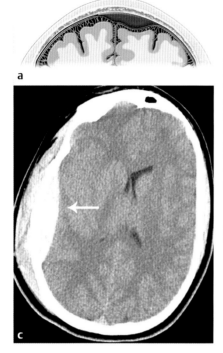

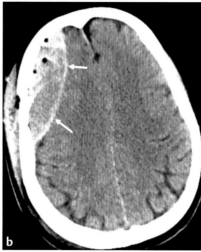

Fig. 3.2 Epidural hematoma. (a) Illustration demonstrating the epidural space between inner table of calvarium and dural matter. (b) Right temporal skull fracture with biconvex epidural hematoma. (c) Right temporoparietal epidural hematoma (*red arrow*).

outer dural layer to the inner table of skull. EDH is often associated with injury to the middle meningeal artery and its branches and thus is most common in the temporoparietal location (75%) (▶ Fig. 3.3).

The expanding hematoma strips dura from the skull but is usually confined to the epidural space and does not cross the suture line (coronal or lambdoid suture) in adults. EDH often, but not always, has a biconvex shape. Venous EDH, on the other hand, results from bleeding from the meningeal or diploic veins or the dural sinuses. Venous EDH, although rare, is most commonly seen in the vertex, posterior fossa, or anterior aspect of the middle cranial fossa (as a result of bleeding from the sphenoparietal sinus). EDH from the sphenoparietal sinus in the anterior middle cranial fossa is usually limited by the sphenotemporal suture laterally and orbital suture medially; it has a benign natural history and rarely requires surgical intervention.[30] Although EDH usually does not cross the suture, that is not the case for vertex venous EDH; near the vertex, periosteum forms the outer layer of the superior sagittal sinus, and it is thus less firmly attached to the sagittal suture, often crossing the midline (*The Fundamentals of Diagnostic Radiology* by Brant and Helms[54] (head injury classification) (▶ Fig. 3.3).

Acute EDH is generally hyperdense, although EDH containing a hypodense area represents unclotted blood, indicating an actively extravasating unclotted blood within the clotted hyperdense blood (the Swirl sign). This is an ominous sign in the acute trauma setting (▶ Fig. 3.4).[31]

Another unique feature of EDH is crossing the tentorium (▶ Fig. 3.5), unlike SDH. One of the common complications related to the posterior fossa venous EDH is venous sinus thrombosis or venous sinus injury. CT venogram is a quick and definitive imaging test to address this clinical situation (▶ Fig. 3.6).

Often EDH is associated with more favorable outcomes compared with subdural hematoma or subarachnoid hemorrhage.

As seen in the Rotterdam Score (▶ Table 3.3), the presence of EDH lowers the score compared with the score when EDH is not present.

3.4.3 Subdural Hematoma

An SDH is a collection of blood between the inner dural layer and arachnoid and is the result of stretching or tearing of cortical veins traversing the subdural space. SDH is often seen after acceleration and deceleration motor-vehicle accident or after a fall. As the brain atrophies, and potential subdural space increases, the chance of stretching and tearing cortical vein increases. SDH is usually crescent-shaped and crosses the suture line, and it usually extends along a much larger space than EDH. SDH is often seen along the tentorium and dural reflection.

Similar to EDH, the presence of a hypodense area within an acute SDH indicates active bleeding (the swirl sign) (▶ Fig. 3.7). Some SDH appears isodense to brain parenchyma. This so-called isodense SDH is seen in patients with disseminated intravascular coagulation, severe anemia, or trauma with arachnoid tear resulting in CSF leaking into SDH (▶ Fig. 3.8). The presence of hematocrit level within SDH can be seen in patients with rebleeding, coagulopathy, or anticoagulation. Occasionally, SDH is bilateral. Smaller SDHs may not be readily visible on the initial CT because of the tamponade effect. A smaller contralateral SDH will rapidly become apparent after the evacuation of a larger hematoma (▶ Fig. 3.9). Diffuse swelling of underlying brain parenchyma is not uncommon in SDH, in such cases, called a complicated SDH. Even a small SDH can therefore lead to a more than expected mass effect or midline shift. A complicated SDH associated with underlying brain injury has a 89% mortality rate compared with a 20% rate for a simple SDH without brain injury.

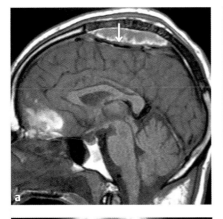

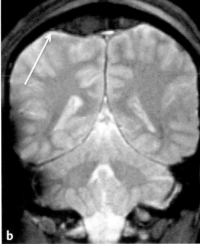

Fig. 3.3 Venous epidural hematoma. (a) T1-weighted sagittal image shows vertex venous epidural hematoma displacing the superior sagittal sinus inferiorly (*short arrow*). (b) Coronal Gradient echo image shows vertex venous epidural hematoma crossing midline over sagittal suture but does not cross the coronal suture (*long arrow*). (c) Coronal FLAIR image shows no underling brain injury.

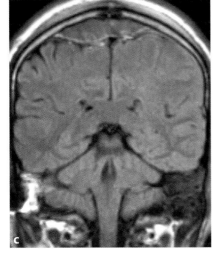

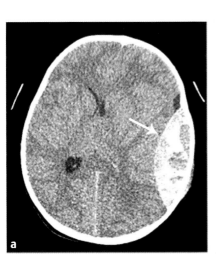

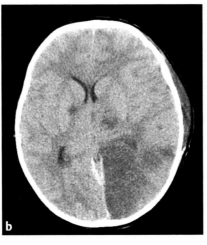

Fig. 3.4 Epidural hemorrhage (EDH) with active extravasation. (a) Active extravasation of EDH with Swirl sign containing the area of hypodensity within the left temporal EDH. (b) Computed tomography performed post evacuation shows area of infarction in the left occipital lobe and thalamus resulting from compression of the left posterior cerebral artery.

3.4.4 Subarachnoid Hemorrhage

An SAH is a collection of blood between the arachnoid and pia mater (▶ Fig. 3.10). Subarachnoid blood extends between the cortical sulci, basilar cistern, sylvian fissures, and interpeduncular cistern. The hemorrhage is usually from the thin layers of the cortical veins passing through the subarachnoid space. Traumatic SAH (tSAH) is frequently seen in patients with skull fracture or brain contusion or is associated with axonal injury.

Often tSAH is seen adjacent to the area of direct impact or contralateral to the site of direct injury. Convexity tSAH is also common among patients after a motor-vehicle collision, often related to TAI. (IVH often results from shearing injury involving the corpus callosum.) Interpeduncular cistern is a common location of pooling of SAH evident on the head CT, as is the atrium of the lateral ventricle for IVH. CT and MRI, in particular using FLAIR or SWI images, are both sensitive in detecting SAH.[32]

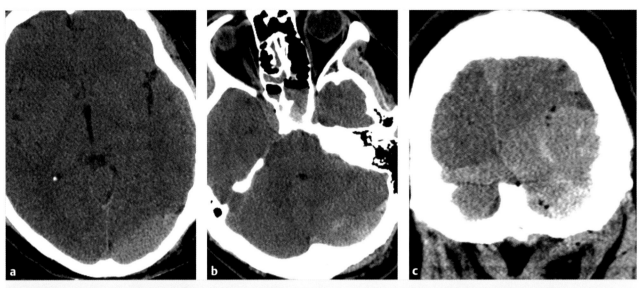

Fig. 3.5 Venous epidural hemorrhage (EDH) in the posterior fossa. Venous EDH extending from supratentorial (a) to infratentorial space (b). This is clearly seen on coronal reformatted image (c).

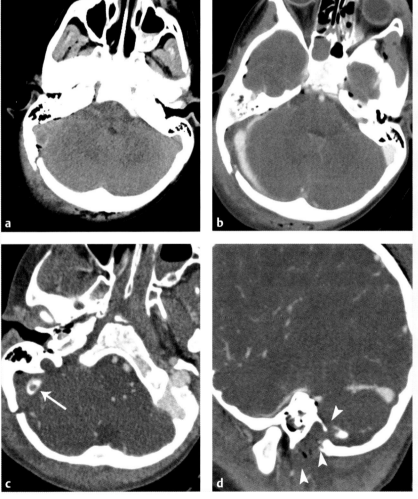

Fig. 3.6 Epidural hematoma (EDH) in the posterior fossa with venous sinus thrombosis. (a) Right occipital fracture with posterior fossa EDH with punctate pneumocephalus. (b) Computed tomography venogram demonstrates displacement of right transverse sinus. (c) Slightly inferiorly, intraluminal thrombus is present (*long arrow*). (d) Sagittal reformatted image shows extension of thrombus into the jugular vein (*short arrows*).

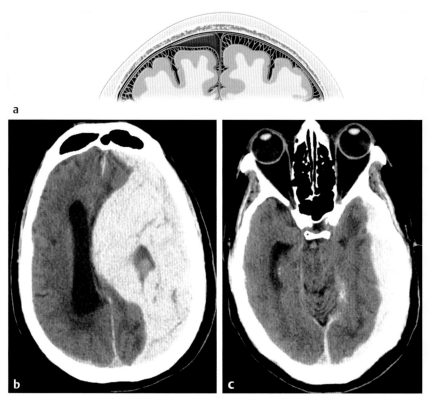

Fig. 3.7 Subdural hemorrhage (SDH) with Swirl sign. (a) Illustration demonstrates the presence of SDH underneath the dura matter, which does not cross the midline. (b) Left SDH extending along the left tentorium with marked midline shift and uncal herniation. Note the ballooning of the left temporal horn. (c) A large left holohemispheric SDH containing the area of hypodensity, indicating active bleeding. Marked compression of the left lateral ventricle and dilatation of the right lateral ventricle, consistent with hydrocephalus.

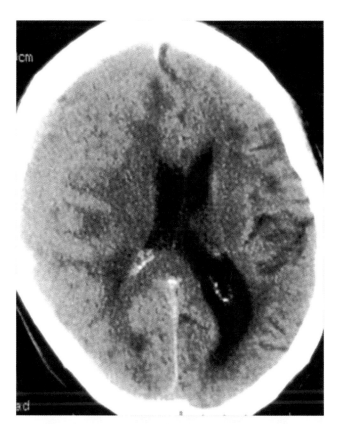

Fig. 3.8 Isodense subdural hemorrhage (SDH). Some SDH is difficult to perceive because of its isodense nature. The patient had profound anemia, which explains the relatively low-density hematoma.

Although in the past tSAH was considered insignificant, recent studies, including the European Brain Injury Consortium, have indicated that the presence of tSAH predicts poor outcomes for TBI patients. Forty-one percent of patients without traumatic SAH achieved a level of good recovery, compared with only 15% of patients with tSAH. Patients with tSAH exhibited lower GCS scores at admission. tSAH is more common in older patients than in younger patients. After adjusting for GCS score at admission and patient age, the presence of tSAH remained a significant predictor for unfavorable outcomes (OR, 2.49; 95% CI, 1.74–3.55; $p < 0.001$).

Another large study conducted in an effort to develop a prognostic model (6-month GOS) based on admission characteristics comprised clinical and imaging data from the International Mission for Prognosis and Analysis of Clinical Trials in TBI (IMPACT) project, including patients with moderate to severe TBI.[33] This study revealed that age, motor score, and pupillary reactivity were significant predictors; prediction was further improved by adding CT findings of tSAH, mass lesion, or signs of increased intracranial pressure. The model also improved by adding secondary insults, such as hypoxia and hypotension.

Hydrocephalus is a late complication of SAH and develops in 15 to 20% of patients with SAH, presumably because of blood interfering with CSF circulation in the acute phase or a reduction in CSF absorption in the chronic stage. Incidence increases with associated IVH. There are substantial variations in the size of the body of lateral ventricles. Enlargement of the temporal horns of the lateral ventricles and third ventricles and effacement of cortical sulci are findings strongly supportive of hydrocephalus (▸ Fig. 3.11). The presence of transependymal CSF flow, a rim of low density along the subependyma (or high intensity on T2 weighted MR) indicates acute hydrocephalus.

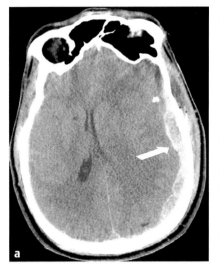

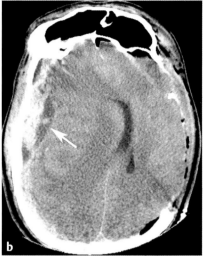

Fig. 3.9 Bilateral subdural hemorrhage (SDH). (a) Initial computed tomography (CT) shows left holohemispheric SDH (*long arrow*) with mild midline shift. The patient underwent evacuation of left SDH. (b) Postevacuation CT reveals development of a large right SDH (*arrowhead*) with a hypodense area of unclotted blood (Swirl sign). Right SDH was not apparent on the preoperative CT. This results in major midline shift.

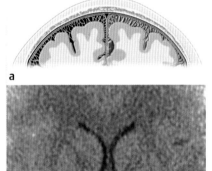

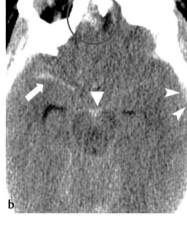

Fig. 3.10 Traumatic subarachnoic hemorrhage (tSAH). (a) Illustration demonstrating subarachnoid space between the arachnoid membrane and pia matter. (b) tSAH in the right sylvian fissure (*arrow*) and interpedincular cistern (*arrowhead*). The patient also has a right frontal contusion and left subdural hematoma (*short arrows*). (c) tSAH in the right sylvian fissure.

Another later complication of SAH is cerebral siderosis, which is deposition of hemosiderin in the leptomeninges.[34] Cerebral siderosis is readily diagnosed on T2-weighted images, where dark T2 signal extends along the surface of the brainstem, cerebellum, or inferior cerebral hemisphere or spinal cord (► Fig. 3.12). Patients show various cranial nerve symptoms, including hearing loss, ataxia, anosmia, and upper motor neuron signs. Hypointensity may extend to involve the cranial nerves I, II, and VIII or upper cervical spinal cord. Atrophy of vermis and cerebellum is also not uncommon.

3.4.5 Contusion

The two broad categories of forces resulting in primary brain parenchymal injury are direct impact force and inertial (acceleration and deceleration, rotational) forces. Direct impact force

results in cerebral contusion, skull fracture, epidural hematoma, and inertial forces result in DAI (discussed later) and intracerebral hematoma. Contusion involves primarily the cortex of the brain because of deformational forces and may extend to subcortical region. These injuries are most often distributed in the expected anatomic locations (► Fig. 3.13).

The following are the common locations of traumatic contusion where the brain rubs against the rough surface of the skull and skull base. These include the anterior temporal lobes against the greater wing of sphenoid bone or anterior clinoid process, the anterior frontal base against the cribriform plate or planum sphenoidale, and the inferior posterior temporal lobe against the petrous ridge (► Fig. 3.14). Less frequent but worth mentioning is the lateral midbrain, where the brainstem is contused against the tentorium cerebelli (► Fig. 3.15). Contusions are often hemorrhagic and appear as a mottled area of

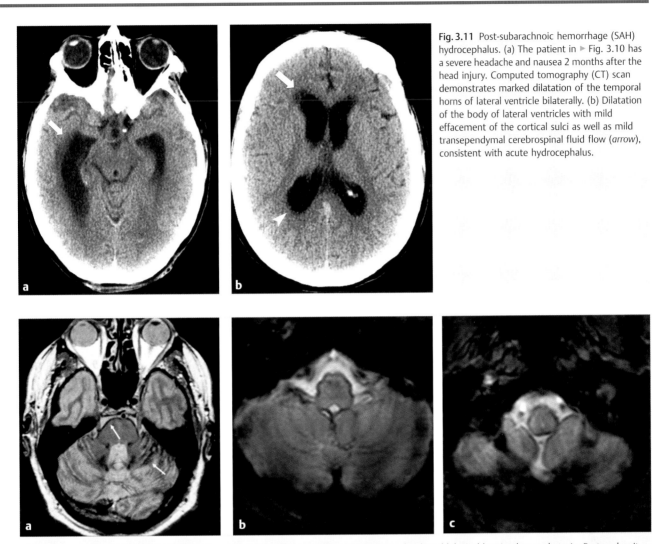

Fig. 3.11 Post-subarachnoic hemorrhage (SAH) hydrocephalus. (a) The patient in ▶ Fig. 3.10 has a severe headache and nausea 2 months after the head injury. Computed tomography (CT) scan demonstrates marked dilatation of the temporal horns of lateral ventricle bilaterally. (b) Dilatation of the body of lateral ventricles with mild effacement of the cortical sulci as well as mild transependymal cerebrospinal fluid flow (*arrow*), consistent with acute hydrocephalus.

Fig. 3.12 Superficial siderosis. (a) Patient after severe traumatic brain injury 2 years ago developed bilateral hearing loss and ataxia. Proton-density image demonstrates a dark signal outlining the arachnid membrane, consistent with the deposition of hemosiderin. (b) Gradient-echo image at the level of the medulla also demonstrates superficial deposition of hemosiderin outlining the surface of medulla and cranial nerves. (c) Superficial siderosis can also be seen at the level of the upper cervical spinal cord.

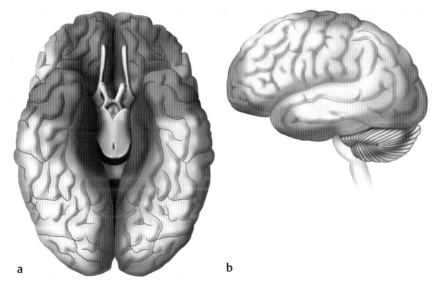

Fig. 3.13 Most common locations of brain contusions. (a) Contusions are most commonly in the base of the frontal lobes, anterior temporal lobes, inferior posterior temporal lobes, and less frequently occipital lobes and posterior frontoparietal convexity. (b) The anterior temporal lobes and inferior frontal lobes (red) are most commonly affected by contusion.

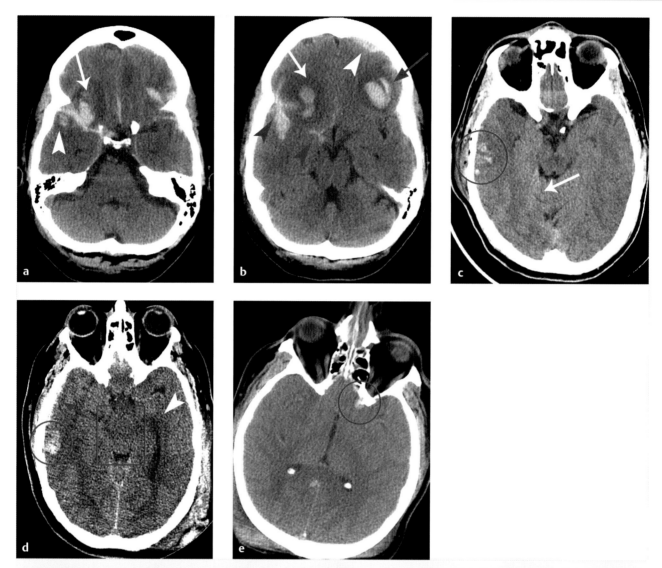

Fig. 3.14 Various contusions. (a) Patient status after a fall demonstrating contusion along the greater wing of sphenoid in the inferior frontal lobes (*arrow*) as well as anterior temporal lobes (*arrowhead*). (b) Large contusions in the base of the frontal lobes with adjacent edema (*arrow*). Note the accompanying left SDH (*arrowhead*) and right SAH along the sylvian fissures and suprasellar cistern (*arrowheads*). (c) Right temporal contusion with mixed-density hemorrhage adjacent to the subgaleal hematoma (*circle*). A small SDH along the right tentorium (*arrow*) is also present. (d) Different patient with posterior right temporal contusion (*circle*) with small SDH (*arrow*). Note the mass effect and compression on the midbrain (*square*) as well as enlargement of contralateral (left) lateral ventricle (*arrowhead*). (e) Patient with large right parietal subgaleal hematoma with small contusion along the left sphenoid wing (*circle*).

heterogeneous hyperdensity on CT; the lesion is characterized by mixed blood and injured brain tissue. Nonhemorrhagic contusions may not be readily visible on the initial head CT, although in a few days, the surrounding edema becomes more prominent (▶ Fig. 3.16). It is important to differentiate contusion from intracerebral hematoma associated with TBI, which is a large collection of blood. Intracerebral hematoma is due to rupture of parenchymal blood vessels, often caused by rotational force rather than by direct impact.

Patients with contusions are less likely to lose consciousness compared with those with DAI. Once contusion and surrounding edema causes mass significant effect and compression of adjacent brain tissue, surgical evacuation is often indicated. Follow up imaging study in the chronic stage often reveals area of encephalomalacia or related Wallerian degeneration.

3.4.6 Diffuse (Traumatic) Axonal Injury

DAI or TAI is referred to as shearing injury or microhemorrhage. Those axonal injury lesions are small (smaller than 5 mm), scattered white matter lesions, and they can be hemorrhagic or nonhemorrhagic. Some use the term *DAI* to describe more than three axonal injury lesions. Axonal injury is often due to rotational deceleration forces and ensuring shear-strain deformation at the interface between tissues of different densities and is thus common in the subcortical gray and white matter junction. As a result, axonal injury is most common in the frontal subcortical white matter, corona radiate, corpus callosum, internal capsule, and dorsal brainstem (▶ Fig. 3.17). Long-tract fibers are more prone to axonal injury, such as medial longitudinal fasciculus, medial lemniscus, superior cerebellar

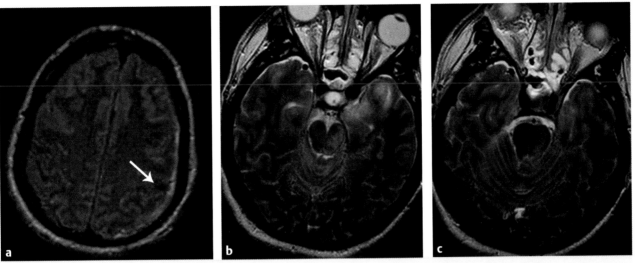

Fig. 3.15 Brainstem contusion. After a fall, the patient underwent brain magnetic resonance imaging. Fluid-attenuated inversion recovery (FLAIR) shows presence of traumatic subarachnoid hemorrhage (SAH) over the bilateral frontoparietal convexity, left greater than right, with a small left subdural hemorrhage (a). T2 weighted images of lower slices shows focal contusion in the left medial temporal lobe and the left lateral midbrain (b) and left lateral pons (c). This is most likely contusion of brainstem up against the tentorium cerebelli.

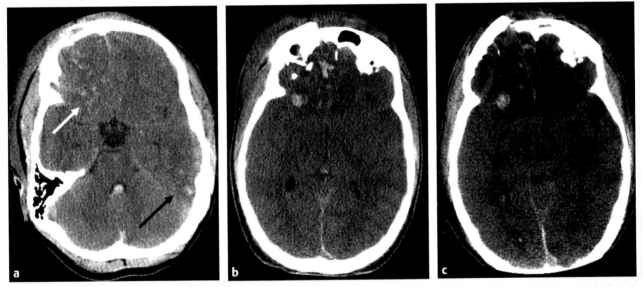

Fig. 3.16 Delayed edema with contusion. (a) Patient after motorcycle collision has a right frontal comminuted fracture with large area of right frontal contusion (*white arrow*) and posterior left temporal contusion (*black arrow*), with additional intraventricular hemorrhage in the fourth ventricle. (b) Computed tomography (CT) scans 12 hours after the initial CT demonstrates increasing edema surrounding the right fontal contusion as well as effacement of cortical sulci and small left subdural hemorrhage. (c) CT scan 24 hours after the initial CT demonstrate progression of edema surrounding contusion in the left frontal lobe as well as the left posterior inferior temporal lobe.

peduncle, and corticospinal (pyramidal) tracts. High-force deceleration and rotational force are responsible for DAIs and thus are most common in patients who have sustained a high speed motor-vehicle accident.

Although DAI was once believed to occur only in fatal cases of TBI, DAI has also been seen in moderate and mTBI patients. Some consider DAI to be a misnomer because shearing injury is not necessarily diffuse but rather multifocal, thus favoring the term *traumatic* axonal injury, or TAI. As imaging techniques advance, DAI or TAI is being more frequently detected

and diagnosed currently compared with the past.[35] MRI, in particular with GRE images, is far superior in revealing DAI or TAI lesions compared with CT (▶ Fig. 3.18). Moreover, SWI is reported to be 6 times more sensitive for detecting microhemorrhage associated with shearing injury compared with GRE images.[36]

At a pathological level, rapid acceleration and rotational deformation forces cause mechanical injury of the sites of different tissue density. The initial injury after stretch occurs at the nodes of Ranvier, which is a short interval between the

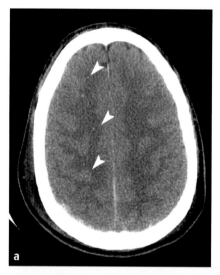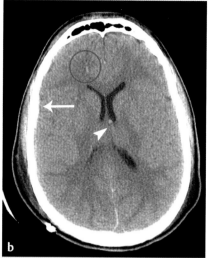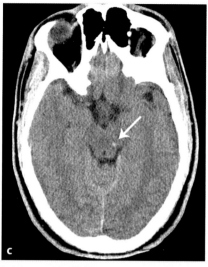

Fig. 3.17 Diffuse axonal injury (DAI). (a) Computed tomography scan of a patient after a high-speed motor-vehicle collision shows multiple small foci of hemorrhagic shearing injury along the right subcortical white matter (*arrowhead*). (b) Additional axonal injury in the right subcortical white matter (*circle*) as well as left fornix (*arrowhead*), one of the common locations for DAI. Note the small right subdural hemorrhage (*arrow*). (c) Image at the midbrain of the same patient shows a focal DAI involving the left dorsolateral midbrain (*arrow*).

processes of oligodendrocytes (▶ Fig. 3.19). This type of injury results in a defect in the axonal membrane, leading to an impairment of axonal transport. Subsequent swelling of the axon creates discrete bulb formation that accumulates transported proteins, causing further influx of calcium and iron, as well as glutamate dysregulation, which initiates the secondary cascade of cell damage. When the axon continues to swell, eventually it becomes disconnected and pulls back toward the cell body. This forms a so-called retraction bulb, which is a pathological hallmark of axonal injury.

Axonal injury results in interference with axonal transport—the movement of mitochondria, lipid, protein, and synaptic vesicles from cell body to the axonal tips—which is an essential mechanism of cytoskeletal integrity and survival of neuron. This is one of the plausible mechanisms for the development of neurodegenerative disease after TBI.

Nonhemorrhagic shearing injury lesions are difficult to visualize on CT and are better seen on FLAIR or DWI (▶ Fig. 3.20). The combination of DWI and SWI is the most sensitive imaging technique available for detection of axonal injury (▶ Fig. 3.21). Occasionally, convergent-type axonal injury lesions near the periventricular white matter radiating from the ventricular surface are noted on SWI images. Some investigators have reported that these convergent-type axonal injury lesions are often diffusion negative and may represent diffuse vascular injury involving the medullary veins, resulting in a serpiginous area of convergent signal drop-off on SWI, likely representing venous congestion.[37] This convergent type of shearing injury is often associated with a poor prognosis.

3.4.7 Intracerebral Hematoma

Intracerebral hematoma is a collection of blood (more than 5 mm) resulting from the disruption of parenchymal blood vessels, with minimum surrounding edema (▶ Fig. 3.22). Its pathology differs from that of contusion because it represents hemorrhage into relatively normal brain tissue. Intracerebral hematomas are often seen in the frontotemporal white matter and occasionally in the basal ganglia or other subcortical gray matter.

Although patients with intracerebral hematoma may remain lucid, mass effect from hematoma may increase in a few days, which potentially causes delayed neurologic symptoms. Intracerebral hematomas seen in the basal ganglia or thalamus are due to disruption of small perforating vessels. Hemorrhage in the subcortical gray matter is considered severe head injury and associated with a poor prognosis.

3.4.8 Brainstem Injury

Brainstem injury is divided into primary injury and secondary injury. The most common primary brainstem injury is DAI and in the dorsolateral aspect of midbrain and pons. Superior cerebellar peduncle and medial lemnisci are most susceptible to DAI (▶ Fig. 3.23). A secondary brainstem injury is called Duret hemorrhage, which is an intracerebral hemorrhage resulting from descending transtentorial herniation.[38] The generally accepted theory for Duret hemorrhage is that the brainstem is pushed inferiorly, stretching perforating arteries, whereas the basilar artery is relatively immobile along the clivus. The brainstem is pushed side-by-side, stretching the mesencephalon and upper pons in an anterior-posterior direction, which further stretches the perforating arterial branches from the basilar artery (▶ Fig. 3.24). Duret hemorrhage is usually near midline in the midbrain tegmentum or pons. Some authorities, however, debate whether the Duret hemorrhage could be venous in origin, secondary to venous thrombosis and hemorrhage. Duret hemorrhage is considered an ominous prognostic sign.

Another secondary brainstem injury occurs in the setting of uncal herniation resulting from the presence of a large intracerebral hematoma or subdural fluid collection. Uncal herniation forces the midbrain to shift and rotate so that the

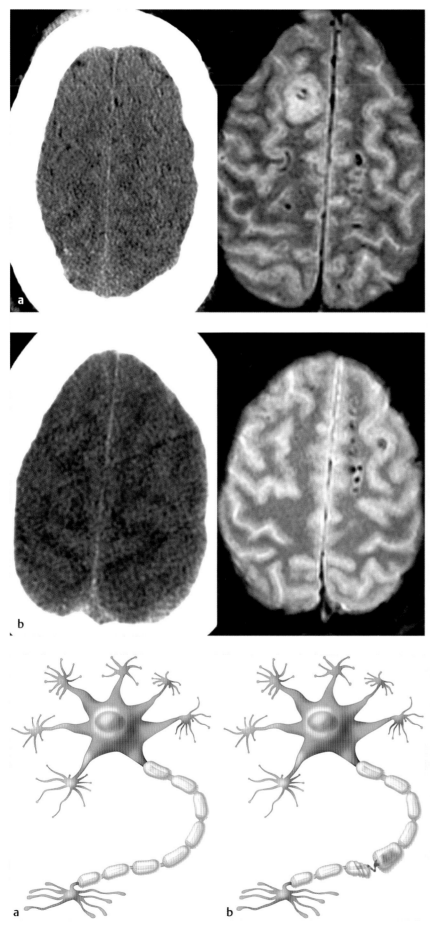

Fig. 3.18 Diffuse axonal injury (DAI) computed tomography (CT) vs. gradient echo (GRE). (a) Patient status post motor-vehicle collision underwent CT and magnetic resonance imaging on the same day. Many of the DAI lesions on GRE images are difficult to detect on noncontrast CT. (b) Numerous foci of DAI in the left frontal subcortical white matter is difficult to appreciate on non-contrast head CT.

Fig. 3.19 Illustration of diffuse axona injury. (a) Normal illustration of neuron consists of neuron's cell body, axon, which is a nerve fiber, and axonal terminal. Electric impulses from the cell body are conducted through the axon. Axons are surrounded by myelin sheath, which is composed of oligodendrocytes in the central nervous system. Gaps in the myelin sheath are called nodes of Ranvier and allow rapid mode of electrical impulse propagation. (b) Axonal injury often takes place at the nodes of Ranvier by the stretching and rotational forces. Subsequent swelling of axon creates discrete bulb formation accumulating transported protein. This is called retraction bulb, a pathological hallmark of axonal injury.

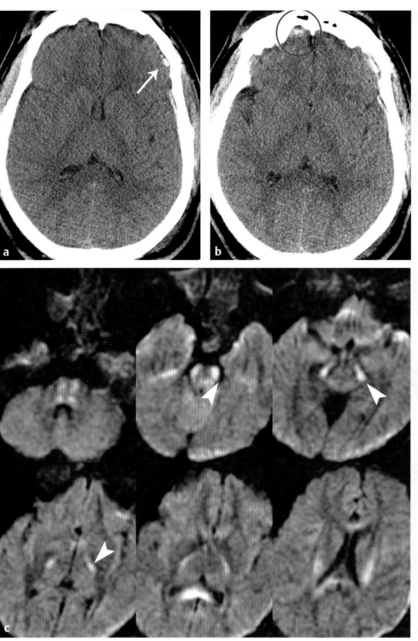

Fig. 3.20 Diffuse axonal injury (DAI). Status post motor-vehicle collision. Low Glasgow Coma Scale despite only small left subdural hemorrhage (*arrow*) and right frontal contusion (*circle*). Images through corpus callosum (a) and internal capsule (b) are unremarkable. (c) Diffusion-weighted images demonstrate restricted diffusion along bilateral corticospinal tract (*arrowheads*) and splenium of the corpus callosum, indicating DAI.

contralateral cerebral peduncle is forced against the contralateral tentorial incisum (▶ Fig. 3.25). If this happens, hemiparesis is ipsilateral to the side of injury or hematoma.[39,40] This phenomenon is called Kernohan-Woltman notch syndrome.

3.4.9 Pituitary or Hypothalamic Injury

It has been recognized that after a moderate to severe TBI patients suffer from varying degrees of pituitary hormone dysfunction.[41] In particular, growth hormone dysfunction (poor sleep and low energy) has been speculated to contribute to some of the post-traumatic symptoms, including social isolation and limited executive function.[42,43] Another study found the pituitary and gonadal dysfunction among severe TBI adult victims.[44] A study investigating soldiers after blast injury revealed that patients with anterior pituitary dysfunction had a higher incidence of facial and skull fractures as well as cognitive function abnormality.[45] Professional boxers and other contact-sports athletes showed more cerebellar and vermian atrophy, pituitary and hippocampal atrophy, the presence of cavum septum pellucidum, and dilated perivascular spaces.

Meta-analysis of adulthood TBI study, however, failed to demonstrate the difference in hypothalamic-pituitary-adrenal axis dysregulation between trauma patients and nontrauma patients.[46] However, subgroup analyses showed increased cortisol suppression after the low-dose dexamethasone suppression test in trauma patients compared with nontrauma subjects. A larger study is necessary to provide a higher level of concrete evidence.

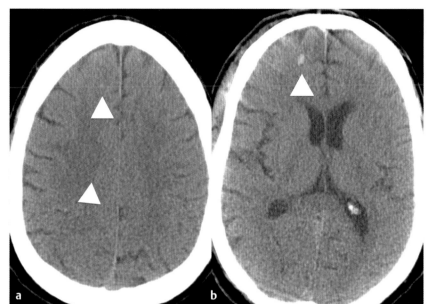

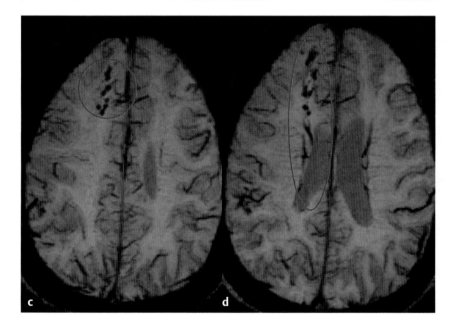

Fig. 3.21 Diffuse axonal injury computed tomography versus susceptibility-weighted imaging. CT images of a patient with head injury show a focus of hemorrhagic shearing injury in the right inferior frontal white matter (*arrowhead*) (a,b). SWI images (c,d) demonstrate many more foci of shearing injury in the right frontal subcortical white matter (*oval*).

3.4.10 Thalamus and Deep Gray Matter Injury

It has been suggested that TBI findings are seen not only in subcortical white matter, but also in deep gray matter structures, such as the thalamus (▶ Fig. 3.26). Several recent group comparison studies suggest that the thalamus could harbor significant traumatic injury, as evidenced by reduced cerebral blood flow, mean kurtosis values, and increased iron deposition.[47–49] Another study analyzing apparent diffusion coefficient (ADC) values of superficial and deep gray matter found that superficial and deep white matter revealed significantly higher ADC values in the deep gray matter among patients with unfavorable outcomes.[50]

Secondary TBI lesions, including cisternal compression, midline shift, and mass effect or herniation, as well as cerebral edema and loss of autoregulation, are discussed in Chapter 4,

Pathophysiology of Traumatic Brain Injury and Impact on Management.

3.4.11 Chronic Sequelae of Traumatic Brain Injury

Over the past several decades, medical and surgical care of TBI has dramatically improved, resulting in a large number of patients with long-term sequelae of TBI. The vast majority of people suffering from moderate to severe TBI have chronic neurobehavioral sequelae, including cognitive deficits, personality changes, and dementia. Certain cognitive domains are typically impaired after TBI, such as executive function, attention, short-term memory and learning, processing information, and language.[51] Personality changes often seen among TBI victims are apathy, impulsivity, irritability, and affective instability.

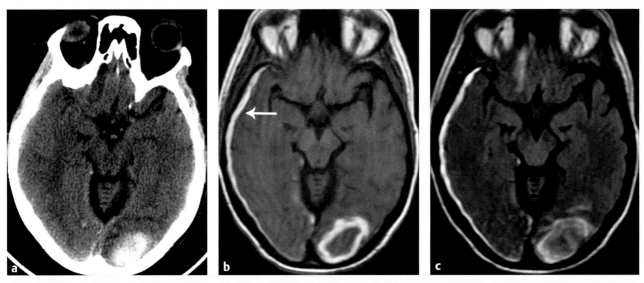

Fig. 3.22 Cerebral hematoma. (a) A computed tomographic image of a patient status post fall shows a focal homogeneous density hematoma in the left occipital lobe with minimum surrounding edema. (b) T1-weighted axial image shows a small right sudural hemorrhage extending along the right tentorium (*arrow*), as well as subacute hematoma. (c) Minimum surrounding edema of left occipital hematoma on fluid-attenuated inversion recovery (FLAIR) image (c).

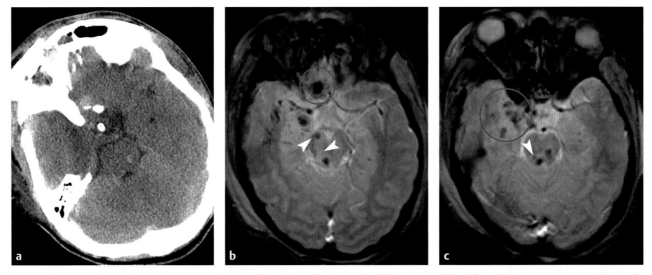

Fig. 3.23 Brainstem axonal injury. (a) Computed tomographic image of a patient who had a motor-vehicle collision demonstrates a punctate area of hemorrhagic shearing injury in the left dorsolateral pons with accompanying right subdural hemorrhage and right frontal depressed fracture. Axial gradient-echo image of the midbrain (b) and pons (c) demonstrates additional foci of shearing injury (*arrowhead*) involving the brainstem, including the right cerebral peduncle, superior cerebellar peduncle, left dorsolateral pons, and right periaqueductal gray matter. Note the contusion involving the medial right temporal lobe and inferior right frontal lobe as well (*circle*).

The brain damage caused by TBI may be diffuse or multifocal. Certain brain regions are thought to be responsible for the high rate of neuropsychiatric illness. These vulnerable and responsible regions include the frontal cortex and subfrontal white matter, the deeper midline structures including the basal ganglia, the rostral brainstem, and the mesial temporal lobes, including the hippocampi (▶ Fig. 3.27). Social and behavioral problems after TBI can be explained to some extent by the regional vulnerability. Recently, some suggest that injury to thalamocortical fibers may account for the loss of executive function among mTBI patients.[47,48]

TBI lesions to the dorsolateral prefrontal cortex and its circuitry impair executive functions, such as working memory, decision making, and problem solving. Injury to the orbitofrontal cortex impairs social behaviors and the capacity to self-monitor and self-correct within a social context. Damage to the anterior cingulate and related circuitry impairs motivated and reward-related behaviors and anger control. Damage to medial temporal regions impairs aspects of memory and the smooth integration of emotional memory with current experience.

In addition to neuropsychiatric illness, interests and attention over the relationship of TBI and dementia have grown. Some

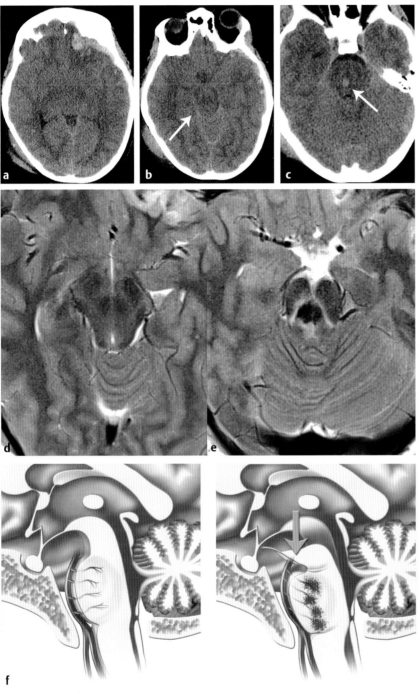

Fig. 3.24 Brainstem Duret hemorrhage. (a) Initial head computed tomogram of a young patient after a pedestrian injury by a car demonstrates left frontal subdural hemorrhage and diffuse effacement of basilar cistern. Note that the midbrain is compressed side-by-side and has an elongated appearance accompanying the effacement of ambient cistern. Image farther down at the level of the pons demonstrates a focal right paramedian hemorrhage, consistent with Duret hemorrhage. (d,e) T2-weighed axial images of the same patient again demonstrate elongated midbrain and a focal hemorrhage in the pons with left frontal contusion and edema. (f) Illustration demonstrates inferior displacement of brainstem (*arrow*) causing stretching of perforating arteries leading to brainstem hemorrhage.

indicated that moderate and severe TBI increased risk of dementia between twofold and fourfold. Many individuals with moderate to severe TBI who have significant impairments in memory and executive function meet the *Diagnostic and Statistical Manual of Mental Disorders*-IV definition of dementia. In addition, patients with chronic traumatic encephalopathy often have metabolic abnormality and aggregation of tau protein and beta-amyloid, features that suggest neurodegenerative disease.[51,52]

Debate continues about whether exposure to a TBI increases the risk of a progressive neurodegenerative dementing disorder such as Alzheimer disease later in life. At present, convincing evidence has not been found to establish the causality that TBI, in particular mTBI, is a risk factor for Alzheimer disease. It is speculated that early clinical onset of Alzheimer disease among TBI survivors relative to noninjured controls is due primarily reduced cognitive reserve.[53]

3.5 Pearls

1. TBI is a major public health problem with significant morbidity and substantial societal costs. The classification based on GCS does not provide mechanistic or pathophysiological information of brain injury and is limited for assessment for

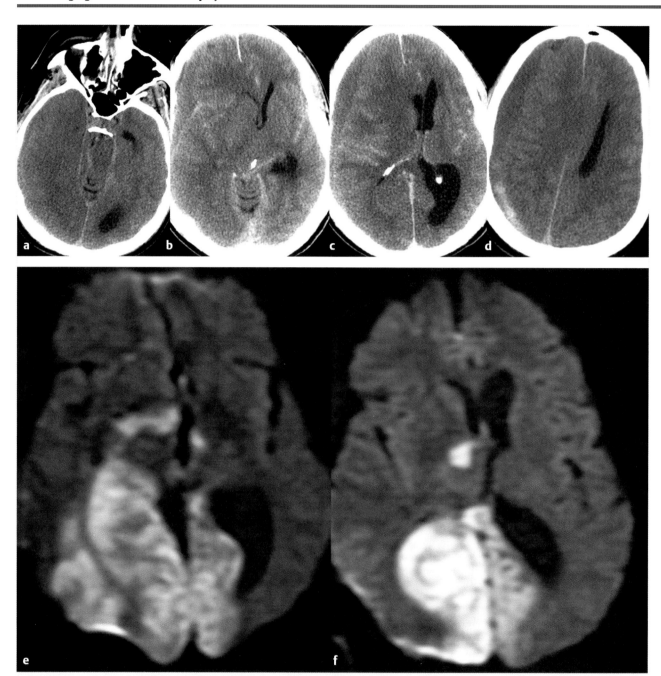

Fig. 3.25 Severe uncal herniation and Kernohan-Woltman notch syndrome. A man working in construction fell 46 feet from the ladder and a few days later had confusion and obtundation. A set of computed tomographic images (a–d) show mixed density right subdural hemorrhage (SDH) with diffuse traumatic subarachnoic hemorrhage (tSAH) as well as severe midline shift and uncal herniation toward left. Dilatation of left lateral ventricle indicates entrapment of the left lateral ventricle likely as a result of compression at the foramen of Monro. Diffusion-weighted image show areas of restricted diffusion in the bilateral occipital lobes and medial thalamus, consistent with bilateral posterior cerebral artery distribution infarction (e,f) (continued).

mTBI. In the acute trauma setting, CT scan remains the first line of imaging study that helps in triaging patients who need emergent intervention from those who can safely observe. Objective assessment of the severity of injury based on CT findings predicts the probability of mortality among TBI patients.

2. Although Brain MR often shows more TBI lesions than CT, the wide clinical adaptation of MR at the acute trauma setting is limited in part due to logistics related to access, required safety process, and higher costs. Given the increasing awareness of biological effects of ionizing radiation from CT, more widespread use of MR among TBI patients is becoming important to accurately assess the extent of injury and presence of DAI/TAI spectrum.

3. There is some debate as to whether or not to repeat head CT routinely for patients with TBI. Routine follow up head CT is more justifiable for patients with severe injury that are sedated or unconscious.

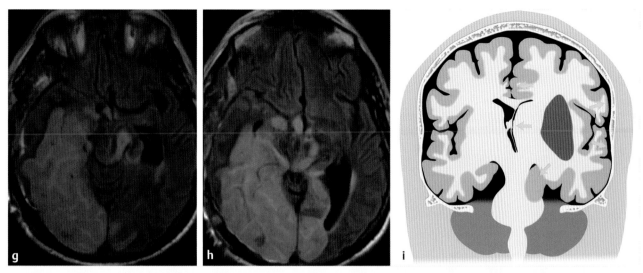

Fig. 3.25 (*continued*) Fluid-attenuated inversion recovery (FLAIR) images at the midbrain demonstrate shift and rotation of midbrain from right uncal herniation. As a result, left midbrain (contralateral side of SDH) shows increased FLAIR signal as a result of compression against the left tentorial edge (g,h). Illustration demonstrates mass effect from a hematoma displacing the uncus hematoma down through the tentorium (uncal herniation) and cingulate gyrus underneath the falx (parafalcian herniation) (i).

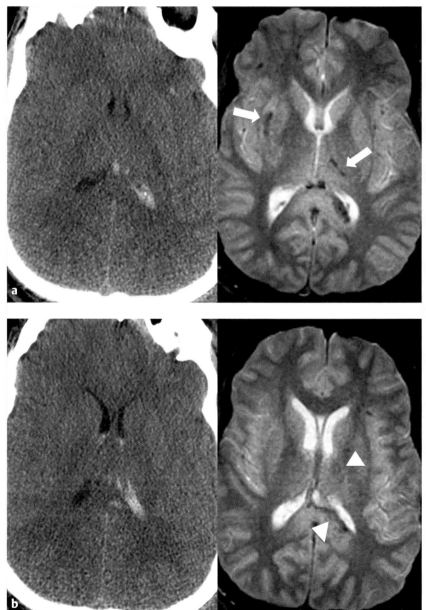

Fig. 3.26 Diffuse axonal injury involving the corpus callosum and thalamus. (a) Computed tomographic (CT) image of a high-speed motor-vehicle collision victim shows intraventricular hemorrhage with a punctate area of shearing injury in the medial left thalamus. Gradient-echo image clearly shows presence of shearing injury in the left thalamus as well as right putamen (*arrow*), not definitely seen on CT. (b) Slightly higher slice of the same patient shows hemorrhagic shearing injury involving the splenium of the corpus callosum as well as the left internal capsule (*arrowhead*).

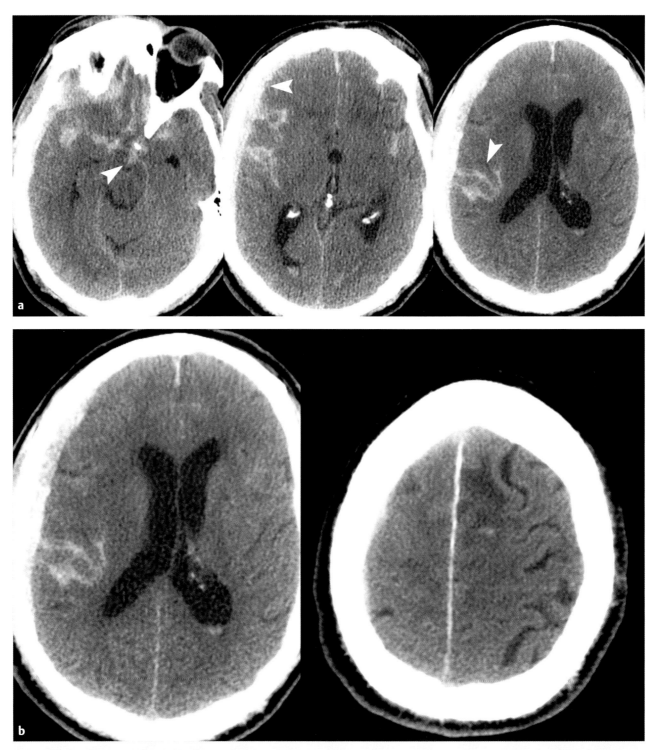

Fig. 3.27 Chronic traumatic encephalopathy. (a) Initial computed tomographic (CT) images of a patient after a motor-vehicle collision demonstrate right subdural hemorrhage (*arrowhead*), traumatic subarachnoid hemorrhage in the bilateral sylvian fissures and basal cistern (*arrow*) as well as contusion involving the frontal lobes bilaterally. (b) (*continued*)

4. Radiologists should be familiar with imaging features of all pathoanatomic types of TBI. Keep in mind that TBI is often associated with vascular damage (i.e. dissection or venous sinus thrombosis/injury). Secondary injury related to cerebral edema or brain herniation and vascular compression could result in ischemic infarction.

5. Patients with poor neurological status despite relatively negative head CT may benefit from brain MR for accurate assessment of traumatic injury in brainstem, deep gray nuclei, as well as DAI/TAI spectrum.

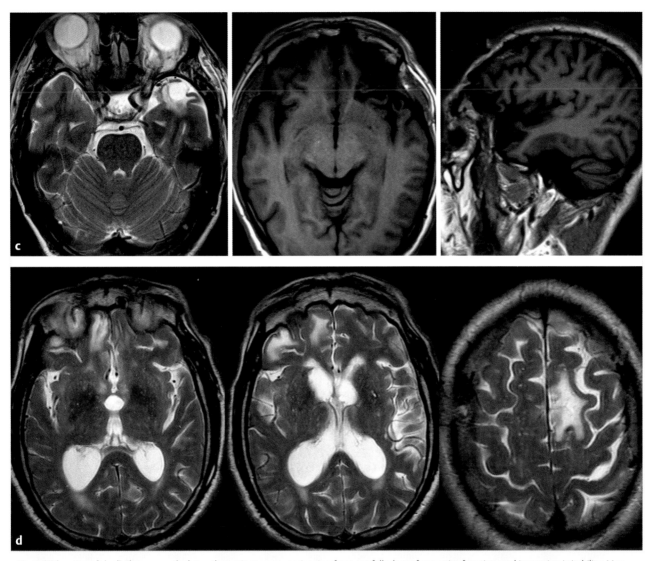

Fig. 3.27 (*continued*) (c,d) Eleven months later, the patient was experiencing frequent falls, loss of executive function, and increasing irritability. Magnetic resonance images show extensive encephalomalacia in the bilateral frontal lobes, anterior temporal lobe, and left frontal convexity and diffuse brain volume loss with ex vacuo dilatation of lateral ventricles.

References

[1] Faul MXL, Wald MM, Coronado VG. Traumatic Brain Injury in the United States: Emergency Department Visits, Hospitalizations, and Deaths. Atlanta, GA: Centers for Disease Control and Prevention, National Center for Injury. Prevention and Control: 2010.

[2] Langlois JA, Kegler SR, Butler JA et al. Traumatic brain injury-related hospital discharges results from a 14-state surveillance system, 1997. MMWR Surveill Summ 2003; 52: 1–20

[3] Taylor BC, Hagel EM, Carlson KF et al. Prevalence and costs of co-occurring traumatic brain injury with and without psychiatric disturbance and pain among Afghanistan and Iraq War Veteran V.A. users. Med Care 2012; 50: 342–346

[4] Koepsell TD, Rivara FP, Vavilala MS et al. Incidence and descriptive epidemiologic features of traumatic brain injury in King County, Washington. Pediatrics. 2011; 128: 946–954

[5] Bazarian JJ, McClung J, Cheng YT, Flesher W, Schneider SM. Emergency department management of mild traumatic brain injury in the USA. Emerg Med J. 2005; 22: 473–477

[6] Jennett B, Teasdale G, Braakman R, Minderhoud J, Knill-Jones R. Predicting outcome in individual patients after severe head injury. Lancet 1976; 1: 1031–1034

[7] Leitgeb J, Mauritz W, Brazinova A et al. Glasgow Coma Scale score at intensive care unit discharge predicts the 1-year outcome of patients with severe traumatic brain injury. Eur J Trauma Emerg Surg 2013; 39: 285–292

[8] Jennett B. The history of the Glasgow Coma Scale: an interview with professor Bryan Jennett. Interview by Carole Rush. Int J Trauma Nurs 1997; 3: 114–118

[9] Saatman KE, Duhaime AC, Bullock R, Maas AI, Valadka A, Manley GT Workshop Scientific Team and Advisory Panel Members. Classification of traumatic brain injury for targeted therapies. J Neurotrauma 2008; 25: 719–738

[10] Barker MD, Whyte J, Pretz CR et al. Application and clinical utility of the Glasgow Coma Scale over time: a study employing the NIDRR Traumatic Brain Injury Model Systems Database. J Head Trauma Rehabil 2013 [epub ahead of print]

[11] Wilson JT, Pettigrew LE, Teasdale GM. Structured interviews for the Glasgow Outcome Scale and the extended Glasgow Outcome Scale: guidelines for their use. J Neurotrauma 1998; 15: 573–585

[12] Tavender EJ, Bosch M, Green S et al. Quality and consistency of guidelines for the management of mild traumatic brain injury in the emergency department. Acad Emerg Med 2011; 18: 880–889

[13] Haydel MJ, Preston CA, Mills TJ, Luber S, Blaudeau E, DeBlieux PM. Indications for computed tomography in patients with minor head injury. N Engl J Med. 2000; 343: 100–105

[14] Stiell IG, Wells GA, Vandemheen K et al. The Canadian CT Head Rule for patients with minor head injury. Lancet 2001; 357: 1391–1396

[15] Smits M, Dippel DW, de Haan GG et al. External validation of the Canadian CT Head Rule and the New Orleans Criteria for CT scanning in patients with minor head injury. JAMA 2005; 294: 1519–1525

[16] Melnick ER, Szlezak CM, Bentley SK, Dziura JD, Kotlyar S, Post LA. CT overuse for mild traumatic brain injury. Jt Comm J Qual Patient Saf 2012; 38: 483–489

[17] Almenawer S, Bogza I, Yarascavitch B et al. The value of scheduled repeat cranial computed tomography following mild head injury: single-center series and meta-analysis. Neurosurgery 2013; 72: 56–62

[18] Connon FF, Namdarian B, Ee JL, Drummond KJ, Miller JA. Do routinely repeated computed tomography scans in traumatic brain injury influence management? A prospective observational study in a level 1 trauma center. Ann Surg 2011; 254: 1028–1031

[19] Thorson CM, Van Haren RM, Otero CA et al. Repeat head computed tomography after minimal brain injury identifies the need for craniotomy in the absence of neurologic change. J Trauma Acute Care Surg 2013; 74: 967–975

[20] Jagoda AS, Bazarian JJ, Bruns JJ Jr. et al. American College of Emergency Physicians. Centers for Disease Control and Prevention. Clinical policy: neuroimaging and decisionmaking in adult mild traumatic brain injury in the acute setting. Ann Emerg Med 2008; 52: 714–748

[21] Lee H, Wintermark M, Gean AD, Ghajar J, Manley GT, Mukherjee P. Focal lesions in acute mild traumatic brain injury and neurocognitive outcome: CT versus 3 T MRI. J Neurotrauma 2008; 25: 1049–1056

[22] Manolakaki D, Velmahos GC, Spaniolas K, de Moya M, Alam HB. Early magnetic resonance imaging is unnecessary in patients with traumatic brain injury. J Trauma. 2009; 66: 1008–1014

[23] Geurts BH, Andriessen TM, Goraj BM, Vos PE. The reliability of magnetic resonance imaging in traumatic brain injury lesion detection. Brain Inj 2012; 26: 1439–1450

[24] Beauchamp MH, Ditchfield M, Babl FE et al. Detecting traumatic brain lesions in children: CT versus MRI versus susceptibility weighted imaging (SWI). J Neurotrauma 2011; 28: 915–927

[25] Scheid R, Preul C, Gruber O, Wiggins C, von Cramon DY. Diffuse axonal injury associated with chronic traumatic brain injury: evidence from T2*-weighted gradient-echo imaging at 3 T. AJNR Am J Neuroradiol 2003; 24: 1049–1056

[26] Maas AI, Hukkelhoven CW, Marshall LF, Steyerberg EW. Prediction of outcome in traumatic brain injury with computed tomographic characteristics: a comparison between the computed tomographic classification and combinations of computed tomographic predictors. Neurosurgery. 2005; 57: 1173–1182

[27] Chastain CA, Oyoyo UE, Zipperman M et al. Predicting outcomes of traumatic brain injury by imaging modality and injury distribution. J Neurotrauma 2009; 26: 1183–1196

[28] Yuh EL, Mukherjee P, Lingsma HF et al. TRACK-TBI Investigators. Magnetic resonance imaging improves 3-month outcome prediction in mild traumatic brain injury. Ann Neurol 2013; 73: 224–235

[29] Muñoz-Sánchez MA, Murillo-Cabezas F, Cayuela-Domínguez A, Rincón-Ferrari MD, Amaya-Villar R, León-Carrión J. Skull fracture, with or without clinical signs, in mTBI is an independent risk marker for neurosurgically relevant intracranial lesion: a cohort study. Brain Inj. 2009; 23: 39–44

[30] Gean AD, Fischbein NJ, Purcell DD, Aiken AH, Manley GT, Stiver SI. Benign anterior temporal epidural hematoma: indolent lesion with a characteristic CT imaging appearance after blunt head trauma. Radiology 2010; 257: 212–218

[31] Al-Nakshabandi NA. The swirl sign. Radiology 2001; 218: 433

[32] Wu Z, Li S, Lei J, An D, Haacke EM. Evaluation of traumatic subarachnoid hemorrhage using susceptibility-weighted imaging. AJNR Am J Neuroradiol 2010; 31: 1302–1310

[33] Maas AI. Standardisation of data collection in traumatic brain injury: key to the future? Crit Care 2009; 13: 1016

[34] Vadala R, Giugni E, Pezzella FR, Sabatin U, Bastianello S. Progressive sensorineural hearing loss, ataxia and anosmia as manifestation of superficial siderosis in post traumatic brain injury. Neurol Sci 2013; 34: 1259–1262

[35] Kim J, Smith A, Hemphill JC III. et al. Contrast extravasation on CT predicts mortality in primary intracerebral hemorrhage. AJNR Am J Neuroradiol 2008; 29: 520–525

[36] Ashwal S, Babikian T, Gardner-Nichols J, Freier MC, Tong KA, Holshouser BA. Susceptibility-weighted imaging and proton magnetic resonance spectroscopy in assessment of outcome after pediatric traumatic brain injury. Arch Phys Med Rehabil 2006; 87 Suppl 2: S50–S58

[37] Iwamura A, Taoka T, Fukusumi A et al. Diffuse vascular injury: convergent-type hemorrhage in the supratentorial white matter on susceptibility-weighted image in cases of severe traumatic brain damage. Neuroradiology 2012; 54: 335–343

[38] Parizel PM, Makkat S, Jorens PG et al. Brainstem hemorrhage in descending transtentorial herniation (Duret hemorrhage). Intensive Care Med 2002; 28: 85–88

[39] McKenna C, Fellus J, Barrett AM. False localizing signs in traumatic brain injury. Brain Inj 2009; 23: 597–601

[40] Zafonte RD, Lee CY. Kernohan-Woltman notch phenomenon: an unusual cause of ipsilateral motor deficit. Arch Phys Med Rehabil 1997; 78: 543–545

[41] De Sanctis V, Sprocati M, Govoni M R, Raiola G. Assessment of traumatic brain injury and anterior pituitary dysfunction in adolescents. Georgian Med News. 2008: 18–23

[42] Czirják S, Rácz K, Góth M. [Neuroendocrine dysfunctions and their consequences following traumatic brain injury] Orv Hetil. 2012; 153: 927–933

[43] Munoz A, Urban R. Neuroendocrine consequences of traumatic brain injury. Curr Opin Endocrinol Diabetes Obes 2013; 20: 354–358

[44] Lee SC, Zasler ND, Kreutzer JS. Male pituitary-gonadal dysfunction following severe traumatic brain injury. Brain Inj 1994; 8: 571–577

[45] Baxter D, Sharp DJ, Feeney C et al. Pituitary dysfunction after blast traumatic brain injury: UK BIOSAP study. Ann Neurol2013;74:527–536

[46] Klaassens ER, Giltay EJ, Cuijpers P, van Veen T, Zitman FG. Adulthood trauma and HPA-axis functioning in healthy subjects and PTSD patients: a meta-analysis. Psychoneuroendocrinology 2012; 37: 317–331

[47] Little DM, Kraus MF, Joseph J et al. Thalamic integrity underlies executive dysfunction in traumatic brain injury. Neurology 2010; 74: 558–564

[48] Tang L, Ge Y, Sodickson DK et al. Thalamic resting-state functional networks: disruption in patients with mild traumatic brain injury. Radiology 2011; 260: 831–840

[49] Grossman EJ, Ge Y, Jensen JH et al. Thalamus and cognitive impairment in mild traumatic brain injury: a diffusional kurtosis imaging study. J Neurotrauma. 2012; 29: 2318–2327

[50] Hou DJ, Tong KA, Ashwal S et al. Diffusion-weighted magnetic resonance imaging improves outcome prediction in adult traumatic brain injury. J Neurotrauma 2007; 24: 1558–1569

[51] Baugh CM, Stamm JM, Riley DO et al. Chronic traumatic encephalopathy: neurodegeneration following repetitive concussive and subconcussive brain trauma. Brain Imaging Behav 2012; 6: 244–254

[52] Blennow K, Hardy J, Zetterberg H. The neuropathology and neurobiology of traumatic brain injury. Neuron 2012; 76: 886–899

[53] Moretti L, Cristofori I, Weaver SM, Chau A, Portelli JN, Grafman J. Cognitive decline in older adults with a history of traumatic brain injury. Lancet Neurol. 2012; 11: 1103–1112

[54] Brant WE and Helms C. Fundamentals of Diagnostic Radiology. 4th edition. Philadelphia: Lippincott Williams & Wilkins.2012; 49–75

4 Pathophysiology of Traumatic Brain Injury and Impact on Management

Kathleen R. Fink

4.1 Introduction

The damage wrought by traumatic brain injury (TBI) is a dynamic process that occurs during many stages, only some of which can be mitigated by medical or surgical intervention. Injury begins at the time of trauma (or even before if the risk factors for injury, such as intoxication, are considered) and continues as the body reacts to the initial injury. This statement applies not only to damage resulting from the TBI itself but also to the sequelae of systemic injury, such as hypotension resulting from hemodynamic shock. This chapter focuses on the mechanism of tissue damage after TBI, including both the primary effects of trauma on the brain and the secondary injuries that can result from the body's response to injury. Although preventative measures, such as wearing protective headgear, can lessen the severity of the primary injury, once the injury has occurred, there is little medical treatment can do to alter or reverse the effects.

Medical or surgical treatment does play a role in diminishing secondary injury. Secondary injury is damage caused by the body's response to the primary insult; that is, the primary injury may be a skull fracture with accumulation of an epidural hematoma. The secondary injury results from mass effect of the hemorrhage, with compression on important structures. Secondary injury also can result from inflammatory mediators that alter metabolism.

Systemic factors also contribute to secondary injury after TBI. These factors include hypoxia, hypothermia, hypotension, and hypercoagulable state.[1] The Brain Trauma Foundation has specific guidelines for addressing the management of these factors,[2] some of which are directly applicable to neuroimaging.

This chapter discusses the mechanism of primary injury to alert radiologists to important imaging findings that may suggest associated injuries or lead to secondary injury. Additionally, this chapter details imaging findings of secondary brain injury, including edema, infarction, and brain herniation. The concept of cerebral autoregulation is introduced. Finally, physiologic monitoring devices used in the intensive care unit for the care of these patients are discussed, with imaging correlates.

4.2 Primary Brain Injury

The effect of primary injury to the brain depends on the nature of the trauma, including the mechanism of injury and the force and direction of impact. Systemic factors, including hypoxia, shock, coagulopathy, and effects of drugs or alcohol, can impact how the primary injury develops.

Injury resulting from a direct blow to the head results from mechanical forces on the skull, underlying vascular structures, and brain parenchyma. Mechanical force to the skull may cause deformation of the calvarium, sometimes resulting in fracture. Compression or tearing of blood vessel walls underlying the

force of impact can result in hemorrhage.[3] The location of the injured vessels will result in the specific pattern of brain injury, including extra-axial or intra-axial hemorrhage. The underlying brain parenchyma may sustain a contusion or laceration. Additional structures underlying the impact zone may also be damaged.

Brain contusions occur on the surface of the brain and result from injury to small vessels and neural tissue (▶ Fig. 4.1). Contusions may be produced by mechanical compression of tissue beneath an area of skull depression caused by mechanical force or by sudden negative pressure when the calvarium snaps back into place.[3] Factors such as whether the head is moving at the time of impact and whether the head is supported (such as against the ground) at impact affect the pattern of contusions.

Although the calvarium provides a good primary defense against blunt trauma to the head, in some cases, the calvarium

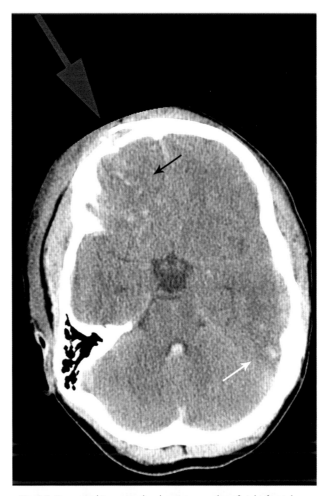

Fig. 4.1 Computed tomography showing sequelae of right frontal impact (*red arrow*) with fractures of the inner and outer table of the frontal sinus, underlying parenchymal contusions (*black arrow*), and contrecoup contusions (*white arrow*).

may also be a means of damage to the brain, such as occurs in the case of contrecoup injury. With sudden deceleration (such as when the skull hits the floor), the inertia of the brain results in a secondary impact of the brain against the opposite inner table of the skull, which can result in hemorrhage of the underlying brain parenchyma and contrecoup contusions (▶ Fig. 4.1). Gliding contusions result when the brain strikes the rigid falx cerebri.

Contusions occur as a result of bleeding within the brain parenchyma. The term *laceration* may be used if the overlying pial membrane is disrupted. Initially, damaged blood vessels result in bleeding into the tissue. Local mass effect or vessel thrombosis can then result in ischemic necrosis.[3] Inflammation results as the body responds to the injured tissue, inciting a leukocytic and lymphocytic response and also an inflammatory cytokine response. Damaged tissue may undergo apoptosis or necrosis.[4] With time, the body removes the damaged tissue, leaving reactive gliosis. The imaging appearance and characteristic locations of brain contusions are discussed further in Chapter 3, Neuroimaging of Traumatic Brain Injury.

At a cellular level, the mechanism of brain parenchymal injury is due to excitotoxicity, mediated via excessive release of excitatory neurotransmitters, including glutamate.[4,5] Extracellular glutamate binds *N*-methyl-*d*-aspartate and AMPA receptors and allows sodium and calcium influxes into the cell. Calcium influx then results in activation of calcium-dependent enzymes, resulting in further cell damage.[4] Mitochondrial dysfunction also plays a role.[6]

Damage to extra-axial blood vessels also results in TBI. Laceration to the meningeal arteries can result in an epidural hematoma, and laceration to the middle meningeal artery in particular can result in rapid accumulation of epidural hematoma with associated mass effect on the underlying brain. Less commonly, epidural hematomas result from injury to the venous sinuses.

Subdural hematomas are caused by laceration of bridging veins from the brain surface to the dura. As a result of direct bleeding, subdural hematomas also can occur in conjunction with adjacent cerebral contusions or lacerations[7,8] or as a result of laceration of a cortical artery or branch.[8–10] Unlike patients with epidural hematomas, those with subdural hematomas commonly sustain associated injuries to the underlying brain parenchyma, which may explain why they experience less favorable outcomes despite early decompressive surgery.[7]

Critical structures within the cranial vault may be damaged by a direct impact, for example, the cochlea (▶ Fig. 4.2a,b). In some cases, the primary injury may spare the brain, but the injury may put the brain at risk for further injury. For example, as discussed in Chapter 10, Maxillofacial Trauma, a frontal sinus fracture extending through an inner table may increase the risk for subsequent brain infection. An arterial injury may result in a rapidly expanding hematoma, compressing surrounding brain structures, or in downstream infarction (▶ Fig. 4.2c–e). Injury to the transverse sinus may result in epidural hematoma (▶ Fig. 4.2f,g) and risk subsequent venous sinus thrombosis and venous infarction. Thus, it is important to consider not only what structures are damaged but also how that injury may put the patient at risk for subsequent complications.

In some cases, there is a rotational component of force applied to the brain. Shear, tensile, and compressive strains on the brain tissue may result in axonal injury. This torsional component can disrupt the fine structures of the brain, resulting in diffuse axonal injury.[3] Damage to axons is a complex process that depends on the type and duration of mechanical trauma and may occur by different mechanisms.[11] The imaging manifestations of diffuse axonal injury may be minor, especially as seen by CT, with the extent of injury evident only by histologic review. The imaging findings of diffuse axonal injury are discussed in Chapter 3, Neuroimaging of Traumatic Brain Injury.

4.3 Secondary Brain Injury

Secondary brain injury occurs after the primary insult as a result of the physiologic response of the brain to injury. The primary culprits behind secondary brain injury are mass effect, brain swelling, and ischemia.

Brain swelling after TBI occurs as a result of cellular edema and is associated with elevated intracranial pressure (ICP).[12] The onset of cerebral edema is variable and may occur late. Certain populations, for example, children, appear more susceptible to severe cerebral edema after TBI.[13] If severe, cerebral edema can result in brain herniation and put the patient at risk for the attendant complications (discussed later in this chapter). CT findings of cerebral edema include small ventricles and subarachnoid spaces, including compression or effaced perimesencephalic (basilar) cisterns (▶ Fig. 4.3).[13]

Brain herniation occurs when mass effect from either a focal mass lesion, such as a hematoma, or generalized increased brain volume, as in the case of cerebral edema, pushes the brain against and around the dural structures that are in place normally to hold the brain in position. Depending on the location of the additional mass, the pattern of herniation will vary.

4.3.1 Subfalcine Herniation

Subfalcine herniation occurs with mass effect from a frontal or parietal lesion and is commonly associated with acute subdural hematoma. Subfalcine herniation occurs when the cingulate gyrus is pushed beneath the rigid falx cerebri (▶ Fig. 4.4). Subfalcine herniation is best measured by assessing for midline shift on the axial image. A line should be drawn from the anterior to the posterior leaves of the falx. The distance between this line and the septum pellucidum is a reliable measure of midline shift. Although the falx is a rigid structure, the falx will deflect, given enough pressure (▶ Fig. 4.4). When severe, or when the location of mass is more inferior, midline shift may be best measured at the level of the third ventricle.

Subfalcine herniation is common and may be well tolerated by patients in whom mass effect has developed over time, such as in the case of brain tumor. When acute, subfalcine herniation can have significant complications and require emergent surgical decompression. Signs of significant herniation include entrapment of the lateral ventricles. This usually first affects the contralateral side and occurs when there is compression of the foramen of Monro, thereby blocking egress of cerebrospinal fluid (CSF) into the third ventricle. There is subsequent enlargement of the entrapped lateral ventricle, which may be best seen by evaluating the size of the temporal horns and comparing to the size of the sulci (▶ Fig. 4.4).

Vascular complications of subfalcine herniation also occur when there is compression of the ipsilateral anterior cerebral

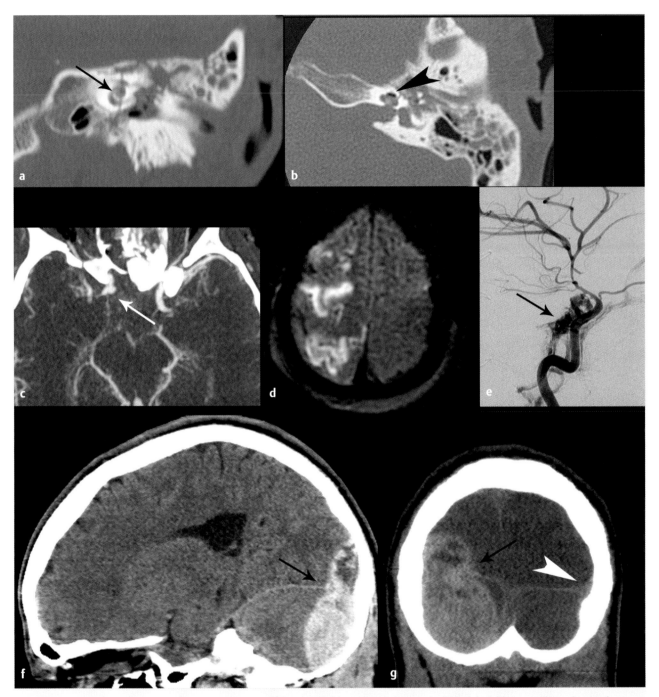

Fig. 4.2 Direct mechanical trauma in three patients. Coronal (a) and axial (b) computed tomography (CT) of the left temporal bone showing fracture line traversing the cochlea (*black arrow*) with pneumolabyrinth (*black arrowhead*) axial CT angiogram (c) shows right internal carotid artery pseudoaneurysm (*white arrow*) related to severe displaced skull-base fracture (not shown), resulting in infarcts [diffusion-weighted imaging magnetic resonance imaging (MRI)] (d). High-flow carotid-cavernous fistula developed within 1 week (e) (*black arrow*). Sagittal (f) and coronal (g) CT shows posterior fossa epidural hematoma (EDH) resulting from surgically proven sigmoid and transverse sinus laceration. Overlying skull fracture is not shown. Note the relationship of the EDH (*black arrow*) to the expected location of the transverse sinus (normal contralateral sinus marked with *white arrowhead*). (g).

artery between the herniating brain and the falx cerebri. If not relieved, this type of herniation may result in infarct (▶ Fig. 4.5). Even without a frank large vessel territory infarct, the presence of midline shift has been associated with a decreased cerebral metabolic rate of oxygen.[14]

4.3.2 Downward Tentorial Herniation

Tentorial herniation occurs when there is downward pressure on the brain against the tentorium cerebelli, ultimately resulting in downward displacement of the brain through the

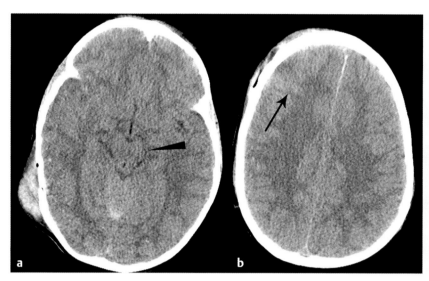

Fig. 4.3 Cerebral edema. Axial computed tomography in a 4-year-old child shows diffuse effacement of the sulci and basilar cisterns (a) (*arrowhead*), consistent with cerebral edema. Note the traumatic convexal subarachnoid hemorrhage (b) (*arrow*).

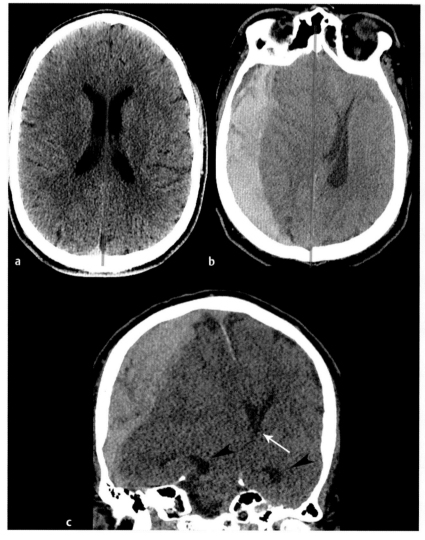

Fig. 4.4 Subfalcine herniation resulting from acute subdural hematoma. Normal computed tomographic imaging (CT) (a) demonstrates midline septum pellucidum, with line drawn from the anterior to the posterior attachment of the falx cerebri. Subfalcine herniation on axial CT (b), showing midline shift (*red lines*). Coronal reformat (c) demonstrates leftward herniation under the deflected falx cerebri. Note the mass effect on the foramina of Monro (*white arrow*) and dilation of the temporal horns of the lateral ventricles (*arrowheads*), out of proportion to sulci, indicating obstructive hydrocephalus.

tentorial incisura. If the mass effect is predominantly temporal, the first structure to herniate will be the uncus, a medially directed bulge of tissue along the mesial temporal lobe (▶ Fig. 4.6).

To assess for uncal herniation, evaluate the position of the uncus with respect to the suprasellar cistern. Whereas medial placement of the uncus alone may indicate impending uncal herniation, when severe, the uncus is clearly medially deviated and effaces the lateral margin of the suprasellar cistern (▶ Fig. 4.6). Clinically, uncal herniation may be marked by dilatation of the ipsilateral pupil ("blown pupil"), caused by

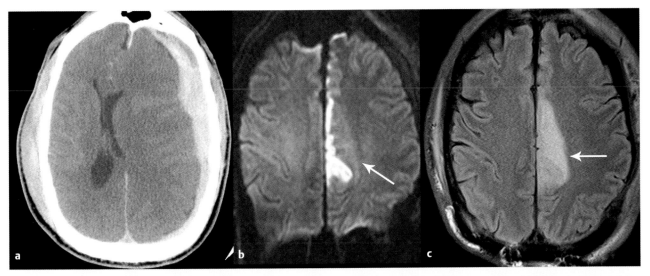

Fig. 4.5 Anterior cerebral artery infarct that is due to subfalcine herniation. Computed tomography (CT) at presentation (a) demonstrates acute left subdural hematoma with significant subfalcine herniation. The patient was immediately taken to surgery and decompressed but developed left anterior cerebral artery infarct evident on diffusion-weighted imaging (b) and fluid-attenuated inversion recovery (FLAIR) (c) sequence.

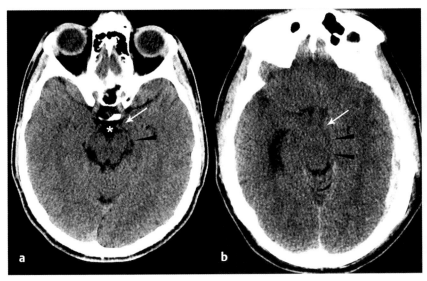

Fig. 4.6 Uncal herniation resulting from acute subdural hemorrhage. Normal computed tomography (CT) (a) demonstrates the normal configuration of the uncus (*arrow*) and ambient cistern (*arrowhead*). Note that the suprasellar cistern is patent (*). Uncal herniation on CT (b) manifests as medial displacement of the uncus (*arrow*), effacement of the ambient cisterns (*arrowhead*), and suprasellar cisterns. Note enlargement of the contralateral temporal horn of the lateral ventricle, consistent with entrapment.

compression of the ipsilateral third nerve against the free edge of the tentorium.

Central transtentorial herniation occurs as the result of more central or more severe mass effect (▶ Fig. 4.7); it may follow subfalcine herniation.[15] For central transtentorial herniation, one or both parahippocampal gyri may slip inferiorly past the tentorial margin. To assess for central transtentorial herniation, evaluate the ambient cistern, the CSF space surrounding the midbrain. Young patients in general will have more brain parenchyma and smaller CSF spaces than older adults, but even in children there should be some CSF evident surrounding the brainstem. When mild, cisterns may only be compressed (i.e. narrowed), but with progressive herniation, basilar cisterns become completed effaced (i.e., absent) (▶ Fig. 4.7).

Significant tentorial herniation can cause compression of the adjacent midbrain, which may be deviated away from the side of herniation.[16] The contralateral cerebral peduncle will be

compressed against the opposite side of the tentorium. If severe, transtentorial herniation will cause compression of the midbrain in the transverse dimension.[16]

With sufficient mass effect, the entire brainstem may be pushed downward, causing traction on the structures and fiber tracts of the brainstem. Traction on the perforating arteries arising from the basilar artery may result in tearing of these vessels with development of Duret hemorrhages in the midbrain and upper pons (▶ Fig. 4.8).[17] This type of hemorrhage is a sign of grave prognosis.

Tentorial herniation may also result in vascular complications. The posterior cerebral artery can be compressed between the herniating brain and the tentorium.[15] If not relieved, posterior cerebral artery territory infarct will develop (▶ Fig. 4.8 and ▶ Fig. 4.9). Uncal and transtentorial herniation may rarely result in noncommunicating hydrocephalus through compression of the cerebral spinal drainage pathways, including the cerebral aqueduct and basilar subarachnoid cisterns.

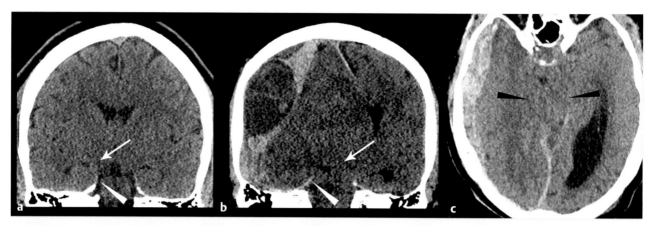

Fig. 4.7 Transtentorial herniation due to acute subdural hematoma (SDH) with hyperacute components. Normal coronal computed tomography (a) demonstrates normal position of the parahippocampal gyrus above tentorium cerebelli (*arrowhead*). With large acute and hyperacute SDH (b), there is medial and downward shifting of the right parahippocampal gyrus (*white arrow*) over the free edge of the tentorium (*white arrowhead*). Axial image (c) demonstrates complete effacement of the basilar cisterns with narrowing of the midbrain in the transverse dimension (*black arrowheads*).

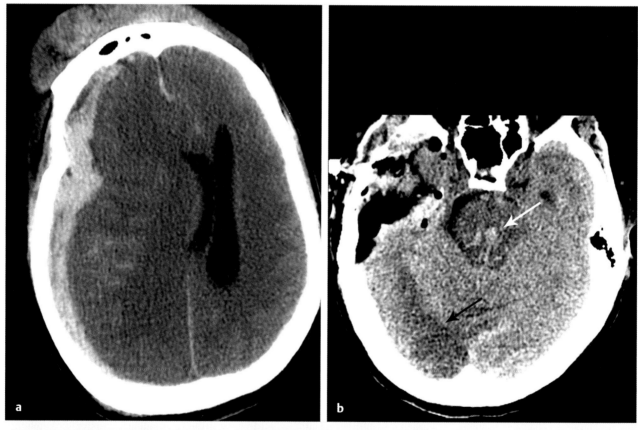

Fig. 4.8 Duret hemorrhage. Computed tomography at initial consultation (a) demonstrates large right subdural hematoma with severe subfalcine herniation. Transtentorial herniation was also present. After surgical decompression (b), hemorrhage in the central pons developed (*white arrow*), consistent with Duret hemorrhage. Note also the developing right posterior cerebral artery territory infarction (*black arrow*), also a complication of transtentorial herniation.

4.3.3 Upward Tentorial Herniation

Brain tissue may also herniate superiorly through the tentorial incisura. This kind of herniation occurs when there is mass effect in the posterior fossa, either from cerebellar mass lesion, such as hematoma, tumor, or infarct, or because of extra-axial hematoma. There is resultant herniation of the cerebellar vermis and cerebellar hemispheres through the tentorial incisura. Upward tentorial herniation appears on imaging as effacement of the quadrigeminal plate cistern (▶ Fig. 4.10).[18] Sagittal images may best demonstrate the cerebellar tissue herniating superiorly. When severe, obstructive hydrocephalus may occur.

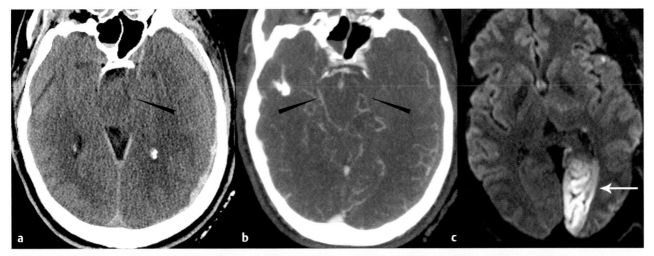

Fig. 4.9 Posterior cerebral artery (PCA) infarct due to transtentorial herniation. Computed tomography (CT) at presentation (a) demonstrates acute left subdural hematoma with transtentorial hernation (*arrowhead*). CT angiography obtained to exclude blunt cerebrovascular injury (b) demonstrates mass effect on the posterior cerebral arteries as they course around the midbrain (*arrowheads*). MRI three days later (c) demonstrates acute left PCA infarct.

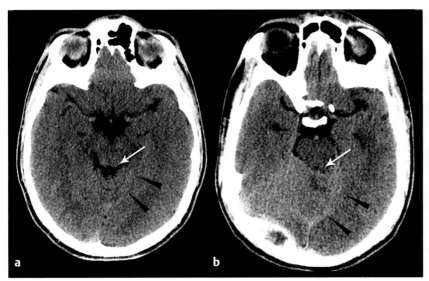

Fig. 4.10 Upward transtentorial herniation. Normal computed tomography CT (a) shows the expected configuration of the quadrigeminal plate cistern (*white arrow*) and tentorial incisura (*black arrowheads*). Note the normal cerebellar folia medially. In upward transtentorial herniation (b), the quadrigeminal plate cistern is compressed (*white arrow*), and the midbrain tectum is mildly compressed. The cerebellar folia are edematous and pressing up though the tentorial incisura (*black arrowheads*). Upward tentorial herniation in this case is due to the posterior fossa epidural hematoma shown in ▶ Fig. 4.2d.

4.3.4 Tonsillar Herniation

Tonsillar herniation occurs with mass effect in the posterior fossa, resulting in downward displacement of the cerebellar tonsils through the foramen. As with upward tentorial herniation, tonsillar herniation may result from posterior fossa mass/hematoma, edema, or extra-axial hematoma. On axial images, tonsillar herniation is evident as crowding of the foramen magnum. Sagittal images are extremely helpful in confirming this finding. A line drawn from the basion (tip of the clivus) to the opisthion (inferior margin of the occipital bone) demarcates the foramen magnum. Normally, the cerebellar tonsils lie above or up to 5 mm below this line but may end more inferiorly in children.[19]

The differential diagnosis of tonsillar herniation includes cerebellar tonsillar ectopia, a condition referring to the cerebellar tonsils terminating below the foramen magnum in the absence of mass effect. This condition can be incidental or occur in the setting of a Chiari I malformation.[20] Thus, if tonsils are low

lying, careful assessment for associated mass lesion causing this herniation acutely is required.

4.3.5 Cerebral Ischemia

Global cerebral ischemia occurs after TBI as a result of systemic hypotension or hypoxemia; ensuring adequate cerebral perfusion to meet the metabolic demands of the brain is a central tenet of caring for patients with TBI. Systemic hypotension may be caused by shock from other injuries and has been shown to worsen the outcome from severe TBI.[21] The Brain Trauma Foundation recommends avoiding systolic blood pressure < 90 mm Hg,[22] although higher blood pressure targets may be indicated.[23]

Although the Brain Trauma Foundation guidelines also recommend avoiding hypoxia (partial pressure arterial oxygen, or PaO_2, lower than 60 mm Hg or oxygen saturation lower than 90%),[22] supratherapeutic oxygenation has also been associated with a greater number of in-hospital deaths.[24] The effects of

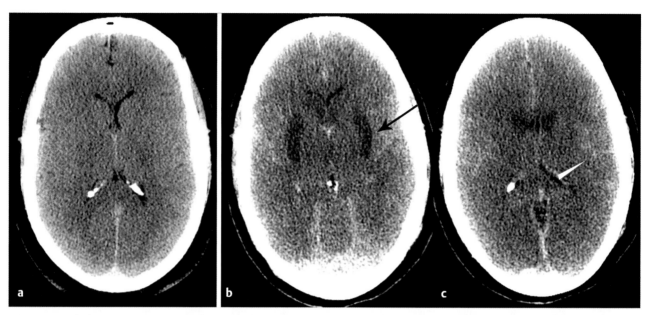

Fig. 4.11 Cerebral anoxia. At presentation (a), computed tomography shows equivocal loss of gray-white differentiation and cerebral edema, manifested as sulcal effacement and small ventricles. Fifteen hours later (b,c), repeat scan confirms cerebral anoxia, with development of basal ganglia infarctions (*black arrow*). Note pseudosubarachnoid hemorrhage (*arrowhead*) resulting from increased conspicuity of the pia arachnoid due to decreasing density of the adjacent brain parenchyma.

hypoxemia may not be easily rectified simply by maintaining arterial oxygenation and may be due on a cellular level to impaired mitochondrial function.[6] Optimizing cerebral oxygenation to match cerebral metabolic needs in brain-injured patients remains an area of ongoing research.

Global cerebral anoxia can become evident by imaging. On CT, cerebral anoxia manifests as brain edema, with effacement of sulci and basilar cisterns and loss of gray-white differentiation (▶ Fig. 4.11).[25] Infarcts may develop in the basal ganglia and watershed distributions.[25] The reversal sign is sometimes seen in severe anoxic or ischemic brain injury, particularly in children, and refers to relatively decreased attenuation of cerebral cortex on CT compared to the normal attenuation cerebellum, thalami, and brainstem.[26] On magnetic resonance imaging (MRI), global cerebral anoxia manifests as increased diffusion-weighted imaging signal in the basal ganglia or cortex,[27] with subsequent development of increased T2/fluid-attenuated inversion recovery (FLAIR) signal in these structures. Often global anoxia is a diffuse process that manifests with bilaterally symmetric findings that may be difficult to recognize.

Cerebral ischemia after TBI may also occur as focal vessel territory infarctions. As described already, vessel infarcts can occur as part of brain herniation syndromes, including anterior cerebral artery territory infarctions secondary to direct arterial compression during subfalcine herniation and posterior cerebral artery territory infarctions secondary to transtentorial herniation. Vessel territory infarctions may also occur secondary to direct vascular injury, as in the case of blunt cerebrovascular injury, discussed in Chapter 7, or as the result of fat embolism in the setting of long-bone fractures.

4.3.6 Hydrocephalus

Hydrocephalus occasionally occurs acutely after TBI or more commonly in a delayed fashion. Acute obstructive hydrocepha-

lus is uncommon after TBI and is associated with intraventricular hemorrhage[28,29] and basilar traumatic subarachnoid hemorrhage (SAH).[3] In these cases, hydrocephalus likely results from obstruction of the CSF outflow pathways by hematoma.[30] Mass effect on the CSF outflow pathway can also cause acute hydrocephalus and may occur in the setting of brain herniation, such as with obstruction of the basilar cisterns with transtentorial herniation or obstruction and entrapment of a single lateral ventricle in the setting of subfalcine herniation. Posterior fossa mass lesions, such as epidural hematoma or cerebellar hemorrhage, may result in acute obstructive hydrocephalus attributable to focal mass effect on the fourth ventricle.

Chronic communicating hydrocephalus also occurs after trauma, particularly in the setting of SAH or intraventricular hemorrhage. Although the exact pathophysiology of the development of chronic communicating hydrocephalus is still uncertain, fibrosis in the subarachnoid spaces has been proposed, as has proliferation of arachnoid cap cells.[30] Regardless, the end result seems to be impaired resorption of CSF. The development of post-traumatic hydrocephalus is associated with worse clinical outcome,[31,32] and surgical shunting may be indicated.

Ventricular dilatation also develops after TBI as a result of cerebral atrophy, and it can be difficult to differentiate this from true hydrocephalus. Ventricular dilatation develops commonly in the first 3 to 6 months after TBI, reported in 30 to 50% or more of patients with severe TBI.[31–33] Hydrocephalus requiring shunting is much less common, reported in around 5% of all patients and 18 to 45% of patients with ventriculomegaly[32–34] but may be higher,[31] as the indications for shunting remain under debate.

Ventricular enlargement can be detected by comparing ventricular size at presentation with subsequent scans (▶ Fig. 4.12). Signs of hydrocephalus include enlargement of the temporal horns of the lateral ventricles, a distended appearance of the frontal horns of the lateral ventricles, with normal or effaced

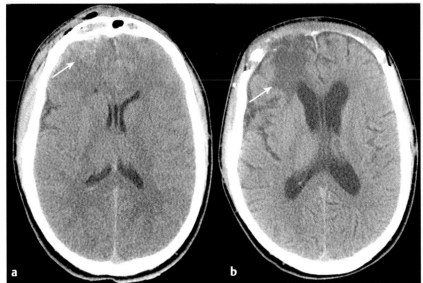

Fig. 4.12 Atrophy after severe traumatic brain injury. Computed tomography at presentation (a) and 6 weeks later (b) in a patient with severe traumatic brain injury demonstrates interval sulcal widening and ventricular dilatation. There is no periventricular edema. Additionally, note gliosis at the site of the right frontal parenchymal contusions (*white arrow*) and sequelae of decompressive surgery. The patient did not exhibit clinical signs of hydrocephalus.

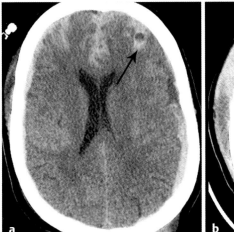
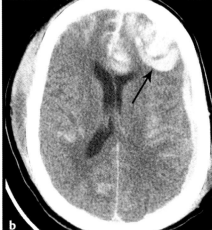

Fig. 4.13 Delayed traumatic intracerebral hemorrhage. Computed tomography (CT) at presentation (a) demonstrates acute bilateral subdural hematoma, subarachnoid hemorrhage, and left frontal contusion (*arrow*). Repeat CT four hours later (b) demonstrates an interval increase in the size of the frontal contusion (*arrow*), also termed "blossoming."

cerebral sulci.[33] Although not always present, periventricular lucency, suggesting periventricular edema or transependymal flow of CSF, supports the diagnosis of hydrocephalus.[31,33] Conversely, in cases of cerebral atrophy, commensurate dilatation of the sulci and fissures should also be present.

4.3.7 Delayed Traumatic Intracerebral Hematoma

Delayed traumatic intracerebral hematoma refers to a posttraumatic hemorrhage that may not be evident on initial imaging or to progressive enlargement of a hemorrhage evident on initial imaging. The classic example is blossoming of cerebral contusions (▶ Fig. 4.13),[35] although delayed appearance of epidural hematomas also occurs.[36] Development of delayed hemorrhages occurs more frequently in patients with coagulopathy at presentation, such as abnormal PT, PTT, or platelet count.[37]

It is important to obtain repeat imaging in patients with neurologic deterioration because this may demonstrate progression of bleeding or another finding that requires surgical intervention.[38] In the absence of neurologic decline, routine repeat computed tomography (CT) scan in the evaluation of minimal or

mild head injury is likely not indicated,[38,39] although the evidence is less clear in patients with severe TBI.[38,40]

4.3.8 Loss of Autoregulation

Cerebral autoregulation is the physiologic process by which the body maintains adequate cerebral blood flow to support cerebral perfusion despite changes in cerebral perfusion pressure, defined as difference between mean arterial pressure and ICP. Autoregulation also prevents excessive cerebral blood flow during arterial hypertension, which could lead to elevated ICP related to increased cerebral blood volume. The optimum strategy to support cerebral perfusion in TBI patients depends in part on whether cerebral autoregulation is intact or impaired.

In the absence of autoregulation, the cerebrovascular system is unable to compensate for changes in blood pressure. In patients with impaired autoregulation, maintaining constant adequate cerebral perfusion pressure may be vital to reducing secondary injury. For example, if autoregulation is impaired and cerebral perfusion pressure falls, cerebral blood flow will also decrease, potentially causing ischemia. Conversely, a sudden increase in cerebral perfusion pressure may lead to rapidly rising cerebral blood

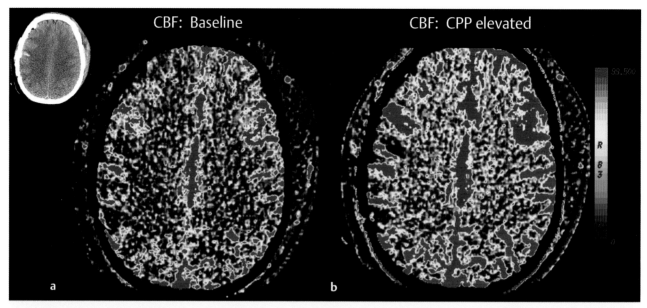

Fig. 4.14 Severe traumatic brain injury in a patient with refractory elevation of intracranial pressure. Computed tomography (CT; inset) demonstrates cerebral edema and subarachnoid hemorrhage. Perfusion CT, cerebral blood flow (CBF) maps before (a) and after (b) elevation of the cerebral perfusion pressure. Note the generalized increase in cerebral blood flow in response to blood pressure elevation, indicating impairment of cerebral autoregulation.

flow, possibly contributing to hemorrhage or edema.[41] Thus, patients with impaired autoregulation may benefit more from ICP-lowering therapy than from aggressive cerebral perfusion pressure support, whereas patients with intact autoregulation may tolerate arterial hypertension to maintain cerebral perfusion.

Although no gold standard is available for use in trauma patients to determine the status of cerebral autoregulation, the use of transcranial Doppler with blood pressure challenge has been widely reported.[42] In this technique, middle cerebral artery flow velocity is measured after blood pressure elevation to determine changes in cerebral vascular resistance. If cerebral autoregulation is intact, cerebral vascular resistance should respond to changes in cerebral perfusion pressure to maintain constant perfusion.

Perfusion CT has also been reported in the evaluation of cerebral autoregulation.[43] Perfusion CT is used at our institution to assess the status of autoregulation in a subset of severely brain-injured patients with elevated ICP refractory to standard treatment. To assess the status of autoregulation, a perfusion scan is obtained at baseline and after elevating the mean arterial pressure by 20 mm Hg during a single sitting.[44] In patients with preserved autoregulation, there is no change in perfusion maps. In patients with impaired autoregulation, the cerebral blood flow increases with blood pressure challenge, reflecting the loss of the body's ability to maintain constant cerebral blood flow (▶ Fig. 4.14).

4.4 Physiologic Monitoring for Traumatic Brain Injury Patients

4.4.1 Intracranial Pressure Monitor

Elevated ICP is associated with increased mortality in severely brain-injured patients.[45] The Brain Trauma Foundation recommends ICP monitoring for all patients with Glasgow Coma Scale score of 8 or lower and an abnormal CT scan. ICP monitoring is also indicated if two of the following criteria are met: age older than 40 years, motor posturing, or systolic blood pressure lower than 90 mm Hg.[46] ICP monitoring allows aggressive reduction in elevated ICP, with a goal of less than 20 mm Hg.[47] Although ICP management remains a central tenet of preventing secondary injury in severely brain-injured patients, a recent study did not find improved outcomes in severely brain injured patients who underwent invasive ICP monitoring compared with those who were managed based on clinical and imaging findings alone.[48] Further research is needed in this area.

Monitoring ICP can be performed by using several different types of monitoring devices. The gold standard is an external ventricular drain (ventriculostomy catheter). Parenchymal ICP monitors are also used, as are extra-axial (subdural, epidural, or subarachnoid) monitors. These devices are discussed further in Chapter 6, Postoperative Imaging of Traumatic Brain Imaging.

4.4.2 Brain Oxygenation Monitoring

Brain oxygenation monitoring is another way to assess for secondary cerebral ischemia after TBI. In the past, jugular venous oxygen saturation monitoring was used, and there is some evidence that episodes of venous desaturation are associated with worse outcomes.[49] Jugular venous oxygen saturation is measured via a venous catheter inserted into the jugular vein with the tip in the jugular bulb.[50] Imaging studies will show an intravenous catheter passing superiorly into the internal jugular vein with the tip at or near the skull base.

Newer methods to measure brain oxygenation include placing sensors directly into the brain parenchyma.[51,52] These can measure directly the partial pressure of oxygen in brain tissue, as well as other values such as pH and brain temperature. These probes can also measure ICP. Low values of partial pressure of O_2 in the brain are associated with higher mortality rates.[49,53]

4.5 Conclusion

Traumatic brain injury occurs both at the time of primary insult and in a delayed fashion as the body responds to the primary brain injury. Although medical treatment can do little to mitigate primary injury once it has occurred, intervention may alleviate or prevent the sequelae of secondary injury. The main causes of secondary brain injury include cerebral edema, herniation, and ischemia, and prompt recognition of these conditions allows prompt intervention. Additionally, recognizing complications of TBI, including global anoxic brain injury, infarction, hydrocephalus, and delayed intracranial hemorrhage, may help guide further therapies. Physiologic monitoring and cerebral autoregulation assessment may play a continued role in treating severely brain-injured patients, although ongoing research is needed.

4.6 Pearls

- Tissue injury resulting from brain trauma occurs both at the time of insult (primary injury) and in a delayed fashion (secondary injury). The pattern of primary injury should alert the radiologist to potential subsequent complications.
- Secondary injury results primarily from cerebral edema, herniation, and ischemia and is worsened by hypoxia and hypotension, among other factors.
- Cerebral herniation syndromes are important indicators of the need for aggressive medical or surgical intervention and may result in infarcts if not relieved.
- Delayed hydrocephalus may occur after TBI and must be differentiated from cerebral atrophy.
- Monitoring of ICP is a key component of the management of TBI patients.

References

[1] McHugh GS, Engel DC, Butcher I et al. Prognostic value of secondary insults in traumatic brain injury: results from the IMPACT study. J Neurotrauma 2007; 24: 287–293

[2] Bratton SL, Chestnut RM, Ghajar J et al. Brain Trauma Foundation. American Association of Neurological Surgeons. Congress of Neurological Surgeons. Joint Section on Neurotrauma and Critical Care, AANS/CNS. Guidelines for the management of severe traumatic brain injury. VI. Indications for intracranial pressure monitoring. J Neurotrauma 2007; 24 Suppl 1: S37–S44

[3] Blumbergs PC. Neuropathology of Traumatic Brain Injury. Youmans Neurological Surgery. Philadelphia, PA: Saunders/Elsevier; 2011.

[4] Andriessen TMJC, Jacobs B, Vos PE. Clinical characteristics and pathophysiological mechanisms of focal and diffuse traumatic brain injury. J Cell Mol Med 2010; 14: 2381–2392

[5] Bullock R, Zauner A, Woodward JJ et al. Factors affecting excitatory amino acid release following severe human head injury. J Neurosurg 1998; 89: 507–518

[6] Verweij BH, Muizelaar JP, Vinas FC, Peterson PL, Xiong Y, Lee CP. Impaired cerebral mitochondrial function after traumatic brain injury in humans. J Neurosurg. 2000; 93: 815–820

[7] Dolinskas CA, Zimmerman RA, Bilaniuk LT, Gennarelli TA. Computed tomography of post-traumatic extracerebral hematomas: comparison to pathophysiology and responses to therapy. J Trauma 1979; 19: 163–169

[8] Matsuyama T, Shimomura T, Okumura Y, Sakaki T. Acute subdural hematomas due to rupture of cortical arteries: a study of the points of rupture in 19 cases. Surg Neurol. 1997; 47: 423–427

[9] Shenkin HA. Acute subdural hematoma: review of 39 consecutive cases with high incidence of cortical artery rupture. J Neurosurg 1982; 57: 254–257

[10] Dalfino JC, Boulos AS. Visualization of an actively bleeding cortical vessel into the subdural space by CT angiography. Clin Neurol Neurosurg 2010; 112: 737–739

[11] Farkas O, Povlishock JT. Cellular and subcellular change evoked by diffuse traumatic brain injury: a complex web of change extending far beyond focal damage. Prog Brain Res 2007; 161: 43–59

[12] Marmarou A, Signoretti S, Fatouros PP, Portella G, Aygok GA, Bullock MR. Predominance of cellular edema in traumatic brain swelling in patients with severe head injuries. J Neurosurg 2006; 104: 720–730

[13] Bruce DA, Alavi A, Bilaniuk L, Dolinskas C, Obrist W, Uzzell B. Diffuse cerebral swelling following head injuries in children: the syndrome of "malignant brain edema". J Neurosurg 1981; 54: 170–178

[14] Valadka AB, Gopinath SP, Robertson CS. Midline shift after severe head injury: pathophysiologic implications. J Trauma. 2000; 49: 1–10

[15] Plum F, Posner JB. The Diagnosis of Stupor and Coma, Volume 19 of Contemporary Neurology Series. 3, illustrated ed: New York: Oxford University Press; 1982.

[16] Osborn AG. Diagnosis of descending transtentorial herniation by cranial computed tomography. Radiology. 1977; 123: 93–96

[17] Parizel PM, Makkat S, Jorens PG et al. Brainstem hemorrhage in descending transtentorial herniation (Duret hemorrhage). Intensive Care Med 2002; 28: 85–88

[18] Osborn AG, Heaston DK, Wing SD. Diagnosis of ascending transtentorial herniation by cranial computed tomography. AJR Am J Roentgenol 1978; 130: 755–760

[19] Smith BW, Strahle J, Bapuraj JR, Muraszko KM, Garton HJL, Maher CO. Distribution of cerebellar tonsil position: implications for understanding Chiari malformation. J Neurosurg 2013; 119: 812–819

[20] Barkovich AJ, Wippold FJ, Sherman JL, Citrin CM. Significance of cerebellar tonsillar position on MR. AJNR Am J Neuroradiol 1986; 7: 795–799

[21] Fearnside MR, Cook RJ, McDougall P, McNeil RJ. The Westmead Head Injury Project outcome in severe head injury: a comparative analysis of pre-hospital, clinical and CT variables. Br J Neurosurg 1993; 7: 267–279

[22] Bratton SL, Chestnut RM, Ghajar J et al. Brain Trauma Foundation. American Association of Neurological Surgeons. Congress of Neurological Surgeons. Joint Section on Neurotrauma and Critical Care, AANS/CNS. Guidelines for the management of severe traumatic brain injury. I. Blood pressure and oxygenation. J Neurotrauma 2007; 24 Suppl 1: S7–S13

[23] Brenner M, Stein DM, Hu PF, Aarabi B, Sheth K, Scalea TM. Traditional systolic blood pressure targets underestimate hypotension-induced secondary brain injury. J Trauma Acute Care Surg 2012; 72: 1135–1139

[24] Rincon F, Kang J, Vibbert M, Urtecho J, Athar MK, Jallo J. Significance of arterial hyperoxia and relationship with case fatality in traumatic brain injury: a multicentre cohort study. J Neurol Neurosurg Psychiatry 2013

[25] Kjos BO, Brant-Zawadzki M, Young RG. Early CT findings of global central nervous system hypoperfusion. AJR Am J Roentgenol 1983; 141: 1227–1232

[26] Han BK, Towbin RB, De Courten-Myers G, McLaurin RL, Ball WS, Jr. Reversal sign on CT: effect of anoxic/ischemic cerebral injury in children. AJR Am J Roentgenol. 1990; 154: 361–368

[27] Arbelaez A, Castillo M, Mukherji SK. Diffusion-weighted MR imaging of global cerebral anoxia. AJNR Am J Neuroradiol 1999; 20: 999–1007

[28] Fleischer AS, Huhn SL, Meislin H. Post-traumatic acute obstructive hydrocephalus. Ann Emerg Med 1988; 17: 165–167

[29] LeRoux PD, Haglund MM, Newell DW, Grady MS, Winn HR. Intraventricular hemorrhage in blunt head trauma: an analysis of 43 cases. Neurosurgery. 1992; 31: 678–685

[30] Massicotte EM, Del Bigio MR. Human arachnoid villi response to subarachnoid hemorrhage: possible relationship to chronic hydrocephalus. J Neurosurg 1999; 91: 80–84

[31] Marmarou A, Foda MA, Bandoh K et al. Posttraumatic ventriculomegaly: hydrocephalus or atrophy? A new approach for diagnosis using CSF dynamics. J Neurosurg 1996; 85: 1026–1035

[32] Mazzini L, Campini R, Angelino E, Rognone F, Pastore I, Oliveri G. Posttraumatic hydrocephalus: a clinical, neuroradiologic, and neuropsychologic assessment of long-term outcome. Arch Phys Med Rehabil 2003; 84: 1637–1641

[33] Gudeman SK, Kishore PR, Becker DP et al. Computed tomography in the evaluation of incidence and significance of post-traumatic hydrocephalus. Radiology. 1981; 141: 397–402

[34] Denes Z, Barsi P, Szel I, Boros E, Fazekas G. Complication during postacute rehabilitation: patients with posttraumatic hydrocephalus. Int J Rehabil Res. 2011; 34: 222–226

[35] Fukamachi A, Nagaseki Y, Kohno K, Wakao T. The incidence and developmental process of delayed traumatic intracerebral haematomas. Acta Neurochir (Wien). 1985; 74: 35–39

[36] Domenicucci M, Signorini P, Strzelecki J, Delfini R. Delayed post-traumatic epidural hematoma: a review. Neurosurg Rev. 1995; 18: 109–122

[37] Maegele M. Coagulopathy after traumatic brain injury: incidence, pathogenesis, and treatment options. Transfusion. 2013; 53 Suppl 1: 28S–37S

[38] Brown CVR, Zada G, Salim A et al. Indications for routine repeat head computed tomography (CT) stratified by severity of traumatic brain injury. J Trauma 2007; 62: 1339–1345

[39] Sifri ZC, Homnick AT, Vaynman A et al. A prospective evaluation of the value of repeat cranial computed tomography in patients with minimal head injury and an intracranial bleed. J Trauma 2006; 61: 862–867

[40] da Silva PSL, Reis ME, Aguiar VE. Value of repeat cranial computed tomography in pediatric patients sustaining moderate to severe traumatic brain injury. J Trauma. 2008; 65: 1293–1297

[41] Rangel-Castilla L, Gasco J, Nauta HJW, Okonkwo DO, Robertson CS. Cerebral pressure autoregulation in traumatic brain injury. Neurosurg Focus 2008; 25: E7.

[42] Panerai RB. Assessment of cerebral pressure autoregulation in humans—a review of measurement methods. Physiol Meas 1998; 19: 305–338

[43] Wintermark M, Chiolero R, Van Melle G et al. Cerebral vascular autoregulation assessed by perfusion-CT in severe head trauma patients. J Neuroradiol 2006; 33: 27–37

[44] Peterson E, Chesnut RM. Static autoregulation is intact in majority of patients with severe traumatic brain injury. J Trauma 2009; 67: 944–949

[45] Saul TG, Ducker TB. Effect of intracranial pressure monitoring and aggressive treatment on mortality in severe head injury. J Neurosurg 1982; 56: 498–503

[46] Bratton SL, Chestnut RM, Ghajar J et al. Brain Trauma Foundation. American Association of Neurological Surgeons. Congress of Neurological Surgeons. Joint Section on Neurotrauma and Critical Care, AANS/CNS. Guidelines for the management of severe traumatic brain injury. VI. Indications for intracranial pressure monitoring. J Neurotrauma. 2007; 24 Suppl 1: S37–S44

[47] Juul N, Morris GF, Marshall SB, Marshall LF The Executive Committee of the International Selfotel Trial. Intracranial hypertension and cerebral perfusion pressure: influence on neurological deterioration and outcome in severe head injury. J Neurosurg. 2000; 92: 1–6

[48] Chesnut RM, Temkin N, Carney N et al. A trial of intracranial-pressure monitoring in traumatic brain injury. N Engl J Med 2012; 367: 2471–2481

[49] Bratton SL, Chestnut RM, Ghajar J et al. Brain Trauma Foundation. American Association of Neurological Surgeons. Congress of Neurological Surgeons. Joint Section on Neurotrauma and Critical Care, AANS/CNS. Guidelines for the management of severe traumatic brain injury. X. Brain oxygen monitoring and thresholds. J Neurotrauma 2007; 24 Suppl 1: S65–S70

[50] Goetting MG, Preston G. Jugular bulb catheterization: experience with 123 patients. Crit Care Med 1990; 18: 1220–1223

[51] Gupta AK, Hutchinson PJ, Al-Rawi P et al. Measuring brain tissue oxygenation compared with jugular venous oxygen saturation for monitoring cerebral oxygenation after traumatic brain injury. Anesth Analg. 1999; 88: 549–553

[52] Hoelper BM, Alessandri B, Heimann A, Behr R, Kempski O. Brain oxygen monitoring: in-vitro accuracy, long-term drift and response-time of Licox- and Neurotrend sensors. Acta Neurochir (Wien). 2005; 147: 767–774

[53] Stiefel MF, Spiotta A, Gracias VH et al. Reduced mortality rate in patients with severe traumatic brain injury treated with brain tissue oxygen monitoring. J Neurosurg. 2005; 103: 805–811

5 Pediatric Head Trauma

Jonathan O. Swanson and Jeffrey P. Otjen

5.1 Introduction

Pediatric head trauma is a major public health concern in the United States. It is a leading cause of acquired disability in children and accounts for more than 50,000 hospital admissions annually and a billion dollars in health care expenditure.[1,2] The mechanism of head trauma varies by age; in those younger than 1 year, abusive head trauma is a major cause, and for those older than 1 year and less than 4 years, falls are the leading cause. Children older than 14 years are often the victims of motor-vehicle collisions.[2,3] In the following sections, we identify and discuss issues related to radiologic evaluation of pediatric head trauma. We discuss general issues such as radiation dose, the identification of patients who need computed tomography (CT), broad issues such as birth trauma and nonaccidental trauma, and some more specific entities that are unique to children in the setting of trauma.

5.2 The Need for Head CT

After major head or multisystem trauma, noncontrast head CT is routinely used to evaluate for intracranial and calvarial injury. As in adults, head CT is considered the imaging study of choice in the acute phase after traumatic brain injury (TBI) to identify the presence and extent of structural damage. The head CT also provides essential diagnostic information for triage and cerebral resuscitation and generates immediate implications for surgical intervention.

For minor trauma, there is no widely accepted guideline in use. Efforts have been made with some success to define clinical decision-making guidelines. A guideline published in 2009 based on a large multicenter prospective patient population can be used to identify children at low risk for clinically significant injury.[4] In children younger than 2 years, this low-risk group includes patients with Glasgow Coma Scale (GCS) 14 or 15; who do not have signs of basilar skull fracture; who do not have a history of loss of consciousness or vomiting, severe headache, or severe mechanism of injury. In children older than 2 years with a GCS of 14 or 15, no CT is recommended for those without palpable skull fracture, occipital or parietal scalp hematoma, less than 5 seconds' loss of consciousness, or altered mental status.

The Canadian Assessment of Tomography for Childhood Head injuries (CATCH) guidelines were published in 2010 to identify signs or symptoms in children aged 0 to 16 years with a minor head injury who should get a CT and are undergoing prospective validation.[5] CATCH comprises a list of seven entities, any of which should trigger a CT:

High risk (need for neurosurgical intervention):
1. GCS lower than 15 at 2 hours after injury
2. Suspected open or depressed skull fracture
3. Worsening headache
4. Irritability on examination.

Moderate risk (CT abnormality of brain injury):
1. Signs of basilar skull fracture (hemotympanum, "raccoon eyes," CSF otorrhea or rhinorrhea)
2. Large boggy scalp hematoma
3. Dangerous mechanism (motor-vehicle collision, fall of more than 3 feet or more than five stairs, fall from bike without a helmet)

The first four criteria are high-risk factors and have a 100% sensitivity and 70% specificity for predicting the need for neurosurgical intervention. The last three criteria are moderate risk factors and have a 98% sensitivity and 50% specificity for predicting brain injury on CT.

5.3 Protocol and Dose

Because the head CT is the imaging study of choice for evaluating for TBI, the radiologist must be aware of the risk associated with pediatric radiation exposure. Children are inherently more sensitive to radiation than are adults, and radiation has greater potential to cause harm as children have more time to develop any delayed effects.[6,7] Age is the most important factor when considering the effect of radiation exposure: children are up to 10 times more sensitive to radiation than adults, and the youngest neonates are more sensitive than the older child.[8] The "as low as reasonably achievable," or ALARA, principle (originally promulgated from the 1950s through the 1970s for nuclear reactor personnel safety[9–11]) has become a tenet of medical radiation safety: the lowest possible dose of radiation should be administered to achieve diagnostic results. In some cases, this means forgoing an examination altogether or substituting an examination without ionizing radiation such as ultrasound or magnetic resonance imaging (MRI). In the acute trauma setting, nonionizing alternatives are not always possible. At a minimum, however, doses should be minimized and monitored.

Most facilities now have pediatric protocols in place for higher radiation examinations, particularly CT. Decreasing the milliamperes and performing helical rather than pure axial CT (as is commonly used with the adult head CT) are examples of ways to reduce dose in the acute setting. Customizing protocols in conjunction with subspecialties should also be considered, such as using a half or quarter dose CT (by decreasing milliamperes) for routine follow-up of patients where fine anatomic detail is not imperative. Examples include examinations for evaluating ventriculoperitoneal shunt placement, revision, or malfunction; preoperative fiducial scans; or postcraniofacial distraction cases. Alternative image reconstruction methods to filtered back-projection are being developed and evaluated; such methods have the potential to significantly reduce dose for all CT examinations. A more complete review is beyond the scope of this paper, but Zachariah et al discuss pediatric specific and general factors, such as centered patient positioning, shielding, filtering, and others.[12]

5.4 Typical Traumatic Findings

Many findings in children who have suffered head trauma mirror the common findings in adults. In a recent evaluation of initial CT findings in pediatric TBI, parenchymal lesions (including contusion, hematoma, and hemorrhagic shear) were found to be most the common injuries.[13]

Subdural hematomas tend to be crescentic and do not respect sutures, but they do respect the midline (▶ Fig. 5.1). Epidural hematomas are usually convex and respect sutures, with a tendency to grow over the course of hours (▶ Fig. 5.2). An underlying fracture is present in almost all cases. Subarachnoid hemorrhage is often scattered or diffuse and seen within the cerebral sulci (▶ Fig. 5.3 and ▶ Fig. 5.4). Hemorrhagic contusions are often seen acutely, and the underlying damage is often greater in extent than that seen on initial imaging (▶ Fig. 5.5). Shear injury is often difficult to appreciate on CT, and MRI will often better detect small foci of injury, T2* and inversion recovery sequences being particularly sensitive (▶ Fig. 5.6).[14] With more severe trauma, multiple findings are often present (▶ Fig. 5.7).

The presence of nonfused skull sutures in children adds some complexity to the evaluation of the injured child. CT is an excellent tool for fracture identification, and the ability to reconstruct images in a multitude of ways augments the examination

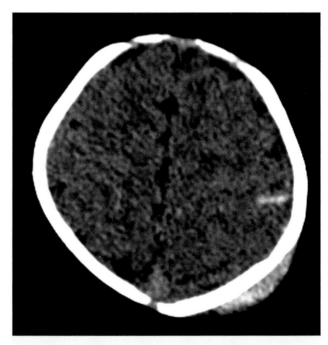

Fig. 5.1 Noncontrast axial computed tomography showing layering high-density material in a left holohemispheric distribution representing a subdural hemorrhage in a 21-month-old child after a fall. The midline shift is an important finding.

Fig. 5.3 Axial image from noncontrast computed tomography in a 4-week-old infant after being dropped 4 feet onto a hardwood floor. There is a single focus of high-density material in a left posterior frontal gyrus consistent with a small amount of subarachnoid blood.

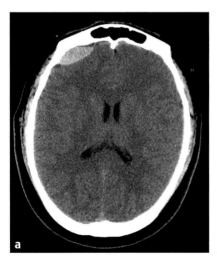

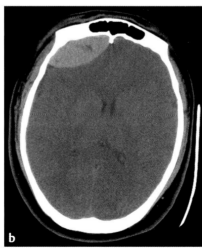

Fig. 5.2 (a) Axial image from noncontrast computed tomography (CT) showing lentiform high-density material in the right frontal area with some mass effect on the underlying gyri typical of an epidural hematoma in this adolescent after being hit in the head with a discus. (b) Three hours later, there is increasing size of the epidural hematoma with increased mass effect on the underlying parenchyma.

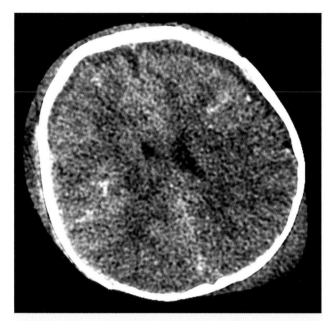

Fig. 5.4 Axial image from noncontrast computed tomography in a 5-month-old child dropped from 15 feet. Diffuse high-density material is seen within the sulci consistent with subarachnoid blood. Subdural fluid collections are also seen, along with scalp hematoma.

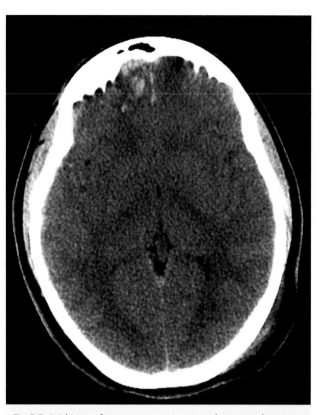

Fig. 5.5 Axial image from noncontrast computed tomography in an adolescent struck on the back of the head showing right frontal intraparenchymal blood consistent with hemorrhagic contusion from a coup-contrecoup mechanism.

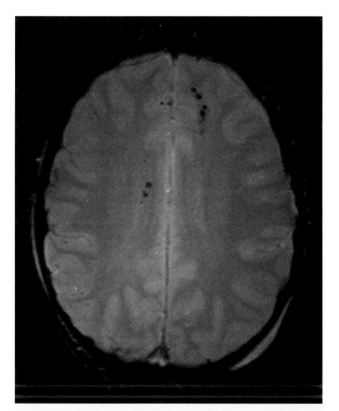

Fig. 5.6 Magnetic resonance imaging gradient recalled echo axial image in a 16-year-old trauma patient showing multiple punctuate foci of blooming signal dropout in the bilateral frontal and right corpus callosum. These are consistent with foci of hemorrhage and can be seen with diffuse axonal injury. Left posterior scalp swelling indicates the site of impact.

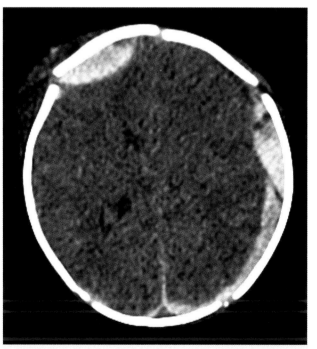

Fig. 5.7 Axial image from noncontrast computed tomography showing bilateral epidural high-density collections and posterior left subdural collection, as well as more subtle diffuse subarachnoid blood in a 1-day-old infant after a difficult forceps assisted delivery.

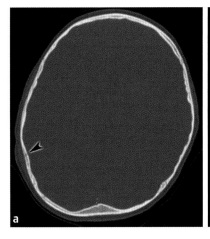
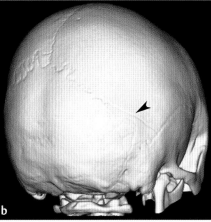

Fig. 5.8 (a) Axial bone reconstruction from non-contrast computed tomography in a 5-year-old boy who fell backward, hitting his head on concrete. There is a very subtle nondisplaced fracture of the posterior parietal bone (*arrowhead*) with overlying scalp swelling that is well seen on three-dimensional surface-rendering images (b) as a linear fracture extending obliquely from the midright lambdoidal suture to the squamosal suture (*arrowhead*). The fracture does not have the characteristic zigzag of normal suture and was not present on the contralateral side.

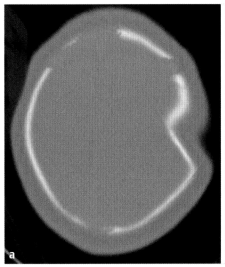
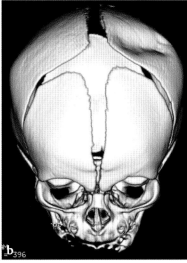

Fig. 5.9 (a) Axial noncontrast head computed tomographic image showing a prominent indentation but no cortical disruption of the left parietal bone in a 6-day-old infant. No history of trauma could be elicited, and the child was otherwise healthy. (b) Three-dimensional surface-rendered image shows the depression to advantage.

significantly, particularly for fractures in axial plane. In addition to the standard axial bone and soft tissue reconstructions, volumetric or surface-rendered three-dimensional images can be useful (▶ Fig. 5.8). Multiplanar reformats and maxiumum intensity projection reconstructions have been shown to add accuracy.[15]

5.5 Pediatric Specific Traumatic Findings

Although children are susceptible to the common types of head trauma seen in adults, some entities are seen exclusively in children. Incomplete or bowing-type fractures are called "ping-pong" fractures, as they have been likened to a dented table tennis ball (▶ Fig. 5.9).

Growing skull fractures (▶ Fig. 5.10) are rare complications that develop after fracture or transdural surgery in the younger patient population, usually in those younger than 3 years.[16] Approximately 1% of skull fracture cases will develop this complication.[17] Also known as leptomeningeal cysts, they are thought to be due to transmission of cerebrospinal fluid (CSF) pulsations through a compromised dura.[18] These can be purely cystic, containing only CSF, but often will contain herniated cerebral

contents (pseudoencephalomeningocele).[19] Underlying porencephaly or encephalomalacia is common. Depending on the extent of calvarial coverage, these patients can have a growing hard lump or a soft lump, which may pulsate. These lumps will enlarge over time, and surgical treatment is required to repair the calvarial defect and underlying dural defect.

A common confounder in the evaluation of young children with head trauma is the relatively common finding of enlarged extra axial CSF spaces, often seen during the evaluation of macrocephaly. A variety of terms have been applied to this finding or similar findings, the most prevalent being *benign external hydrocephalus* and *subdural hygroma*, despite the subarachnoid location.[20] The hallmark features are children less than 3 years with enlargement of subarachnoid CSF spaces seen usually in the frontal and intrahemispheric areas. Bridging veins can be seen on MRI or high frequency cranial ultrasound if the fontanelle is open (▶ Fig. 5.11). The fluid should follow the density or signal of CSF on all imaging modalities. This condition can be idiopathic, acquired, or familial. Benign familial macrocephaly is an autosomal dominant condition in families with incomplete penetrance. There is debate in the literature regarding whether these children are prone to subdural hemorrhage with minor or even no known trauma.[20,21]

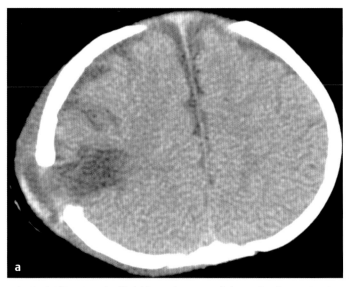

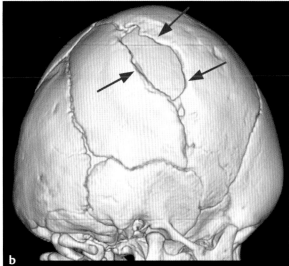

Fig. 5.10 This 5-month-old child was the victim of abusive head trauma at 2 months of age that resulted in a parietal skull fracture and parenchymal contusion (not shown). Follow-up axial noncontrast CT (a) shows an area of low-density encephalomalacia protruding through a prominent skull defect at the site of prior fracture. Surface-rendered three-dimensional image (b) shows the bone defect situated within the fracture line (*arrows*) consistent with a leptomeningeal cyst and pseudomyelomeningocele.

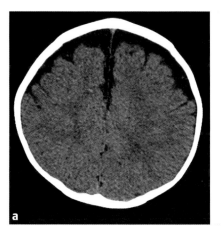

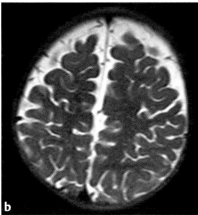

Fig. 5.11 (a) Axial noncontrast head computed tomography image in an infant being evaluated for macrocephaly. This shows prominent low-density frontal fluid collections but no other abnormality. (b) T2 magnetic resonance imaging shows vessels traversing this space, confirming them as subarachnoid.

5.6 Abusive Head Trauma (Nonaccidental Head Injury)

Child abuse is a leading cause of injury and death in young children in the United States, and growing recognition has led to the creation of Child Abuse Pediatrics as a U.S. board-certified specialty.[22,23] In 2010, more than 120,000 children were physically abused in the United States, and more than 1500 children died as a result.[24–26] Most of the morbidity and mortality resulting from abuse are due to head trauma.[27,28]

A clinical suspicion from a referring provider may prompt an evaluation for nonaccidental trauma. An absent history, one that does not match the injuries, or a changing history can commonly be seen. On other occasions, findings on radiologic examination may be the first indication of abuse, and it is incumbent on the radiologist to alert the providers so that a full evaluation is undertaken.

The biomechanics of abusive head trauma have been evaluated using forensic, animal, and computer models. Controversy persists regarding exact trauma mechanisms and injury pattern. Whereas the exact form of abuse is often never known, shaking alone, shaking with impact, or direct blow should prompt evaluation of all forms of injury.[29–31]

No radiologic findings are pathognomonic for abusive head trauma, and imaging may be normal,[32] but studies have shown that certain injury patterns are highly suspicious. Highly suspicious findings include subdural hemorrhages of different ages, cerebral ischemia, diffuse axonal injury, and retinal hemorrhages. Any finding suggesting multiplicity of events should also raise suspicion. Almost every form of intracranial traumatic pathology has been described in abusive head trauma, including subdural, epidural, subarachnoid, and parenchymal hemorrhage; ischemia; skull fracture; diffuse axonal injury; edema; contusion; and hydrocephalus; subdural hemorrhage is the most common.[33–36] Skull fractures are more common in accidental trauma, although multiple, complex, or stellate skull fractures are often seen in the nonaccidental trauma (▶ Fig. 5.12). Ischemia in the setting of pediatric trauma is a poor prognostic factor and is found significantly more commonly in abuse than in nonabuse cases.[35,37] MRI may also identify retinal hemorrhage, although this is an insensitive imaging finding (▶ Fig. 5.13).[38]

When evaluating subdural hematomas, certain characteristics are more common in abuse. Multilayered hematomas or those of distinctly different ages are more specific for abuse (▶ Fig. 5.14). Intrahemispheric hematomas or those under the tentorium are more commonly seen in abuse, as are bilateral subdural hematomas and isolated chronic subdural hematomas.[36,39,40]

Radiologic mimics of abusive head trauma have been described. Hyperacute subdural hematomas are of mixed density because of incompletely clotted blood, but on follow-up, they homogenize within hours.[41] Benign external hydrocephalus is commonly seen in nonabused young children, and these children may be more susceptible to spontaneous subdural hemorrhage or hemorrhage with minor accidental trauma.[42,43] Glutaric aciduria and other metabolic and congenital conditions also predispose to subdural hematoma.[41,44,45] Birth-related intracranial hemorrhage can be seen, usually resolving by 4 weeks of age.[28] A more complete list of potential mimics is beyond the scope of this text. Given the potentially devastating outcome of abuse, and the relative rarity of seeing the alternative pathology, it is recommended that a full evaluation be performed, ruling out potential mimics of abusive trauma as clinically indicated.

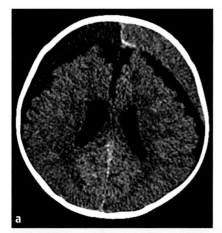

Fig. 5.12 Surface-rendered three-dimensional image from a noncontrast head CT in a 1-month-old infant with a complex skull fracture. Linear defects radiate from the central left parietal bone in a stellate pattern originating from the site of the injury.

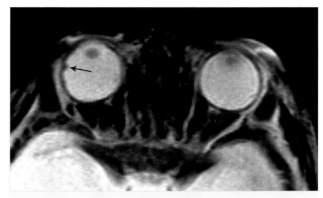

Fig. 5.13 Gradient echo image from a magnetic resonance image in a 5-week-old victim of abusive head trauma and retinal hemorrhages on ophthalmologic examination. Subtle low-intensity foci of retinal contour abnormality (*arrow*) suggest retinal hemorrhage.

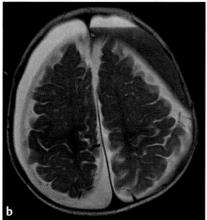
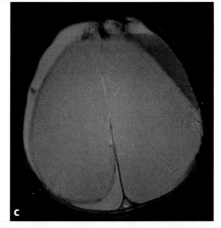

Fig. 5.14 Images from a 5-month-old victim of abusive head trauma. (a) Axial noncontrast head computed tomography shows bilateral subdural fluid collections of different densities suggesting different stages of evolution. (b) T2 magnetic resonance image (MRI) showing layering blood products in the left frontal subdural space and significant right subdural fluid. (c) Gradient echo MRI again shows the left layering blood products, along with low-density material coating the dura on the right consistent with older blood products and hemosiderin.

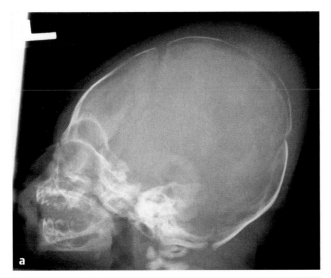

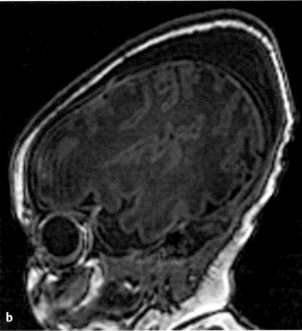

Fig. 5.15 (a) Lateral radiograph of a newborn with significant calvarial deformity showing prominent posterior soft tissue swelling after a prolonged vaginal birth, consistent with caput succedaneum. (b) Sagittal T1 magnetic resonance imaging (MRI) showing simple scalp fluid. The MRI was performed to evaluate for hypoxic brain injury.

5.7 Birth Trauma

Trauma to the head is rare in the setting of a normal delivery. A difficult delivery can lead to extreme maneuvers to deliver the child, and the risk of head trauma is increased.[46] The cephalohematoma and the more serious subgaleal hematoma can be seen, mimicking the more frequent and benign atraumatic caput succedaneum. Differentiating between these entities is usually done by physical examination, but in equivocal cases imaging may be required.

Caput succedaneum is a serosanguineous scalp infiltrate or fluid collection seen most commonly as a result of prolonged pressure on the presenting portion of the infant's head against a dilated cervix (▶ Fig. 5.15). It crosses suture lines and resolves within days, usually without sequelae, although occasionally hair loss and skin necrosis are seen.[47]

A cephalohematoma is the most common form of birth trauma (▶ Fig. 5.16).[48] A subperiosteal collection of blood is bound by the relatively tight connection between bone and periosteum; on examination, it is firm and respects suture boundaries. This limits the size of the hematoma, and large volumes are rare. These usually resolve without sequelae, but a minority will calcify or become incorporated into the underlying bone with subsequent mild deformity (▶ Fig. 5.17). Rarely, these become infected, leading to abscess and osteomyelitis.[49]

The subgaleal space is a potential space with the capacity to allow a hemodynamically significant amount of blood to collect, not bound by sutures (▶ Fig. 5.18). Hypotension, shock, and death can result. These are associated with vacuum extraction devices[50] and are more often seen with larger infants and primiparous mothers. In addition to hematomas, even more rare complications of vacuum extraction have been described, such as iatrogenic encephaloceles.[51]

Intracranial hemorrhages have been described after deliveries; these are generally small and resolve without sequelae. These are significantly more common after vaginal delivery compared with cesarean delivery and are seen in up to 26% of births.[52]

5.8 Mild Traumatic Brain Injury

Mild traumatic brain injury (mTBI), often used synonymously with concussion, is defined as blunt trauma with or without transient loss of consciousness. The neurologic examination is normal, and GCS is 15, but mild cognitive and psychological

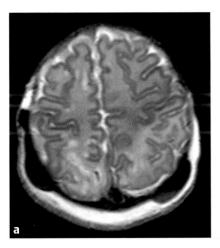

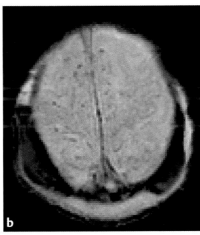

Fig. 5.16 T2-weighted (a) and gradient echo (b) magnetic resonance images from newborn after traumatic birth show hypointense scalp fluid collections consistent with subperiosteal blood in cephalohematoma.

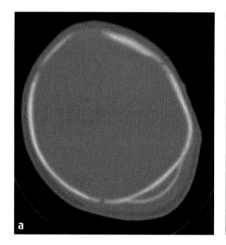

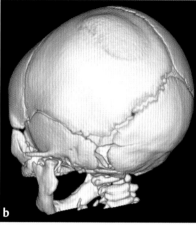

Fig. 5.17 Noncontrast computed tomographic images in a 1-month-old infant with a bump on the back of the head and history of cephalohematoma. Axial image (a) shows a rim calcified collection in the left parietal area. The size and distribution are well demonstrated on the three-dimensional surface-rendered images (b).

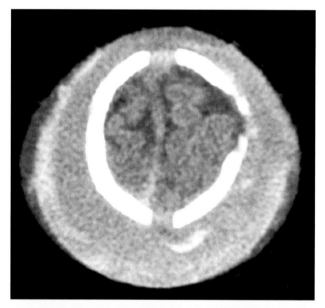

Fig. 5.18 Axial image from a noncontrast head computed tomography in a 12-hour-old newborn after cardiopulmonary arrest and resuscitation, with subsequent fatal hypoxic brain injury. The patient was born after lengthy vacuum-assisted delivery. A large heterogeneously dense fluid collection was seen around the vertex not respecting suture boundaries consistent with subgaleal hemorrhage

deficits can be present and persistent over time, especially in the setting of repetitive trauma. This type of injury is being increasingly recognized as a major health issue in the pediatric population.[53,54] In children, bicycle falls, sports, and motor-vehicle collisions (after 15 years old) are the most common causes.[55,56] If patients with mTBI seek medical care, they often will not undergo neuroimaging, as most modalities are insensitive to any pathology.

Pediatric studies are lacking, but some adult studies have shown, with higher-field-strength MRI (1.5 teslas (T) and higher), a minority of patients with a history of concussion have detectable injury, usually taking the form of microhemorrhages in the setting of diffuse axonal injury (▶ Fig. 5.6).[14]

Diffusion tensor imaging to evaluate decreased regional fractional anisotropy has recently been studied as a way of quantifying white matter changes associated with concussions, but its clinical application is not yet defined.[57,58]

5.9 Prognostic Importance of the Initial Head CT

Associations exist between findings on the initial head CT in the trauma setting and quality of life after the injury. The most important prognostic findings that lead to decreased quality of life were effacement of the basal cisterns, intraventricular hemorrhage, parenchymal injury, midline shift greater than 5 mm, and the presence of subdural hematomas thicker than 3 mm.[13] These characteristics are similar but not identical to outcomes shown to predict poor outcomes in adults.[59]

5.10 Conclusion

Pediatric head trauma is a major cause of morbidity and mortality with distinct epidemiologic factors, clinical characteristics, and imaging features compared with adult populations. The differences in clinical presentation have necessitated the development and validation of criteria for acute neuroimaging specific to children. Traumatic head injury imaging findings are often similar to those seen in adults; however, there are entities that are unique to young patients of which the radiologist must be aware.

Recognition of common birth-related intracranial and extracranial injuries will help guide the radiologist and clinician to proper treatment and follow-up. Knowledge of the clinical scenario, including the birth history, is important, particularly if abuse is suspected. Although accidental and abusive head traumas have overlapping imaging features, certain findings may direct strongly toward one cause. Although no single finding is 100% specific for abuse, multiple complex skull fractures, subdural hemorrhages of different stages, and a history that does not fit with the imaging findings should prompt further evaluation.

There is increasing awareness of radiation's effects on children, and monitoring radiation doses is important. New CT technology will likely reduce but not eliminate this concern in the future. This concern should not deter from rapid imaging in the trauma setting given the significant value of information to be gained. An initial early head CT in the setting of trauma allows appropriate triage and resuscitation direction, defines the extent of injury, and also gives important prognostic information about eventual quality of life. MRI is increasingly important for neurologic evaluation, but the lengthy examination, sedation requirement, and relative difficulty of access can be prohibitive.

References

[1] Schneier AJ, Shields BJ, Hostetler SG, Xiang H, Smith GA. Incidence of pediatric traumatic brain injury and associated hospital resource utilization in the United States. Pediatrics. 2006; 118: 483–492

[2] Guice KS, Cassidy LD, Oldham KT. Traumatic injury and children: a national assessment. J Trauma 2007; 63 Suppl: S68–S86

[3] McCarthy ML, Serpi T, Kufera JA, Demeter LA, Paidas C. Factors influencing admission among children with a traumatic brain injury. Acad Emerg Med 2002; 9: 684–693

[4] Kuppermann N, Holmes JF, Dayan PS et al. Pediatric Emergency Care Applied Research Network (PECARN). Identification of children at very low risk of clinically-important brain injuries after head trauma: a prospective cohort study. Lancet. 2009; 374: 1160–1170

[5] Osmond MH, Klassen TP, Wells GA et al. Pediatric Emergency Research Canada (PERC) Head Injury Study Group. CATCH: a clinical decision rule for the use of computed tomography in children with minor head injury. CMAJ 2010; 182: 341–348

[6] Kleinerman RA. Cancer risks following diagnostic and therapeutic radiation exposure in children. Pediatr Radiol. 2006; 36 Suppl 2: 121–125

[7] American Academy of Pediatrics. Committee on Environmental Health. Risk of ionizing radiation exposure to children: a subject review. Pediatrics 1998; 101: 717–719

[8] Hall EJ. Introduction to session I: helical CT and cancer risk. Pediatr Radiol 2002; 32: 225–227

[9] Rogers L, Dunster HJ, Polyani C, Stevens DJ. Implications of Commission Recommendations that Doses be Kept as Low as Readily Achievable in Protection TlCoR, ed. Vol 22. New York: Pergamon Press; 1973:22.

[10] Recommendations of the International Commission on Radiological Protection, ICRP Publication 9. New York: Pergamon Press; 1965:10

[11] Baum JW. ALARA and de minimis concepts in regulation of personnel exposure. American Nuclear Society Topical Conference; 1987; Oak Ridge, TN

[12] Zacharias C, Alessio AM, Otto RK et al. Pediatric CT: strategies to lower radiation dose. AJR Am J Roentgenol. 2013; 200: 950–956

[13] Swanson JO, Vavilala MS, Wang J et al. Association of initial CT findings with quality-of-life outcomes for traumatic brain injury in children. Pediatr Radiol 2012; 42: 974–981

[14] Topal NB, Hakyemez B, Erdogan C et al. MR imaging in the detection of diffuse axonal injury with mild traumatic brain injury. Neurol Res 2008; 30: 974–978

[15] Ringl H, Schernthaner R, Philipp MO et al. Three-dimensional fracture visualisation of multidetector CT of the skull base in trauma patients: comparison of three reconstruction algorithms. Eur Radiol 2009; 19: 2416–2424

[16] Keshavarzi S, Meltzer H, Cohen SR et al. The risk of growing skull fractures in craniofacial patients. Pediatr Neurosurg 2010; 46: 193–198

[17] Ersahin Y, Gülmen V, Palali I, Mutluer S. Growing skull fractures (craniocerebral erosion). Neurosurg Rev 2000; 23: 139–144

[18] Muhonen MG, Piper JG, Menezes AH. Pathogenesis and treatment of growing skull fractures. Surg Neurol 1995; 43: 367–373

[19] Vignes JR, Jeelani NU, Jeelani A, Dautheribes M, Liguoro D. Growing skull fracture after minor closed-head injury. J Pediatr. 2007; 151: 316–318

[20] Zahl SM, Egge A, Helseth E, Wester K. Benign external hydrocephalus: a review, with emphasis on management. Neurosurg Rev 2011; 34: 417–432

[21] Ghosh PS, Ghosh D. Subdural hematoma in infants without accidental or non-accidental injury: benign external hydrocephalus, a risk factor. Clin Pediatr (Phila). 2011; 50: 897–903

[22] Christian CW, Block R Committee on Child Abuse and Neglect. American Academy of Pediatrics. Abusive head trauma in infants and children. Pediatrics. 2009; 123: 1409–1411

[23] Newton AW, Vandeven AM. Child abuse and neglect: a worldwide concern. Curr Opin Pediatr 2010; 22: 226–233

[24] Childhood injuries in the United States. Division of Injury Control, Center for Environmental Health and Injury Control, Centers for Disease Control. Am J Dis Child. 1990; 144: 627–646

[25] Pierce MC, Bertocci G. Injury biomechanics and child abuse. Annu Rev Biomed Eng 2008; 10: 85–106

[26] Herman-Giddens ME, Brown G, Verbiest S et al. Underascertainment of child abuse mortality in the United States. JAMA 1999; 282: 463–467

[27] Case ME, Graham MA, Handy TC, Jentzen JM, Monteleone JA National Association of Medical Examiners Ad Hoc Committee on Shaken Baby Syndrome. Position paper on fatal abusive head injuries in infants and young children. Am J Forensic Med Pathol 2001; 22: 112–122

[28] Chiesa A, Duhaime AC. Abusive head trauma. Pediatr Clin North Am. 2009; 56: 317–331

[29] Couper Z, Albermani F. Mechanical response of infant brain to manually inflicted shaking. Proc Inst Mech Eng H 2010; 224: 1–15

[30] Duhaime AC, Gennarelli TA, Thibault LE, Bruce DA, Margulies SS, Wiser R. The shaken baby syndrome: a clinical, pathological, and biomechanical study. J Neurosurg 1987; 66: 409–415

[31] Roth S, Raul JS, Willinger R. Finite element modelling of paediatric head impact: global validation against experimental data. Comput Methods Programs Biomed 2010; 99: 25–33

[32] Morad Y, Avni I, Benton SA et al. Normal computerized tomography of brain in children with shaken baby syndrome. J AAPOS 2004; 8: 445–450

[33] Keenan HT, Runyan DK, Marshall SW, Nocera MA, Merten DF. A population-based comparison of clinical and outcome characteristics of young children with serious inflicted and noninflicted traumatic brain injury. Pediatrics 2004; 114: 633–639

[34] Vinchon M, de Foort-Dhellemmes S, Desurmont M, Delestret I. Confessed abuse versus witnessed accidents in infants: comparison of clinical, radiological, and ophthalmological data in corroborated cases. Childs Nerv Syst 2010; 26: 637–645

[35] Fujiwara T, Okuyama M, Miyasaka M. Characteristics that distinguish abusive from nonabusive head trauma among young children who underwent head computed tomography in Japan. Pediatrics 2008; 122: e841–e847

[36] Datta S, Stoodley N, Jayawant S, Renowden S, Kemp A. Neuroradiological aspects of subdural haemorrhages. Arch Dis Child 2005; 90: 947–951

[37] Ransom GH, Mann FA, Vavilala MS, Haruff R, Rivara FP. Cerebral infarct in head injury: relationship to child abuse. Child Abuse Negl 2003; 27: 381–392

[38] Altinok D, Saleem S, Zhang Z, Markman L, Smith W. MR imaging findings of retinal hemorrhage in a case of nonaccidental trauma. Pediatr Radiol 2009; 39: 290–292

[39] Sato Y, Yuh WT, Smith WL, Alexander RC, Kao SC, Ellerbroek CJ. Head injury in child abuse: evaluation with MR imaging. Radiology. 1989; 173: 653–657

[40] Feldman KW, Bethel R, Shugerman RP, Grossman DC, Grady MS, Ellenbogen RG. The cause of infant and toddler subdural hemorrhage: a prospective study. Pediatrics 2001; 108: 636–646

[41] Fernando S, Obaldo RE, Walsh IR, Lowe LH. Neuroimaging of nonaccidental head trauma: pitfalls and controversies. Pediatr Radiol 2008; 38: 827–838

[42] McNeely PD, Atkinson JD, Saigal G, O'Gorman AM, Farmer JP. Subdural hematomas in infants with benign enlargement of the subarachnoid spaces are not pathognomonic for child abuse. AJNR Am J Neuroradiol. 2006; 27: 1725–1728

[43] Raul JS, Roth S, Ludes B, Willinger R. Influence of the benign enlargement of the subarachnoid space on the bridging veins strain during a shaking event: a finite element study. Int J Legal Med 2008; 122: 337–340

[44] Köhler M, Hoffmann GF. Subdural haematoma in a child with glutaric aciduria type I. Pediatr Radiol 1998; 28: 582.

[45] Barnes PD. Imaging of nonaccidental injury and the mimics: issues and controversies in the era of evidence-based medicine. Radiol Clin North Am. 2011; 49: 205–229

[46] Swanson AE, Veldman A, Wallace EM, Malhotra A. Subgaleal hemorrhage: risk factors and outcomes. Acta Obstet Gynecol Scand 2012; 91: 260–263

[47] Williams H. Lumps, bumps and funny shaped heads. Arch Dis Child Educ Pract Ed. 2008; 93: 120–128

[48] Hughes CA, Harley EH, Milmoe G, Bala R, Martorella A. Birth trauma in the head and neck. Arch Otolaryngol Head Neck Surg 1999; 125: 193–199

[49] King SJ, Boothroyd AE. Cranial trauma following birth in term infants. Br J Radiol 1998; 71: 233–238

[50] Chadwick LM, Pemberton PJ, Kurinczuk JJ. Neonatal subgaleal haematoma: associated risk factors, complications and outcome. J Paediatr Child Health 1996; 32: 228–232

[51] Jeltema HR, Hoving EW. Iatrogenic encephalocele: a rare complication of vacuum extraction delivery. Childs Nerv Syst 2011; 27: 2193–2195

[52] Looney CB, Smith JK, Merck LH et al. Intracranial hemorrhage in asymptomatic neonates: prevalence on MR images and relationship to obstetric and neonatal risk factors. Radiology 2007; 242: 535–541

[53] Yeates KO. Mild traumatic brain injury and postconcussive symptoms in children and adolescents. J Int Neuropsychol Soc 2010; 16: 953–960

[54] Bazarian JJ, McClung J, Shah MN, Cheng YT, Flesher W, Kraus J. Mild traumatic brain injury in the United States, 1998–2000. Brain Inj 2005; 19: 85–91

[55] Powell JW, Barber-Foss KD. Traumatic brain injury in high school athletes. JAMA 1999; 282: 958–963

[56] Laker SR. Epidemiology of concussion and mild traumatic brain injury. PM&R 2011; 3 Suppl 2: S354–S358

[57] Wozniak JR, Krach L, Ward E et al. Neurocognitive and neuroimaging correlates of pediatric traumatic brain injury: a diffusion tensor imaging (DTI) study. Arch Clin Neuropsychol 2007; 22: 555–568.

[58] Niogi SN, Mukherjee P, Ghajar J et al. Extent of microstructural white matter injury in postconcussive syndrome correlates with impaired cognitive reaction time: a 3 T diffusion tensor imaging study of mild traumatic brain injury. AJNR Am J Neuroradiol 2008; 29: 967–973

[59] Maas AI, Steyerberg EW, Butcher I et al. Prognostic value of computerized tomography scan characteristics in traumatic brain injury: results from the IMPACT study. J Neurotrauma 2007; 24: 303–314

6 Postoperative Imaging of Traumatic Brain Injury

Nicholas D. Krause, Kathleen R. Fink, and Yoshimi Anzai

6.1 Introduction

As described in earlier chapters of this book, traumatic brain injury (TBI) is a major problem in the United States, with 1.5 million head injuries occurring every year. Furthermore, it results in 52,000 deaths per year,[1] with a preponderance of cases occurring in children and younger adults. As a leading cause of death and disability in this younger population, TBI results in a major expense to society. Reducing the degree of disability can have a significant financial impact, reducing both health care costs and resulting in an earlier return to the work. In the past, there was a lack of enthusiasm by many surgeons for operative treatment of TBI, as many believed prognosis was dictated by the inciting incident. An overall lack of high-quality, controlled research in the subject likely contributed to this pessimistic view. However, more recent data have shown that the mortality rate is significantly reduced at centers with aggressive treatment for TBI.[2] An extensive literature review led to the third edition of the "Guidelines for the Surgical Management of Traumatic Brain Injury" in 2006, a joint venture between the Brain Trauma Foundation and the Congress of Neurological Surgeons, which helped outline indications for surgical intervention of TBI.[3]

Given the impact of aggressive treatment and early intervention on the morbidity and mortality rates of TBI, it is paramount that radiologists are familiar with indications for surgery, common surgical interventions, expected postsurgical appearance, and potential complications. The radiology literature focusing on postoperative imaging for TBI patients is scarce. In this chapter, we summarize the imaging findings of various surgical interventions and the expected and unexpected imaging findings of which radiologists, intensive care specialists, or surgeons must be aware.

6.2 Intracranial Pressure Monitors and External Ventricular Drains

Although some patients with moderate or severe TBI are rushed immediately to the operating room, many others will first undergo a trial of nonoperative management, which may include bedside placement of intracranial pressure (ICP) monitors or ventriculostomy catheters. ICP monitor placement is usually indicated for TBI patients with a Glasgow Coma Score (GCS) of less than 8 (i.e., patients who are comatose after their initial injury). They are also placed in patients with a more mildly decreased score (9–12) who may be undergoing procedures that have the potential to affect the ICP.[4] Placement can be done at the bedside in the intensive care unit, and they are usually inserted via a transfrontal approach after burr hole placement (▶ Fig. 6.1). Intraparenchymal hemorrhage at the insertion site is a fairly common occurrence (▶ Fig. 6.2), seen in almost 10% of patients at the authors' institution.[4]

An external ventricular drain (EVD), or ventriculostomy catheter, can also measure ICP but has the advantage of also being able to lower ICP if necessary by draining off cerebrospinal fluid (CSF). An EVD can be placed at the bedside or in the operating room as part of a more extensive procedure. An EVD is most commonly placed via a transfrontal approach, entering the ventricular system at the frontal horn of the lateral ventricle and terminating midline near the foramen of Monro (▶ Fig. 6.3). However, placement can be complicated by concomitant intracranial injuries, as midline shift related to intracranial mass effect may be present, or the ventricles may be slit-like as a result of cerebral edema or swelling.[2] Follow-up computed tomographic examinations should be evaluated for evidence of hemorrhage along the catheter tract (▶ Fig. 6.4) or for suboptimal catheter tract placement (▶ Fig. 6.5), both possible complications to the procedure.

6.3 Subdural Hematomas

Acute subdural hematoma (aSDH) is one of the most common reasons for a TBI patient to undergo surgical intervention. Acute subdural bleeds warrant surgical intervention when they are larger than 10 mm thick or cause more than 5 mm of midline shift.[2] For purely aSDHs, surgical intervention typically involves craniotomy for evacuation. As aSDH often extends over much of one hemisphere, large frontotemporoparietal craniotomies are typically performed for evacuation. Imaging after successful surgery typically shows a significant reduction in the size of the collection and adjacent mass effect, with some expected postcraniotomy changes, including gas, fluid, and a small amount of blood products at the craniotomy site (▶ Fig. 6.6).[5,6]

Treatment of chronic SDHs, as well as acute on chronic SDHs, can be somewhat more complicated. Conservative management may be used for patients with asymptomatic collections with little adjacent mass effect.[2] Given that chronic SDHs often occur in an older population in whom diffuse cerebral volume loss is more prevalent, even moderate-sized collections can have little mass effect on the adjacent brain parenchyma. When treatment is warranted, burr hole drainage is often the first step. Typically, two burr holes are created over the thickest part of the collection, and a drainage catheter is often left temporarily in place. Early imaging often shows only a mild reduction in collection size, with gas replacing some of the previously seen fluid. Complete resolution of the collection and adjacent mass effect often takes weeks to months (▶ Fig. 6.7). For collections that continue to recur after drainage, or for particularly large chronic SDHs, craniotomy may be used, similar to that done for aSDHs.[2] In these cases, prior burr holes may be incorporated into the craniotomy.

When evaluating postoperative imaging studies after either acute or chronic SDH evacuation, attention should be given to rebleeding, which can appear as either an increase in size of the collection or increase in collection density (▶ Fig. 6.8; ▶ Fig. 6.9). Reducing the collection and adjacent mass effect can result in blossoming of other intracranial injuries, such as parenchymal contusions and contralateral subdural collections, and follow-up imaging may demonstrate interval enlargement (▶ Fig. 6.10; ▶ Fig. 6.11).

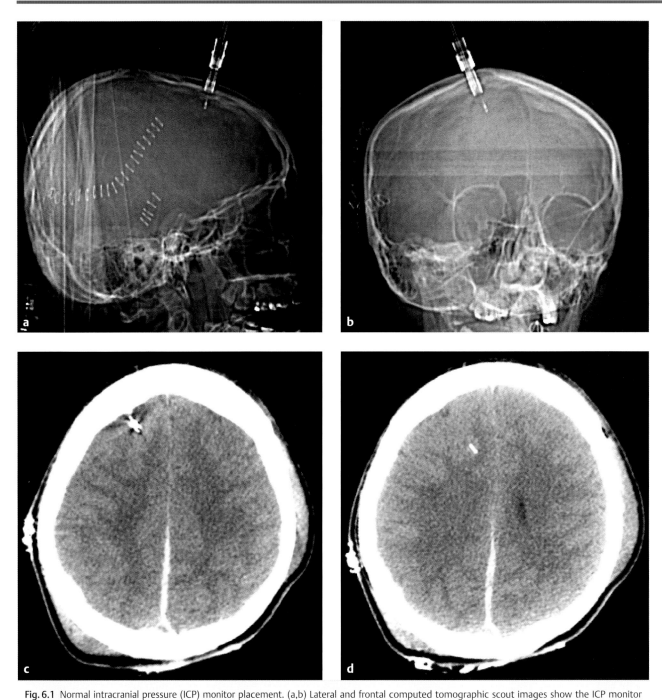

Fig. 6.1 Normal intracranial pressure (ICP) monitor placement. (a,b) Lateral and frontal computed tomographic scout images show the ICP monitor entering in the right frontal region. (c,d) Sequential noncontrast CT images in the same patient show a right frontal approach ICP monitor terminating in the frontal lobe. Parafalcine subdural hematoma is also noted.

Tension pneumocephalus can also occur, as with craniotomies for any reason. In this situation, a large amount of gas collects in the subdural space, compressing the adjacent frontal lobes and causing increased prominence to the interhemispheric fissure, sometimes referred to as the "Mount Fuji" sign (▶ Fig. 6.12).[7,8] Although often asymptomatic, significant pneumocephalus, particularly tension pneumocephalus, may lead to clinical deterioration and is potentially life threatening if untreated. Clinically significant tension pneumocephalus is treated with immediate surgical decompression.[9]

6.4 Epidural Hemorrhages

Epidural hematomas are less common than SDHs after TBI, although prompt identification of the abnormality is crucial, as studies have shown surgical evacuation to be cost-effective in regard to survival and quality of life.[10] It is often helpful to convey three-dimensional measurements of an acute epidural hematoma (aEDH) in a radiologic report, as an aEDH volume of greater than 30 mL is one indication for surgery.[2] Location is also key, as middle cranial fossa collections can compress the brainstem at sizes smaller than 30 mL, leading to lower cutoff criteria for surgical intervention.[11,12] Other factors that are considered include the GCS score, associated mass effect and midline shift, and associated injuries. Up to half of aEDHs treated surgically will have a concomitant intracranial hemorrhage (ICH).[3]

Surgical intervention for an isolated aEDH typically involves a more limited craniotomy compared with aSDH. Often a pronounced decrease in mass effect is seen on immediate postoperative CT studies (▸ Fig. 6.13). As many aEDH are associated with calvarial fractures, elevation and fixation of depressed skull fractures will sometimes be performed at surgery (▸ Fig. 6.14). As concomitant injuries are rather common in the setting of aEDH, close attention to follow-up studies for blossoming of other ICHs, such as parenchymal contusions (▸ Fig. 6.15), is vital.

6.5 Parenchymal Hematomas

Although contusional intraparenchymal hematomas are common in patients after a severe TBI, most are treated nonoperatively. The decision to proceed to surgery may be multifactorial, although common indications include large contusions (> 50 mL), smaller lesions with associated cisternal compression or midline shift greater than 5 mm, neurologic deterioration, and increased ICP refractory to medical management.[2] Compared with aEDH and aSDH, parenchymal contusions have a greater propensity to worsen in the first few days after a traumatic injury or to develop in an area that was previously normal on imaging. This is especially true after surgical intervention for another ICH, where surgical decompression can reduce adjacent mass effect (and associated tamponade of hemorrhage), allowing a parenchymal contusion to enlarge or "blossom" (▸ Fig. 6.11; ▸ Fig. 6.15; ▸ Fig. 6.16).

Some patients are more susceptible to rebleeding, also called progressive hemorrhagic injury (PHI), and these patients may warrant closer postoperative monitoring or imaging.[13] A list of risk factors for rebleeding/PHI follows:

- Coagulopathy
  - Therapeutic anticoagulation
  - Liver disease
  - Thrombocytopenia
  - Elevated prothrombin time/international normalized ratio, partial thromboplastin time, or D-dimer
- Higher-grade initial injuries:
  - Intra-axial hematomas (as opposed to aSDH/aEDH)
  - Midline shift
  - Decreased GCS
  - Nonreactive pupils
- Older age (i.e., > 57 years old)
- Elevated blood glucose

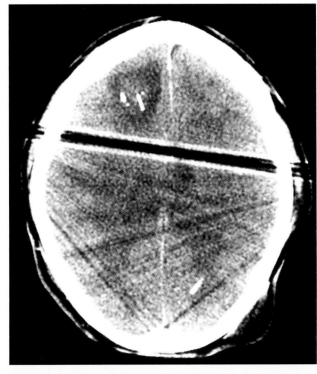

Fig. 6.2 Axial computed tomography image shows extensive edema and a small amount of hemorrhage surrounding a right frontal approach intracranial pressure monitor.

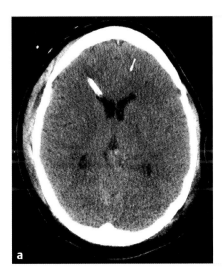
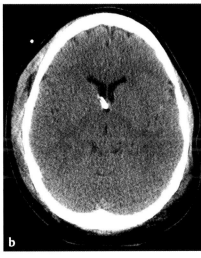

Fig. 6.3 Normal external ventricular drain placement. (a,b) Sequential noncontrast computed tomography shows a right frontal approach intracranial pressure monitor traversing the frontal horn of the right lateral ventricle, terminating near the foramen of Monro.

Given the degree of cerebral swelling associated with parenchymal hematomas warranting operative management, surgical intervention typically involves a decompressive craniectomy (▸ Fig. 6.16; ▸ Fig. 6.17). The goal of a decompressive craniectomy is to allow the brain to swell, herniating out of the craniectomy defect if needed, without concomitant elevated ICP and the associated complications of brain herniation or ischemia.

The location and size of the craniectomy will depend on the location and size of the original hematoma and associated injuries. The bone flap is then stored for later replacement once cerebral swelling has decreased. If the bone flap is unsuitable for reimplantation, a prosthetic flap may also be used.

Posterior fossa hematomas create a unique situation. These injuries are relatively uncommon, usually a result of direct trauma to the occipital region, and can be asymptomatic early, with

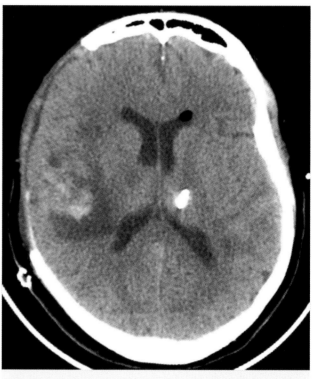

Fig. 6.4 Axial computed tomographic image shows a large amount of edema and hemorrhage surrounding a right frontal approach external ventricular drain in an area that was previously normal by imaging. Hemorrhage extends into the right lateral ventricle. The patient was status postsuboccipital craniectomy for hematoma evacuation.

Fig. 6.5 In a patient status postdecompressive right craniectomy, there is suboptimal placement of a left frontal approach external ventricular drain, with the tip terminating in the left thalamus.

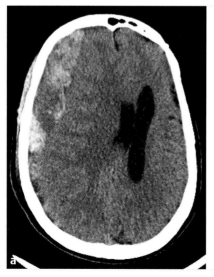
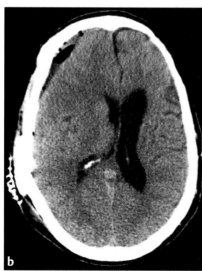

Fig. 6.6 Acute subdural hematoma (aSDH) evacuation by craniotomy. (a) Preoperative computed tomography shows a very large, predominately right frontal aSDH causing marked adjacent mass effect on the right cerebral hemisphere and right lateral ventricle, resulting in subfalcine herniation. (b) Immediately after aSDH evacuation by craniotomy, mass effect and leftward midline shift are markedly improved. Expected postsurgical changes include extra-axial gas, fluid, and minimal residual blood products at the craniotomy site.

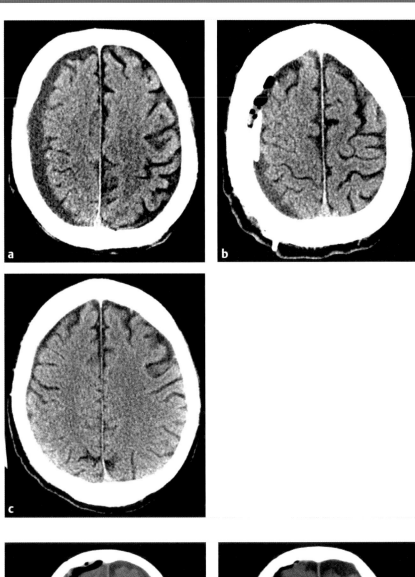

Fig. 6.7 Chronic subdural hematoma (SDH) with delayed improvement post burr hole drainage. (a) Presenting computed tomography shows a small-to-moderate sized chronic right holohemispheric SDH, with only mild adjacent mass effect given the underlying volume loss. (b) Immediately after Burr hole placement, the collection is only mildly decreased in size, with some of the hypodense fluid replaced by gas. A drain was left in the collection. (c) Follow-up head computed tomography performed 6 weeks later shows complete resolution of the SDH.

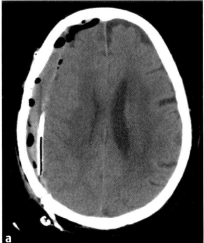
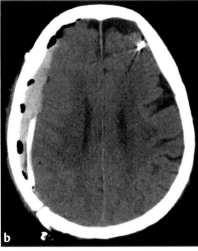

Fig. 6.8 Rebleeding following craniotomy for SDH evacuation. (a) Postcraniotomy computed tomography (CT) shows a small residual right holohemispheric SDH with expected postoperative gas. A drain was left in place. (b) Follow-up CT shows little change in size to the residual collection, although the collection is now hyperdense, suggestive of rebleeding.

a risk of slow progression. With time, mass effect on the fourth ventricle resulting in obstructive hydrocephalus and compression of the brainstem can result in a delayed rapid clinical decline. Indications for surgery include a hematoma with mass effect on the fourth ventricle, cisternal effacement, obstructive hydrocephalus, or clinical decline.[2]

Posterior fossa bleeds are often first treated with EVD placement, although there should be attention on subsequent CT examinations for any evidence of ascending transtentorial herniation, as these patients are at risk. Posterior fossa parenchymal hematomas are typically treated by decompressive suboccipital craniectomies (▶ Fig. 6.18), often with a fairly wide

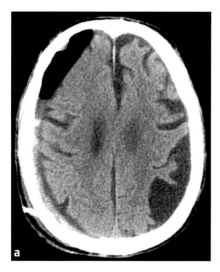

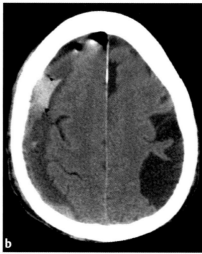

Fig. 6.9 Rebleeding following Burr hole placement for SDH evacuation. (a) Post burr hole placement CT shows a residual right subdural collection containing gas, fluid, and blood products. (b) Follow-up CT shows that the collection has increased in size, with more hyperdense blood products, consistent with rebleeding. Adjacent mass effect has also slightly increased.

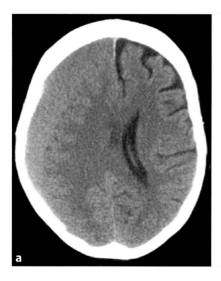

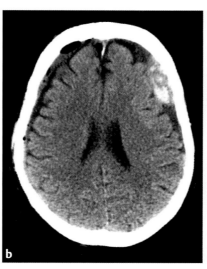

Fig. 6.10 Contralateral subdural hematoma (SDH) enlargement after burr hole placement. (a) Initial computed tomography (CT) scan shows an isodense right SDH with associated mass effect and leftward midline shift. (b) CT performed immediately following right Burr hole placement shows marked reduction in right SDH and associated mass effect, although a contralateral aSDH has developed.

bone flap removed given the propensity of these injures to result in marked swelling.

6.6 Frontal Sinus Injuries

Traumatic injuries to the frontal sinuses, especially those involving both the inner and outer tables, are particularly prone to developing infectious complications, often in a delayed fashion.[14] Because of this risk, these fractures are often treated surgically with frontal sinus cranialization. For this procedure, the inner table of the frontal sinus is completely removed, the remaining sinus mucosa is removed (stripped) or cauterized, and outer table fractures are fixed with plates and screws (▸ Fig. 6.19). Sometimes the remaining defect is filled with autogenous fat, which may be visualized by imaging.

On subsequent images, it is important to evaluate for complications of infection or mucocele formation. Mucoceles can form when there is incomplete removal of the frontal sinus mucosa. Because the frontal sinus ostia are intentionally obstructed as part of this procedure to block communication between the intracranial compartment and the paranasal sinuses, residual mucosa may lead to the development of a mucocele.

Another potential complication of cranialization of the frontal sinus is CSF leak, which may manifest as persistent fluid in the paranasal sinuses with the appropriate clinical history of a salty taste in the mouth or fluid leaking from the nose. Alternatively, persistent communication of the intracranial compartment with the paranasal sinuses may manifest as pneumocephalus.

6.7 Delayed Postoperative Complications

As mentioned earlier in this chapter, imaging studies after surgery for TBI should be evaluated for evidence of rebleeding, evolving mass effect, and any postsurgical complications. TBI patients who undergo surgery should also be closely observed for any signs of infection, as several factors can increase the risk of infection in this population relative to patients who undergo craniotomy or craniectomy for other reasons. Risk factors for infection include penetrating injuries, urgent or emergent surgeries, delayed cranioplasty, and larger bone flaps.[9] Infection can involve the brain parenchyma, the extra-axial space, or the bone flap. As with parenchymal infections from any cause,

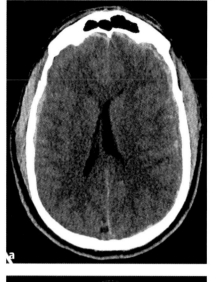

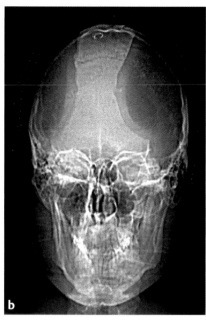

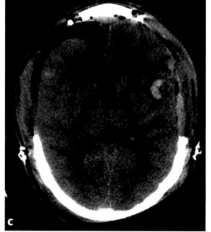

Fig. 6.11 Blossoming contusion after subdural hematoma (SDH) evacuation. (a) In a 23-year-old man status post 30-foot fall, there are bilateral holohemispheric hematomas with adjacent mass effect. (b) Scout image from follow-up computed tomography (CT) scan shows the patient has undergone interval "T-top" bilateral craniectomies. (c) Follow-up CT shows evacuation of subdural collections with blossoming of a left frontal lobe contusion.

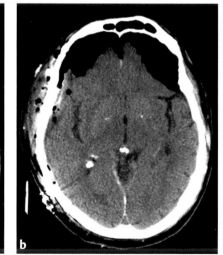

Fig. 6.12 Tension pneumocephalus. (a) Presenting computed tomography shows a right acute subdural hematoma (SDH) with adjacent mass effect. (b) After right craniotomy for SDH evacuation, there is a large amount of pneumocephalus compressing the bilateral frontal lobes, concerning for tension pneumocephalus. The patient was treated nonoperatively.

imaging signs include enhancement (particularly rim enhancement), associated vasogenic edema, and evidence of restricted diffusion on magnetic resonance imaging (▶ Fig. 6.20). Of note, enhancement after TBI must be put in the context of the clinical situation, as an evolving, noninfected hematoma can show enhancement, even rim enhancement, as well as diffusion signal abnormality. It should also be noted that hematomas can become superinfected, with the blood products providing a nutrient rich medium for microorganisms.

The craniotomy bone flap is also prone to infection, as this bone is devascularized. Lytic changes to the bone flap can suggest osteomyelitis; however, this too must be put in context of

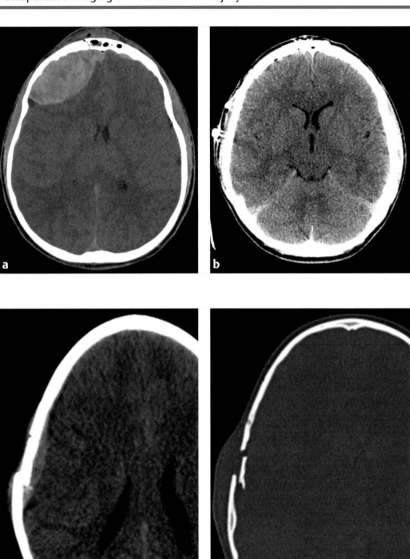

Fig. 6.13 Acute epidural hematoma (aEDH) with evacuation. (a) Initial computed tomography shows a right frontal aEDH with adjacent mass effect. An associated nondisplaced frontal bone fracture is visible. (b) Immediately after surgery, there is complete evacuation of the hematoma with expected minimal postoperative gas and fluid. Adjacent mass effect has dramatically reduced.

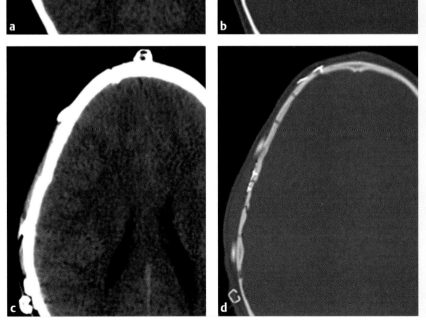

Fig. 6.14 Acute epidural hematoma (aEDH) with depressed skull fracture. (a,b) Presenting computed tomography (CT) shows a relatively small right frontoparietal aEDH with an associated depressed calvarial fracture. (c,d) Postoperative CT shows evacuation of the hematoma with elevation and fixation of the calvarial fracture.

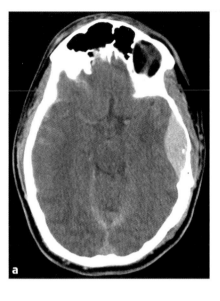

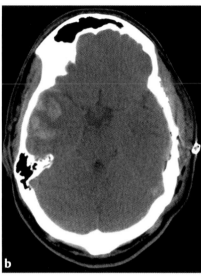

Fig. 6.15 Acute epidural hematoma (aEDH) with blossoming contusion following decompression. (a) Preoperative computed tomography (CT) shows an aEDH in the left temporal region. In the right temporal lobe, there is a suggestion of a small amount of blood, raising concern for a contrecoup contusion. (b) After evacuation of the left temporal region aEDH, marked blossoming of the right temporal hemorrhagic contusion has occurred.

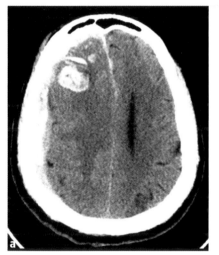

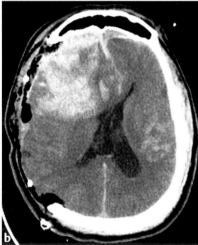

Fig. 6.16 Growing contusion after subdural hematoma (SDH) evacuation. (a) Initial computed tomography (CT) shows a holohemispheric right aSDH and right frontal hemorrhagic contusion. (b) After decompressive craniectomy and evacuation of the aSDH, marked enlargement of the right frontal contusion and mass effect are seen, necessitating an immediate return trip to the operating room. (c) The right frontal hematoma was evacuated in the second operation, with expected gas in the evacuation cavity. Adjacent mass effect is minimally affected.

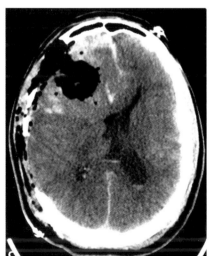

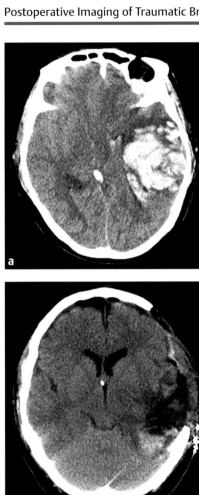

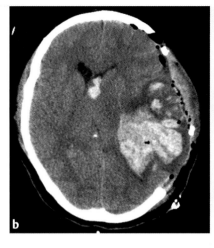

Fig. 6.17 Decompressive craniectomy for left frontotemporal contusion. (a) Initial computed tomography (CT) shows a large left frontotemporal hemorrhagic contusion with adjacent mass effect and diffuse sulcal and cisternal effacement. The patient was brought to the operating room for a decompressive craniectomy and hematoma evacuation. (b) Immediate postoperative CT shows rapid reaccumulation of hemorrhage. The patient was brought back to the operating room for repeat evacuation. (c) Delayed follow-up CT shows expected postoperative gas in the evacuation cavity. Significant improvement is noted in the previously seen cisternal and sulcal effacement with less adjacent mass effect.

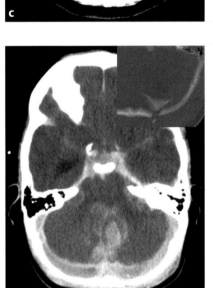

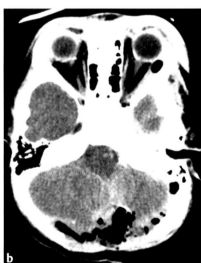

Fig. 6.18 Posterior fossa parenchymal hematoma. (a) This pediatric patient incurred direct occipital trauma from a television. Noncontrast computed tomography shows a cerebellar hemorrhagic contusion and extra axial blood, with displaced occipital bone fracture (inset image). (b) The patient underwent suboccipital decompression with hematoma evacuation.

the clinical scenario, as bone resorption can occur in the absence of infection (▶ Fig. 6.21). Patients with bone flap infection usually have evidence on physical examination of an overlying skin infection. In one recent series of patients who underwent cranioplasty after decompressive craniectomy, 11.6% of patients required subsequent removal of the bone flap because of infec-

tion, and 7.2% of patients required flap augmentation for extensive flap bone resorption without infection.[15]

Another potential complication that can occur days to weeks after surgery for TBI is the development of excess extraventricular CSF, sometimes referred to as external hydrocephalus.[16] External hydrocephalus is more commonly discussed in pediatric

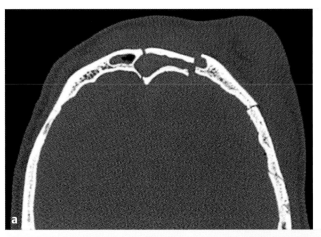

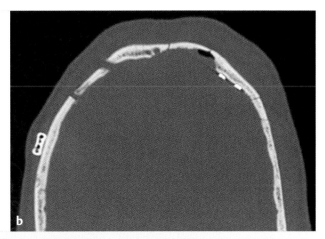

Fig. 6.19 Frontal sinus injury with subsequent cranialization. (a) Presenting maxillofacial computed tomography shows comminuted fractures involving the inner and outer tables of the frontal sinus with mild displacement of some fracture fragments. (b) The patient underwent frontal sinus cranialization, with removal of inner table bone and fixation of fragments with plates and screws.

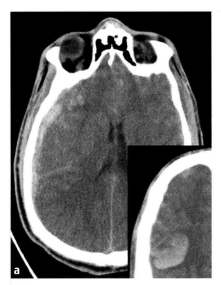

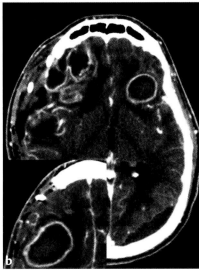

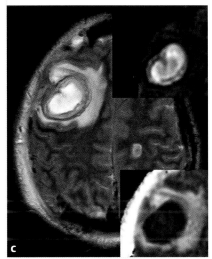

Fig. 6.20 Multiple abscesses following trauma. (a) Noncontrast head computed tomography (CT) at initial assessment shows a right temporal acute subdural hematoma (aSDH) as well as a frontal lobe contusion (inset image). (b) Post-contrast CT performed several weeks later after a decompressive right craniectomy shows multiple rim-enhancing collections, including in the region of the previously seen right frontal hematoma (inset image). White blood cell count showed a significant leukocytosis, and the patient was febrile. (c) Axial T2 magnetic resonance imaging of the brain at the level of the previously seen right frontal hematoma shows a lesion with central hyperintensity, a T2 hypointense rim, and surrounding edema. Diffusion-weighted images (upper right inset) and apparent diffusion coefficient map (lower right inset) show evidence of restricted diffusion. Cultures of the collections were inconclusive, possibly related to multiple courses of antibiotics prior to surgical sampling, although polymerase chain reaction showed evidence of *Mycoplasma* spp.

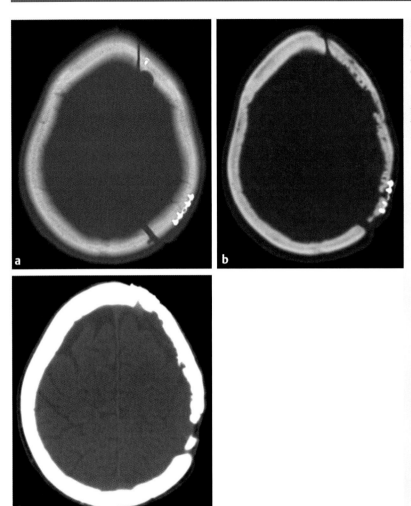

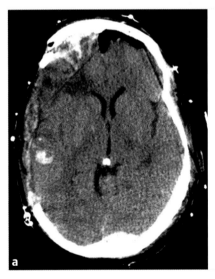

Fig. 6.21 Bone flap resorption. (a) Early postoperative computed tomography (CT) demonstrates an intact autologous cranioplasty. The patient previously had a decompressive craniectomy for an acute subdural hematoma related to an assault. (b,c) Follow-up CT 8 months later shows marked resorption of the bone flap. There was clinically no evidence of infection, and the soft tissue window shows no secondary signs, such as scalp soft tissue swelling or fluid collections.

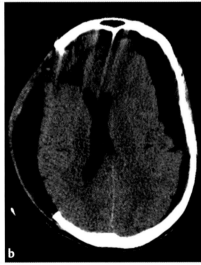

Fig. 6.22 External hydrocephalus. (a) Early postoperative computed tomography demonstrates evolving contusions after right frontotemporal decompressive craniectomy. (b) Several weeks later, the contusions have evolved and are no longer hyperdense, but bilateral cerebrospinal fluid density extra-axial fluid collections have developed, with the left-sided collection causing mass effect and midline shift.

patients, but it can also occur in adults after trauma. In this situation, blood products can impair the resorption of CSF by arachnoid villi, and excess CSF accumulates predominately in the extraventricular space (▸ Fig. 6.22). The collections can be symptomatic and are related to adjacent mass effect.

6.8 Conclusion

Evaluating and caring for patients following surgery for TBI are complex issues, and clinicians depend on imaging studies when formulating care strategies. It is imperative that radiologists who practice in a trauma setting be familiar with the common indications for surgical management, as discussed in this chapter, to appropriately alert clinicians. Knowledge of the common surgeries, their expected postoperative appearances, and possible complications are also crucial. Placing these findings in context with the patient's clinical status is also important, particularly when infection is considered a possibility. Keeping these concepts in mind will help improve imaging interpretation to the many TBI patients in the postoperative setting.

References

[1] Langlois JA, Rutland-Brown W, Wald MM. The epidemiology and impact of traumatic brain injury: a brief overview. J Head Trauma Rehabil 2006; 21: 375–378

[2] Zacko JC, Harris L, Bullock MR. Surgical Management of Traumatic Brain Injury. In: Winn HR, ed. Youmans Neurological Surgery. 6th ed.

[3] Bullock MR, Chesnut R, Ghajar J et al. Guidelines for the surgical management of traumatic brain injury: introduction. Neurosurgery. 2006; 58 S2: 1–3

[4] Blaha M, Lazar D. Traumatic brain injury and haemorrhagic complications after intracranial pressure monitoring. J Neurol Neurosurg Psychiatry 2005; 76: 147

[5] Rastogi H, Bazan C III, da Costa Leite C, Jinkins JR. The posttherapeutic cranium. In: Jinkins JR, ed. Post-therapeutic Neurodiagnostic Imaging. Philadelphia, PA: Lippincott-Raven; 1997: 3–36.

[6] Ross JS. Modic MT Postoperative neuroradiology. In: Little JR, Awad IA, eds. Reoperative Neurosurgery. Baltimore, MD: Williams & Wilkins, 1992: 1–47.

[7] Ishiwata Y, Fujitsu K, Sekino T et al. Subdural tension pneumocephalus following surgery for chronic subdural hematoma. J Neurosurg. 1988; 68: 58–61

[8] Michel SJ. The Mount Fuji sign. Radiology. 2004; 232: 449–450

[9] Sinclair AG, Scoffings DJ. Imaging of the post-operative cranium. Radiographics 2010; 30: 461–482

[10] Pickard JD, Bailey S, Sanderson H, Rees M, Garfield JS. Steps towards cost-benefit analysis of regional neurosurgical care. BMJ 1990; 301: 629–635

[11] Bullock R, Teasdale G. Head injuries—surgical management of traumatic intracerebral hematomas. In: Braakman R, ed. Handbook of Clinical Neurology. Amsterdam: Elsevier; 1990:249–298.

[12] Andrews BT, Chiles BW III Olsen WL, Pitts LH. The effect of intracerebral hematoma location on the risk of brain-stem compression and on clinical outcome. J Neurosurg 1988; 69: 518–522

[13] Yuan F, Ding J, Chen H et al. Predicting progressive hemorrhagic injury after traumatic brain injury: derivation and validation of a risk score based on admission characteristics. J Neurotrauma 2012; 29: 2137–2142[Epub ahead of print]

[14] Sataloff RT, Sariego J, Myers DL, Richter HJ. Surgical management of the frontal sinus. Neurosurgery. 1984; 15: 593–596

[15] Honeybul S, Ho KM. Long-term complications of decompressive craniectomy for head injury. J Neurotrauma 2011; 28: 929–935

[16] Tzerakis N, Orphanides G, Antoniou E, Sioutos PJ, Lafazanos S, Seretis A. Subdural effusions with hydrocephalus after severe head injury: successful treatment with ventriculoperitoneal shunt placement: report of 3 adult cases. Case Rep Med. 2010; 2010: 743–784.

7 Blunt Cerebrovascular Injury

Carrie P. Marder and Kathleen R. Fink

7.1 Mechanisms of Vascular Injury

Penetrating trauma is the most common mechanism for cerebrovascular injury, but injuries to the carotid or vertebral arteries from nonpenetrating trauma are more common than previously suspected, with a reported incidence of approximately 1% among those admitted to the hospital for blunt trauma.[1,2] The rate of blunt cerebrovascular injury (BCVI) increases with the use of more liberal screening criteria and more sensitive imaging tests,[3] indicating there are unrecognized, asymptomatic cases.

Mechanisms of blunt carotid artery injury include direct blows to the neck, intraoral trauma, skull-base fractures involving the carotid canal, severe hyperextension of the neck with contralateral rotation, and hyperflexion.[4,5] The distal extracranial portion of the internal carotid artery is particularly vulnerable to injury during extremes of head motion as a result of stretching of the carotid artery over the lateral masses of C1–C3 or compression between the angle of the mandible and upper cervical spine.[4]

Mechanisms of blunt vertebral artery injury include cervical spinal subluxation, fractures— especially those involving the transverse foramen—and stretch-type injuries caused by lateral bending and axial rotation.[6,7] Motor-vehicle accidents, hanging, strangulation, falls from a height, and sports accidents are frequent causes of BCVI, but injuries also occur in association with seemingly minor trauma, such as chiropractic manipulations. It is controversial whether cerebrovascular injuries occurring with minor trauma are best classified as BCVI or whether these injuries represent part of a spectrum of "spontaneous" cervical artery dissections that may have a different underlying pathophysiology.[8] Additionally, gunshot wounds, although typically associated with penetrating vascular injuries, may also cause BCVI at sites remote from the bullet tract, presumably secondary to extreme neck movements.[9]

7.2 Rationale for Screening

Cerebrovascular injuries from blunt trauma are more common than once suspected, and the outcomes are frequently devastating, with a high risk of stroke and associated morbidity and mortality. Many patients with BCVI are initially asymptomatic, but platelet aggregation and thrombosis at the site of an intimal injury can lead to thromboembolic stroke after a delay of hours to days,[10] or even months to years.[5,11] Accumulating class II and class III evidence indicates that early institution of anticoagulant or antiplatelet therapy reduces the risk of stroke in asymptomatic patients with BCVI and improves neurologic outcomes in symptomatic patients.[12–16] Accordingly, it is crucial to identify those patients at high risk for clinically occult BCVI who can be screened with vascular imaging and treated before they develop strokes.

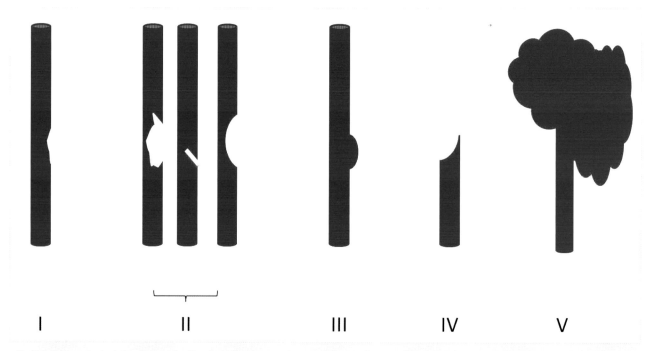

Fig. 7.1 Schematic depicting Denver Grading Scale for blunt cerebrovascular injury (see ▶ Table 7.1 for description).

Table 7.1 The Denver Grading Scale for blunt cerebrovascular injury

Injury Grade	Description
I	Vessel wall irregularity *or* dissection/intramural hematoma with <25% luminal stenosis
II	Intraluminal thrombus *or* raised intimal flap *or* dissection/intramural hematoma with ≥25% luminal stenosis
III	Pseudoaneurysm
IV	Occlusion of a vessel
V	Vessel transection with free contrast extravasation *or* hemodynamically significant arteriovenous fistula

7.3 Indications for Vascular Imaging in Blunt Trauma

Blunt trauma victims require vascular imaging when they have signs or symptoms of BCVI or when they have high risk factors for BCVI, based on the mechanism of injury or associated injury patterns.

7.3.1 Signs and Symptoms

Trauma patients with signs or symptoms attributable to BCVI require emergent diagnostic imaging and prompt treatment of hemorrhages or strokes. Signs and symptoms of BCVI include the following: (1) hemorrhage from the mouth, nose, ears, or face of potential arterial origin; (2) large or expanding cervical hematoma; (3) cervical bruit in a patient under age 50; (4) unexplained focal or lateralizing neurologic deficit, including hemiparesis, transient ischemic attack, vertebrobasilar insufficiency, or Horner syndrome; (5) acute infarct on computed tomography (CT) or magnetic resonance imaging (MRI); and 6) any neurologic deficit inconsistent with CT or MRI findings.[17]

7.3.2 Risk Factors

Relatively inclusive indications for screening of asymptomatic patients were established by the Denver group to identify a larger number of at-risk patients.[13,17-19] The Denver Imaging Criteria are based on injury mechanisms combined with high-risk radiologic or physical examination findings.

These criteria include an injury mechanism capable of producing severe cervical hyperextension with rotation or hyperflexion associated with any of the following: complex mandibular fractures, displaced Le Fort type II or III midface fractures, skull-base fractures involving the carotid canal, closed head injuries with diffuse axonal injury and low GCS score, cervical subluxations or fractures extending to the transverse foramen, any fracture at C1–C3, near-hanging resulting in cerebral anoxia, and seat-belt abrasions with severe swelling or altered mental status. The definition of complex mandible fracture has not been clarified.

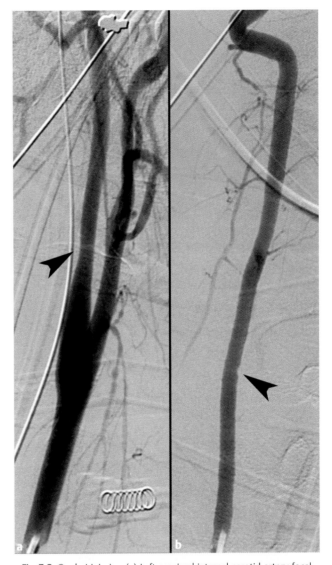

Fig. 7.2 Grade I injuries. (a) Left proximal internal carotid artery focal smooth narrowing of less than 25% just distal to the carotid bulb (*arrowhead*). No visible intimal flap or pseudoaneurysm. (b) Right vertebral artery focal wall irregularity at the level of C6–C7 (*arrowhead*), without stenosis, intimal flap, or pseudoaneurysm.

Subsequent logistic regression analysis identified four independent predictors of carotid artery injury: (1) GCS of 6 or lower, (2) petrous temporal bone fracture, (3) diffuse axonal injury, and (4) Le Fort II or III fractures.[19] A similar analysis showed cervical spine fractures to be an independent predictor of vertebral artery injury.[19] These "high-risk" factors constitute a more restrictive core set of screening criteria, but approximately 20% of the patients screened using the more liberal preceding criteria had none of the independent risk factors. Additionally, a substantial number of cerebrovascular injuries occur in patients who have no associated injuries or classic risk factors and are diagnosed either incidentally or because screening was performed based on clinical suspicion of injury.[18-22]

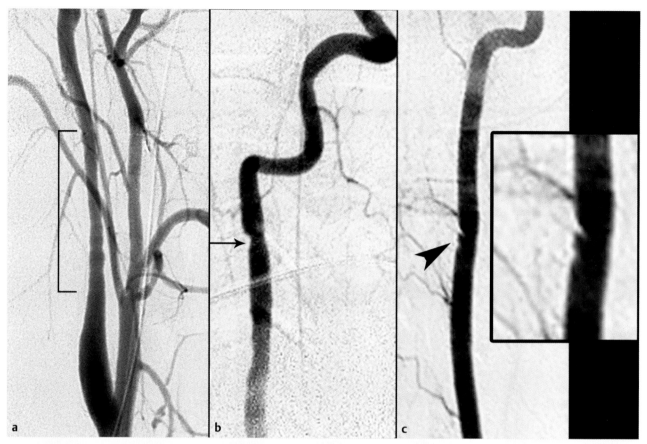

Fig. 7.3 Grade II injuries. (a) Right proximal internal carotid artery long-segment wall irregularity with narrowing of 50% (*bracket*). (b) Right vertebral artery focal-wall irregularity with narrowing of 40% (*arrow*). (c) Right vertebral artery focal-wall irregularity with less than 25% narrowing but with a small visible intimal flap, (*arrowhead* and enlarged, inset).

Accordingly, continued use of broad screening criteria is likely justified to prevent missing treatable injuries.

Because screening is now usually performed noninvasively using CT angiography (CTA), some favor using even broader screening criteria. In patients with an appropriate mechanism of injury, additional proposed criteria include any fracture of the mandible or skull base;[22,23] any cervical spine fracture[2,23] or thoracolumbar spine fracture;[2] any major thoracic trauma;[2,20] any thoracic injury combined with head trauma or any thoracic vascular injury;[22] scalp degloving injuries;[22] and gunshot wounds to the head, face, or neck.[9] Further research is needed to determine the optimal screening criteria to detect the patients not captured by the Denver criteria, as well as to balance the risks and cost of screening with the benefits.

7.4 Screening Modality of Choice

The optimal imaging modality for screening remains another important topic for ongoing investigations. Conventional catheter-based four-vessel digital subtraction angiography (DSA) is the gold standard for diagnosis of BCVI, but it is invasive and consumes time and resources. Duplex ultrasonography, magnetic resonance angiography (MRA), and CTA are noninvasive

diagnostic imaging modalities that have been considered as potential alternatives to DSA.

Ultrasound, although useful for screening the extracranial carotid arteries for atherosclerotic disease, suffers from marked limitations in evaluating the carotid arteries near the skull base, where most carotid injuries occur. Ultrasound is also limited in evaluating the vertebral arteries within the bony vertebral foramen, where most vertebral artery injuries occur. In a large retrospective series of more than 1400 blunt trauma patients screened with ultrasound, eight injuries were missed that resulted in symptomatic neurologic deficits, and the overall sensitivity of the test was only 39%.[24] Ultrasound is therefore not recommended for screening.[16,17]

Although MRA initially held promise as a noninvasive option for screening, in the two series that prospectively compared MRA with DSA, MRA had a sensitivity of only 50 to 75% and a specificity of only 47 to 67%.[25,26] MRA also has practical disadvantages, including long examination times and lack of availability at some centers, and MRA may not be feasible in unstable trauma patients requiring external monitoring equipment. MRA is therefore not recommended for screening at this time.[16,17] MRA may still be an option in patients with contraindications to iodinated contrast or for follow-up of BCVI.

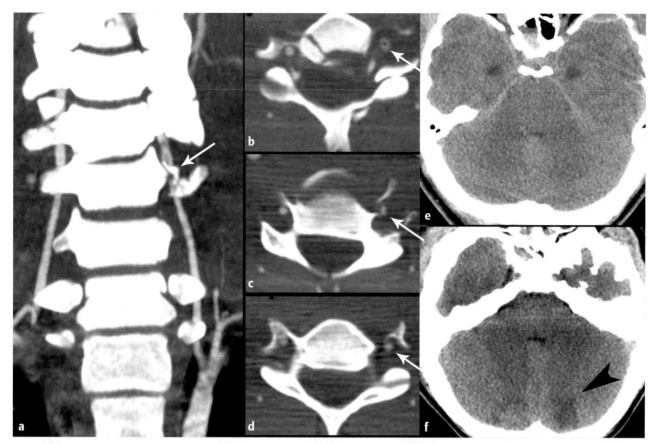

Fig. 7.4 Left vertebral artery grade II injury with visible intraluminal thrombus at level of fracture. Coronal reformat from computed tomographic angiography (CTA) (a) shows fracture involving the left lateral mass and foramen transversarium in close association with the left vertebral artery (*arrow*). Axial CTA source images demonstrate central filling defect in the left vertebral artery (b) (*arrow*), indicating intraluminal thrombus. Artery is narrowed at the level of the fracture (c) (*arrow*) but normal in caliber inferiorly (d). Initial head CT was normal (e), but acute posterior circulation infarcts developed after a delay (f) (*arrowhead*).

Axial fat-saturated proton density or T1-weighted images are useful for demonstrating hyperintense intramural hematoma in subacute dissections, but they are less useful during the acute phase when the signal characteristics of intramural hematoma are inconspicuous. Special techniques such as high-resolution vessel-wall black blood MRI with dedicated neck coils may allow for improved performance of MRI or MRA in the future for diagnosing BCVI.

Early studies comparing CTA with DSA demonstrated poor sensitivity and specificity of CTA, but with the advent of multi-slice detector techniques, CTA has emerged as the screening modality of choice.[17,27–31] CTA has the advantages of being fast, noninvasive, and readily available. Moreover, most trauma patients already require CT scanning. Some controversy remains concerning the accuracy of CTA compared with DSA, with relatively poor sensitivity and specificity reported at some institutions.[32] It has been suggested that some of the variability in the reported accuracy of CTA reflects differences in radiologist experience, subspecialty training, or interpretive abilities.[21,31,33] For example, in the study by Malhotra and colleagues, all the false-negative CTA interpretations occurred in the first half of the study period, indicating that interpretive ability improved

with experience.[34] Additionally, lower-grade injuries are more difficult to detect on CTA compared with DSA,[25] so CTA will have a lower sensitivity in population samples with lower-grade injuries. Strategies for improving the detection of subtle findings on CTA include evaluating each of the four vessels individually, as one would with DSA, and using both source images and multiplanar reconstructions to carefully examine the most commonly injured areas, such as near the skull base and adjacent to fractures of the carotid canals or transverse foramen.[31]

7.5 Classification of Arterial Injuries

The Denver Grading Scale (▶ Fig. 7.1; ▶ Table 7.1) has been widely adopted for classifying traumatic cerebrovascular injuries based on the angiographic appearance of the injured vessel.[18] *Grade I* injuries are defined as irregularity of the vessel wall or a dissection or intramural thrombus causing less than 25% narrowing of the vessel lumen (▶ Fig. 7.2). *Grade II* injuries are defined as a dissection or intramural thrombus causing

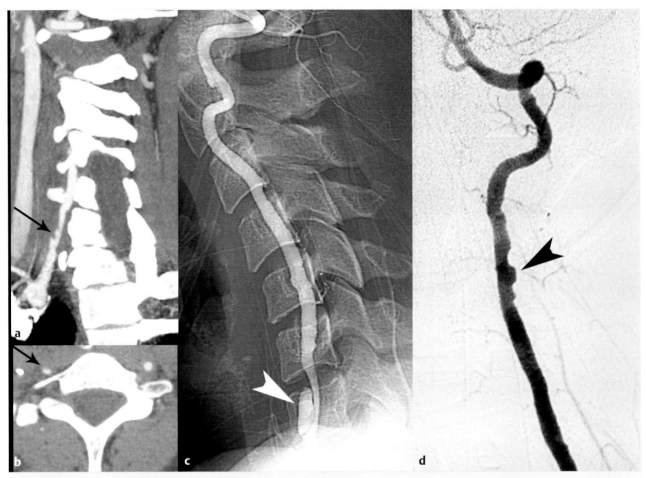

Fig. 7.5 Grade III injuries in two patients. (a,b) Long-segment grade II right vertebral artery injury on computed tomographic angiography (*arrows*) that progressed to pseudoaneurysm on follow-up angiogram (c). Left vertebral artery pseudoaneurysm in a second patient (*arrowhead*). Note the surrounding long segment of vessel-wall irregularity.

luminal stenosis of 25% or greater (▸ Fig. 7.3a,b), or injuries in which a raised intimal flap (▸ Fig. 7.3c) or an intraluminal thrombus (▸ Fig. 7.4) occurs. Grade II injuries also include small, hemodynamically insignificant arteriovenous fistulae.[35]

Grade III injuries are pseudoaneurysms (▸ Fig. 7.5; ▸ Fig. 7.6; ▸ Fig. 7.7), *grade IV* injuries are complete occlusions (▸ Fig. 7.8; ▸ Fig. 7.9), and *grade V* injuries are transections with free extravasation of contrast material (▸ Fig. 7.10; ▸ Fig. 7.11). Grade V injuries also include large, hemodynamically significant arteriovenous fistulae,[35] which sometimes result from complete arterial transection.

For carotid artery injuries, this grading scale has prognostic significance, with higher injury grades corresponding to higher risk of associated stroke.[18] Vertebral artery injuries, which are less common and historically under-recognized, also carry substantial risk for stroke when untreated, but unlike carotid artery injuries, the risk of stroke is independent of injury grade.[7]

7.6 Treatment

The goals of BCVI treatment are to prevent strokes in asymptomatic patients and to limit neurologic complications in patients presenting with cerebral ischemia. Strokes in the setting of BCVI are likely thromboembolic in most cases, although hypoperfusion resulting from severe stenosis or occlusion may also contribute to ischemic infarctions (▸ Fig. 7.6d,e). Anticoagulant and antiplatelet therapies are therefore the mainstay of treatment,[12–15,17] with apparent equivalence between heparin and aspirin or other antiplatelet agents.[36,37] To date, no prospective, randomized controlled trials evaluating the optimal therapy have been reported, and most of the existing retrospective and prospective, nonrandomized trials are necessarily limited by selection bias and other confounding factors.[33]

Choice of treatment depends partially on injury grade. Grade I injuries carry the lowest risk of stroke and are usually managed medically. Grade V injuries, on the other hand, are often fatal and require emergent surgical repair or endovascular treatment. Injuries with progressive luminal narrowing or enlarging pseudoaneurysm on follow-up may also require endovascular stent placement to maintain vessel patency.

Nonmedical treatments include surgery and endovascular interventions. Options for surgical repair include parent vessel ligation, thrombectomy, direct suturing of an intimal injury, replacement of an injured segment with an interposition graft,

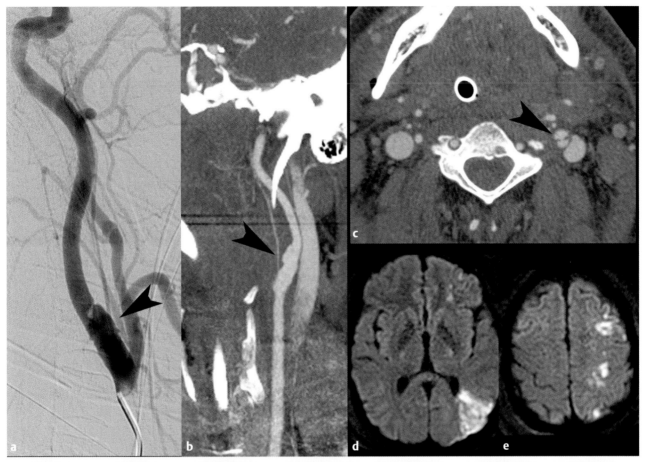

Fig. 7.6 Left proximal internal carotid artery grade III injury. Pseudoaneurysm (arrowheads) with associated raised intimal flap and 70% luminal narrowing on (a) digital subtraction angiography and (b,c) computed tomographic angiography. (d,e) Magnetic resonance imaging diffusion-weighted image shows acute infarcts in the left middle cerebral artery (MCA) and MCA-anterior cerebral artery border-zone territories.

and extracranial-intracranial bypass.[33,38] Because most cerebrovascular injuries occur in surgically inaccessible sites at the skull base, endovascular approaches such as stenting or coil embolization are usually preferred. Long-term use of antiplatelet agents is required after stent placement to avoid stent thrombosis.

Patients without contraindications to anticoagulation with grades I–IV injuries are usually treated initially with heparin, which is given without an initial bolus to limit hemorrhagic complications.[16,17] Repeat imaging after 7 to 10 days of treatment, or after any change in neurologic status, is performed to assess the need for further treatment.[35,39] Most patients with grade I or II injuries require a change in management, as many grade I injuries heal, allowing discontinuation of heparin, and many grade II injuries progress, sometimes requiring endovascular repair.[35,39] Grade III injuries usually do not heal with anticoagulation alone, but follow-up imaging is useful for treatment planning. Grade IV injuries rarely change on follow-up and probably do not require repeat imaging. Patients having a persistent injury on follow-up require continued medical treatment, usually an antiplatelet agent for safer long-term use. Medical treatment is lifelong in the absence of radiographic resolution.

7.7 Venous Injuries

Calvarial fractures that extend to a dural venous sinus or jugular bulb require further evaluation with vascular imaging to assess for venous patency because of the risk for dural venous sinus thrombosis (▶ Fig. 7.12).[40] CT venography (CTV) is the imaging modality of choice, but noncontrast MR venography is a viable alternative for stable patients with contraindications to iodinated contrast. In patients with occlusive dural venous sinus thrombosis, there is risk of developing increased intracranial pressure, hydrocephalus, and venous infarction. Long-term complications theoretically include development of a dural arteriovenous fistula. Optimal treatment of traumatic dural venous sinus thrombosis is unknown. Some patients are treated with anticoagulation, but many are monitored and show resolution or lack of progression without any specific treatment.[40]

Venous outflow obstruction can also occur as a result of external compression by an epidural hematoma (▶ Fig. 7.13), and this is a potential pitfall when evaluating for venous sinus thrombosis on CTV.[41] The presence of an epidural hematoma in the posterior fossa adjacent to an occipital bone fracture extending to the transverse sinus or torcula usually implies traumatic injury to a dural venous sinus.[42,43] In this case, treatment

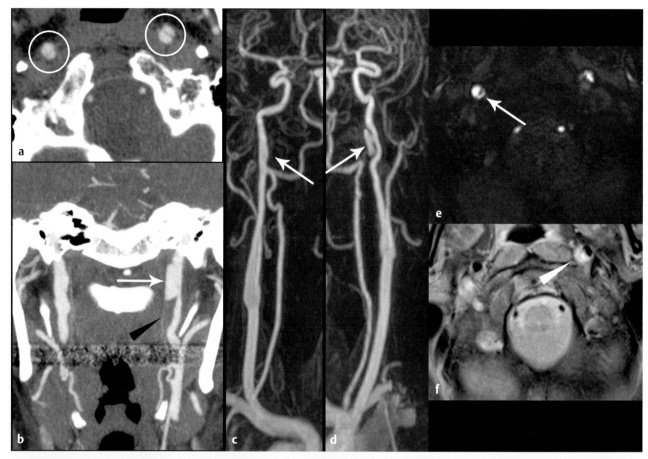

Fig. 7.7 Bilateral grade III internal carotid artery (ICA) injuries at the level of C1–C3. (a) Computed tomography angiographic axial image shows a visible intimal flap in both ICAs, with narrowing of the true lumen (circled). Coronal maximum intensity projection reconstruction (b) better demonstrates aneurysmal dilation bilaterally. Note the large intramural hematoma (*black arrowhead*) just inferior to the large left ICA pseudoaneurysm (*white arrow*). (c,d) Coronal gadolinium-enhanced magnetic resonance angiography (MRA) several months later shows persistent bilateral ICA pseudoaneurysms, larger on the left side. The right ICA injury is more subtle, but an intimal flap is again visible on the axial two-dimensional time-of-flight MRA (e) (*arrow*). Note the narrowing of the true lumen on the left side. (f) Axial fat-saturated proton density image shows hyperintense mural thrombus on the left side (*arrowhead*).

may include hematoma evacuation rather than anticoagulation or observation. Unlike supratentorial epidural hematomas, which are usually associated with injury to the middle meningeal artery, epidural hematomas in the posterior fossa are more likely a result of venous sinus rupture.[42,43]

7.8 Conclusion

Vascular injuries are a potentially devastating sequela of blunt trauma, and early recognition is important to prevent complications. Screening criteria for BCVI are a useful aid in detecting these injuries, although up to 20% of patients with BCVI are not detected using accepted screening criteria. Thus, further research to refine screening criteria is critical.

Venous injuries may also complicate head injury. The pattern and location of injury, particularly fractures and extradural hematomas adjacent to the expected location of major dural venous sinuses, should raise the possibility of venous injury. A high index of suspicion is vital to appropriately direct imaging evaluation.

7.9 Pearls

- BCVI occurs in about 1% of blunt trauma admissions and carries a high risk for stroke.
- Early treatment with anticoagulation likely improves outcomes.
- DSA is gold standard for diagnosis, but multidetector CTA is an accepted screening test.
- Sensitivity of CTA increases with radiologist experience and higher-grade injuries.
- Follow-up imaging at 7 to 10 days changes management for most grade I and II injuries.
- Higher-grade injuries may require surgical or endovascular treatment.
- Skull fractures that extend to a dural sinus can cause venous outflow obstruction by thrombosis or external compression from an epidural hematoma. CTV is the screening test of choice.

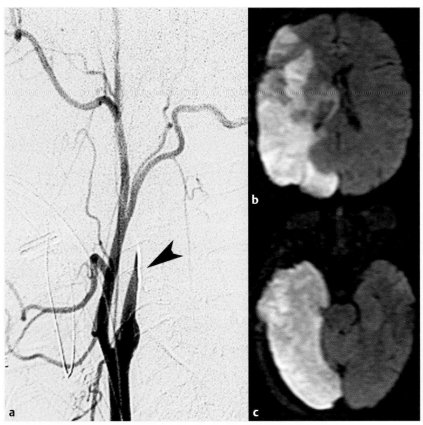

Fig. 7.8 Grade IV carotid injury in a man who presented with stroke 10 days after a fall. (a) Digital subtraction angiography, right common carotid artery injection, shows smooth tapering with complete occlusion of the internal carotid artery (ICA) just beyond the bifurcation (*arrowhead*). (b,c) Diffusion-weighted magnetic resonance imaging shows a large acute infarct in both the right MCA and PCA vascular territories, likely due to a fetal origin of the right posterior cerebral artery (not shown). The anterior cerebral artery territory was supplied by the left ICA across a patent anterior communicating artery (not shown).

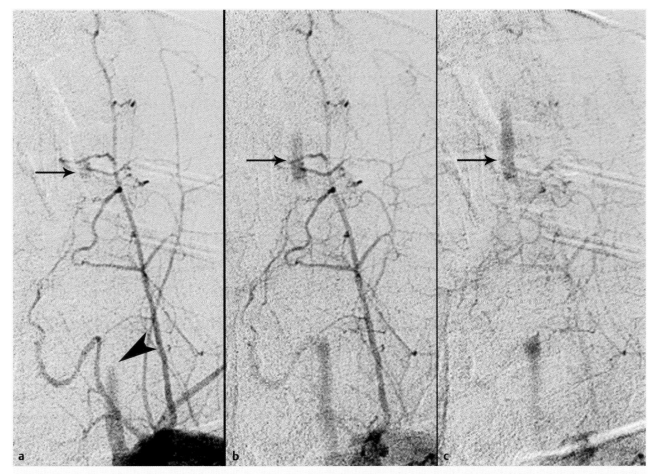

Fig. 7.9 Left vertebral artery grade IV injury. Digital subtraction angiography, arterial phase (a) shows complete occlusion of the left vertebral artery (*arrowhead*), with small early reconstitution (*black arrow*). Delayed images (b,c) show slow reconstitution of the vertebral artery superior to the occlusion from cervical collaterals. No acute infarct was seen on magnetic resonance imaging (not shown).

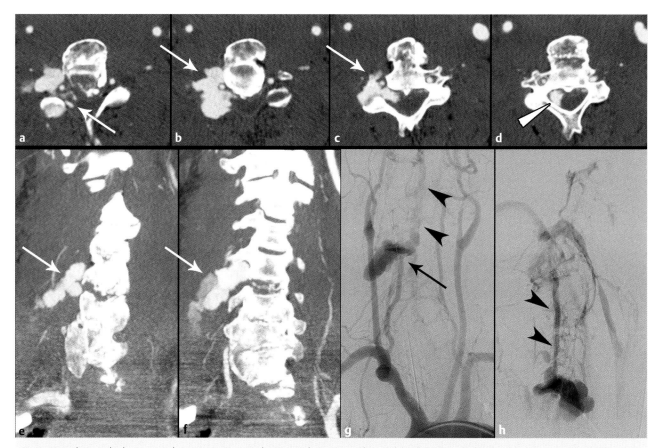

Fig. 7.10 Right vertebral artery grade V injury. Computed tomography angiographic axial (a–d) and coronal (e,f) images demonstrate free extravasation of contrast from a transected right vertebral artery at the level of a C4–C5 fracture-dislocation (*white arrows*). Contrast tracks through the neuroforamen into the epidural space (*arrowhead*) (d). Digital subtraction angiography images (g,h) show a large lobular pseudoaneurysm arising from the right vertebral artery, with no filling of the right vertebral artery above that level (*black arrow*). In the venous phase, contrast tracks within the epidural space and drains into the neck veins, consistent with a post-traumatic spinal epidural arteriovenous fistula (AVF) (*black arrowheads*). Hemodynamically significant AVFs are classified as grade V injuries.

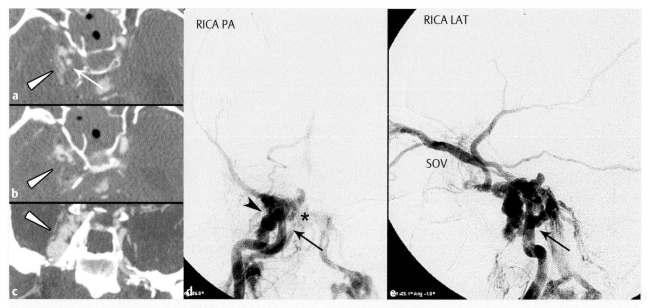

Fig. 7.11 Traumatic right grade V injury with direct carotid-cavernous fistula. Axial computed tomographic angiography (a,b) demonstrates contrast extravasation into the right cavernous sinus (*arrowheads*), demonstrated also on the coronal maximum-intensity projection reformat (c). Note the right internal carotid artery (ICA) fills in (a) but is absent in (b) (*arrow*). Digital subtraction angiography, right ICA injection in the frontal (d) and lateral (e) projection demonstrates right ICA ending at the cavernous sinus (*arrow*) with contrast opacification of the cavernous sinus (*arrowhead*) and venous drainage including via the intercavernous sinus(*) and the superior ophthalmic vein.

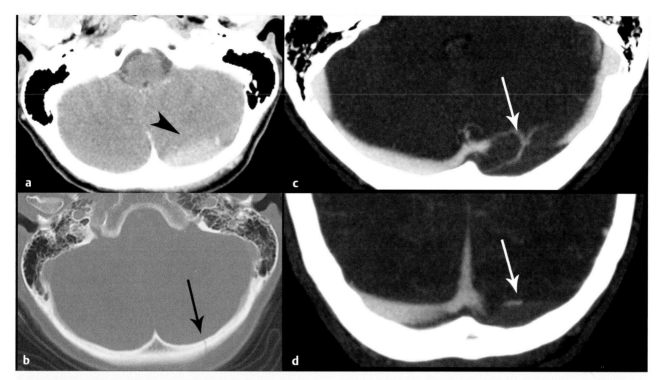

Fig. 7.13 Venous sinus occlusion. Noncontrast computed tomography CT (a,b) demonstrates posterior fossa epidural hematoma (*arrowhead*) (a) with associated occipital bone fracture (*arrow*) (b). CT venography in the axial (c) and coronal (d) plane demonstrates occlusion of the left transverse sinus resulting from extrinsic compression by the hematoma.

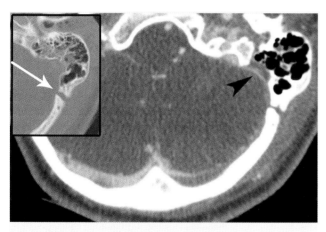

Fig. 7.12 Venous sinus thrombosis. Contrast-enhanced computed tomography demonstrates a filling defect in the left sigmoid sinus (*arrowhead*), indicating intraluminal thrombus. There is an associated skull fracture (*arrow*, inset).

References

[1] Liang T, Plaa N, Tashakkor AY, Nicolaou S. Imaging of blunt cerebrovascular injuries. Semin Roentgenol 2012; 47: 306–319

[2] Franz RW, Willette PA, Wood MJ, Wright ML, Hartman JF. A systematic review and meta-analysis of diagnostic screening criteria for blunt cerebrovascular injuries. J Am Coll Surg 2012; 214: 313–327

[3] Biffl WL. Diagnosis of blunt cerebrovascular injuries. Curr Opin Crit Care 2003; 9: 530–534

[4] Zelenock GB, Kazmers A, Whitehouse WM, Jr et al. Extracranial internal carotid artery dissections: noniatrogenic traumatic lesions. Arch Surg 1982; 117: 425–432

[5] Crissey MM, Bernstein EF. Delayed presentation of carotid intimal tear following blunt craniocervical trauma. Surgery. 1974; 75: 543–549

[6] Nibu K, Cholewicki J, Panjabi MM et al. Dynamic elongation of the vertebral artery during an in vitro whiplash simulation. Eur Spine J 1997; 6: 286–289

[7] Biffl WL, Moore EE, Elliott JP et al. The devastating potential of blunt vertebral arterial injuries. Ann Surg 2000; 231: 672–681

[8] Kim Y-K, Schulman S. Cervical artery dissection: pathology, epidemiology and management. Thromb Res. 2009; 123: 810–821

[9] Steenburg SD, Sliker CW. Craniofacial gunshot injuries: an unrecognised risk factor for blunt cervical vascular injuries? Eur Radiol 2012; 22: 1837–1843

[10] Krajewski LP, Hertzer NR. Blunt carotid artery trauma: report of two cases and review of the literature. Ann Surg 1980; 191: 341–346

[11] Mokri B, Piepgras DG, Houser OW. Traumatic dissections of the extracranial internal carotid artery. J Neurosurg 1988; 68: 189–197

[12] Fabian TC, Patton JH Jr Croce MA, Minard G, Kudsk KA, Pritchard FE. Blunt carotid injury: importance of early diagnosis and anticoagulant therapy. Ann Surg 1996; 223: 513–525

[13] Biffl WL, Moore EE, Ryu RK et al. The unrecognized epidemic of blunt carotid arterial injuries: early diagnosis improves neurologic outcome. Ann Surg 1998; 228: 462–470

[14] Miller PR, Fabian TC, Bee TK et al. Blunt cerebrovascular injuries: diagnosis and treatment. J Trauma 2001; 51: 279–286

[15] Cothren CC, Moore EE, Biffl WL et al. Anticoagulation is the gold standard therapy for blunt carotid injuries to reduce stroke rate. Arch Surg 2004; 139: 540–546

[16] Bromberg WJ, Collier BC, Diebel LN et al. Blunt cerebrovascular injury practice management guidelines: the Eastern Association for the Surgery of Trauma. J Trauma 2010; 68: 471–477

[17] Biffl WL, Cothren CC, Moore EE et al. Western Trauma Association critical decisions in trauma: screening for and treatment of blunt cerebrovascular injuries. J Trauma 2009; 67: 1150–1153

[18] Biffl WL, Moore EE, Offner PJ, Brega KE, Franciose RJ, Burch JM. Blunt carotid arterial injuries: implications of a new grading scale. J Trauma 1999; 47: 845–853

[19] Biffl WL, Moore EE, Offner PJ et al. Optimizing screening for blunt cerebrovascular injuries. Am J Surg 1999; 178: 517–522

[20] Stein DM, Boswell S, Sliker CW, Lui FY, Scalea TM. Blunt cerebrovascular injuries: does treatment always matter? J Trauma 2009; 66: 132–144

[21] Burlew CC, Biffl WL. Imaging for blunt carotid and vertebral artery injuries. Surg Clin North Am 2011; 91: 217–231

[22] Burlew CC, Biffl WL, Moore EE, Barnett CC, Johnson JL, Bensard DD. Blunt cerebrovascular injuries: redefining screening criteria in the era of noninvasive diagnosis. J Trauma Acute Care Surg .2012; 72: 330–339.

[23] Berne JD, Cook A, Rowe SA, Norwood SH. A multivariate logistic regression analysis of risk factors for blunt cerebrovascular injury. J Vasc Surg 2010; 51: 57–64

[24] Mutze S, Rademacher G, Matthes G, Hosten N, Stengel D. Blunt cerebrovascular injury in patients with blunt multiple trauma: diagnostic accuracy of duplex Doppler US and early CT angiography. Radiology 2005; 237: 884–892

[25] Biffl WL, Ray CE, Jr, Moore EE, Mestek M, Johnson JL, Burch JM. Noninvasive diagnosis of blunt cerebrovascular injuries: a preliminary report. J Trauma. 2002; 53: 850–856

[26] Miller PR, Fabian TC, Croce MA et al. Prospective screening for blunt cerebrovascular injuries: analysis of diagnostic modalities and outcomes. Ann Surg 2002; 236: 386–395

[27] Bub LD, Hollingworth W, Jarvik JG, Hallam DK. Screening for blunt cerebrovascular injury: evaluating the accuracy of multidetector computed tomographic angiography. J Trauma 2005; 59: 691–697

[28] Biffl WL, Egglin T, Benedetto B, Gibbs F, Cioffi WG. Sixteen-slice computed tomographic angiography is a reliable noninvasive screening test for clinically significant blunt cerebrovascular injuries. J Trauma 2006; 60: 745–752

[29] Berne JD, Reuland KS, Villarreal DH, McGovern TM, Rowe SA, Norwood SH. Sixteen-slice multi-detector computed tomographic angiography improves the accuracy of screening for blunt cerebrovascular injury. J Trauma. 2006; 60: 1204–1210

[30] Eastman AL, Chason DP, Perez CL, McAnulty AL, Minei JP. Computed tomographic angiography for the diagnosis of blunt cervical vascular injury: is it ready for primetime? J Trauma 2006; 60: 925–929

[31] Utter GH, Hollingworth W, Hallam DK, Jarvik JG, Jurkovich GJ. Sixteen-slice CT angiography in patients with suspected blunt carotid and vertebral artery injuries. J Am Coll Surg 2006; 203: 838–848

[32] Goodwin RB, Beery PR, II, Dorbish RJ et al. Computed tomographic angiography versus conventional angiography for the diagnosis of blunt cerebrovascular injury in trauma patients. J Trauma 2009; 67: 1046–1050

[33] Fusco MR, Harrigan MR. Cerebrovascular dissections: a review. Part II: blunt cerebrovascular injury. Neurosurgery. 2011; 68: 517–530

[34] Malhotra AK, Camacho M, Ivatury RR et al. Computed tomographic angiography for the diagnosis of blunt carotid/vertebral artery injury: a note of caution. Ann Surg. 2007; 246: 632–643

[35] Biffl WL, Ray CE, Jr, Moore EE et al. Treatment-related outcomes from blunt cerebrovascular injuries: importance of routine follow-up arteriography. Ann Surg. 2002; 235: 699–707

[36] Edwards NM, Fabian TC, Claridge JA, Timmons SD, Fischer PE, Croce MA. Antithrombotic therapy and endovascular stents are effective treatment for blunt carotid injuries: results from longterm followup. J Am Coll Surg 2007; 204: 1007–1015

[37] Cothren CC, Biffl WL, Moore EE, Kashuk JL, Johnson JL. Treatment for blunt cerebrovascular injuries: equivalence of anticoagulation and antiplatelet agents. Arch Surg 2009; 144: 685–690

[38] Nunnink L. Blunt carotid artery injury. Emerg Med (Fremantle) 2002; 14: 412–421

[39] Franz RW, Goodwin RB, Beery PR, II, Hari JK, Hartman JF, Wright ML. Postdischarge outcomes of blunt cerebrovascular injuries. Vasc Endovascular Surg. 2010; 44: 198–211

[40] Delgado Almandoz JE, Kelly HR, Schaefer PW, Lev MH, Gonzalez RG, Romero JM. Prevalence of traumatic dural venous sinus thrombosis in high-risk acute blunt head trauma patients evaluated with multidetector CT venography. Radiology. 2010; 255: 570–577

[41] Zhao X, Rizzo A, Malek B, Fakhry S, Watson J. Basilar skull fracture: a risk factor for transverse/sigmoid venous sinus obstruction. J Neurotrauma 2008; 25: 104–111

[42] Garza-Mercado R. Extradural hematoma of the posterior cranial fossa. Report of seven cases with survival. J Neurosurg 1983; 59: 664–672

[43] Khwaja HA, Hormbrey PJ. Posterior cranial fossa venous extradural haematoma: an uncommon form of intracranial injury. Emerg Med J. 2001; 18: 496–497

8 Penetrating Traumatic Brain Injury

Robert Linville and Wendy A. Cohen

8.1 Introduction

The remarkable Phineas Gage, a railroad foreman in 1848, was fortunate to survive an accidental transcranial impalement with his tamping iron, a metal bar more than an inch in diameter and about 3.5 feet long (used to compact sand over a rock-breaking explosive charge). The accidental missile entered lateral to Mr. Gage's face and exited through his superior cranium. The case is notable for, among other things, how improbable his survival was. Even in the modern setting, penetrating traumatic brain injuries are frequently catastrophic. Modern computed tomography (CT) has become an essential tool for characterizing similar injuries (the first radiograph would not be invented until decades after Mr. Gage's death in 1860, although Ratiu and Talos recently redemonstrated the injury quite well).[1] Both acute and follow-up imaging of such injuries is standard of care for diagnosis, assessment of the need for intervention, prognosis, and related complications. Considerations for imaging after penetrating traumatic brain injury are discussed here, including special consideration of gunshot wounds (GSWs) to the head and wood impalement, the latter because of the significant risk of misdiagnosis with CT imaging.

8.2 Acute Imaging

As with all head trauma, the initial imaging study of choice for a penetrating injury is a noncontrast CT of the head.[2–4] This evaluation should include evaluation of the frontal and lateral scout views (▶ Fig. 8.1). Scouts are particularly important in the case of GSW because they provide general orientation to the injury and localization of metallic fragments. Plain radiographs of the head are of limited usefulness.[4,5]

In assessing penetrating injury, regardless of cause, the location of all large bone fragments and foreign material should be noted.[6] Any superficial injuries with possible intracranial extension should be assessed carefully for the presence of pneumocephalus.[3] Intracranial injuries may include herniation (uncal, subfalcine, upward and downward transtentorial), cisternal effacement, ventricular compression, and parenchymal injury. Identification of hemorrhage in any intracranial space is important for both the possible mass effect and the identification of any significant vascular injury (▶ Fig. 8.2).[7]

With penetrating head trauma, computed tomography angiography (CTA) of the head and neck is frequently valuable, particularly when the suspected injury is close to cervical or intracranial vasculatures. It is considered by the American College

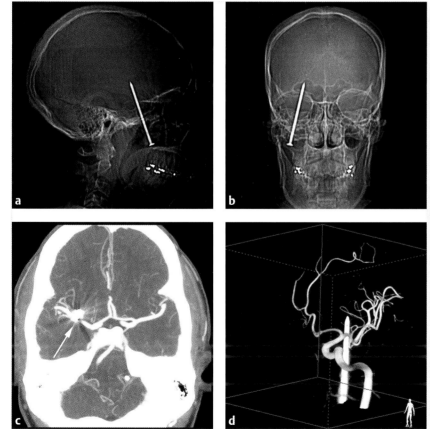

Fig. 8.1 Severe jaw pain and normal neurologic examination 24 hours after an unsuspected injury sustained while using a nail gun: (a,b) Scout images from the computed tomography (CT) show the nail that entered under his zygoma, passed through the mouth, and penetrated the brain. (c) The nail is visible immediately anterior to the right M1 segment (*arrow*) on the CT angiogram maximum intensity reconstruction. (d) Three-dimensional rotational angiographic reconstruction from the right posterior oblique view shows the nail passing in close proximity to the M1 segment of the middle cerebral artery. Vascular structures were also normal on follow-up angiography following removal of the nail.

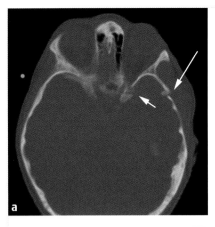

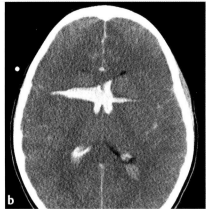

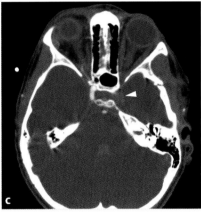

Fig. 8.2 Seven-year-old boy with a penetrating knife wound to the head: (a) There was disruption of the squamosal portion of the left temporal bone (*long arrow*) and fracture of the left anterior clinoid (*short arrow*). (b) Axial noncontrast computed tomography (CT) shows diffuse brain edema and diminished gray-white differentiation. Blood was present in the wound tract and passed through both lateral ventricles. (c) CT angiogram revealed no flow in the left cavernous internal carotid artery (*arrowhead*). The patient had no spontaneous movement, and care was withdrawn.

of Radiology that the appropriate criteria is as "usually appropriate," at seven of nine on a nine-point scale of appropriateness. By comparison, the noncontrast head CT has a nine in nine recommendation strength.[4] If the CTA is not obtained at the time of original imaging, recommendation for CTA or conventional angiography should be made when there appears to be risk of injury to any major vessels.[3,5–8] This is true when the bullet, nail, knife, umbrella, chopstick, or other object passes through or adjacent to the skull base, the carotid siphons, or any of the named intracranial vessels, including the dural venous sinuses.[5,6] The CTA is essential for preoperative planning before any attempted removal of an impaled object or missile.

The CTA may also be recommended at subsequent intervals to assess for arterial vasospasm.[7] In a series of 33 patients with penetrating gunshot wounds to the head, 14 demonstrated evidence of middle cerebral artery vasospasm by transcranial Doppler criteria (performed 0 to 33 days after injury). These findings were also significantly associated with the presence of subarachnoid hemorrhage on the initial head CT evaluation.[9]

Skull-base injuries have a high likelihood of vascular injury, of cranial nerve injury, and of cerebrospinal fluid (CSF) leak. In Shindo and coleagues' series of 43 patients with GSW to the head involving the temporal bone, 51% demonstrated facial nerve injury, and 33% demonstrated vascular injury. Six of 43 patients (14%) also suffered a CSF leak.[10] A CSF leak is important to identify for a number of reasons, including the increased risk of infection: as high as 31% in patients with a known post-traumatic CSF leak.[11] CT cisternography may be the most appropri-

ate and sensitive technique for identifying a fistula or leak,[5,12] although the utility of radionuclide cisternography has also been demonstrated.[13] Magnetic resonance (MR) cisternography is difficult in the acute penetrating trauma patient because MR imaging may be contraindicated if the retained metallic object is ferromagnetic.

In the acute setting of penetrating injury, MR imaging is rarely used. It is certainly to be avoided whenever any part of the penetrating object(s) may contain ferromagnetic material, given the risk of significant migration of metal fragments while the patient is within the magnet. Although most bullets in civilian penetrating brain injury do not contain ferromagnetic material, the inevitable lack of certainty about this limits MR use.[5] MR can be more sensitive than CT for retained wood,[14,15] although this may depend on how long the wood has been present. At the time of initial injury, wood is usually near air density. Wood may become hydrated with increasing time in place, making its identification with either CT or MR easier.[16]

Conventional angiography is the gold standard for assessment of vascular injury, both for acute vascular injury and for late-developing complications. It is essential in the diagnosis and characterization of traumatic intracranial aneurysms and arteriovenous fistulae (▶ Fig. 8.3 and ▶ Fig. 8.4). This modality is also superior to CT in the presence of metal because of the presence of streak artifact on CT. Additional indications for conventional angiography include evidence of arterial extravasation and unexpected delayed hemorrhage.[7,8]

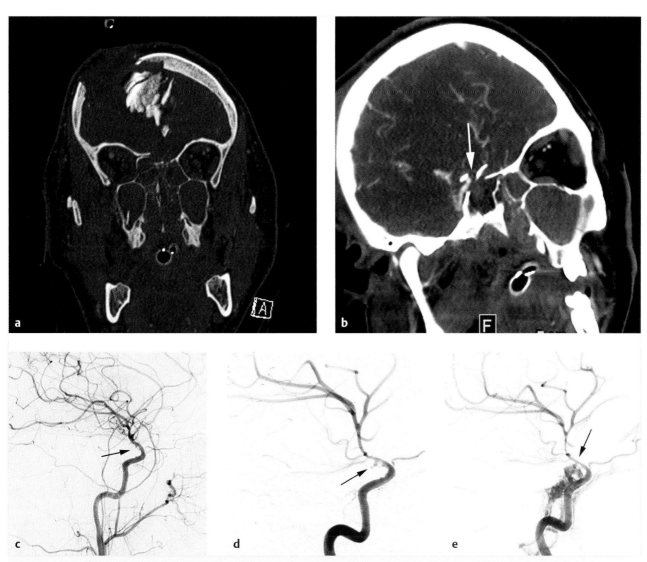

Fig. 8.3 An 18-year-old patient after a high-speed motor-vehicle collision with complex skull-base fractures, depressed frontal bone fractures and right internal carotid artery (RICA) injury: (a) Initial coronal computed tomography (CT) reformation demonstrates a fracture of the planum sphenoidale with upward displacement of the bone as well as massive inward displacement of the frontal bone into the cranial cavity. (b) Oblique coronal maximum-intensity projection from the initial CT angiogram shows the anatomic proximity of the fracture in the planum sphenoidale to the RICA (*white arrow*). (c) RICA injection from the catheter angiogram on admission demonstrates a narrowed and irregular supraclinoid segment of the RICA consistent with a dissection (*black arrow*). The irregularity was concerning for a pseudoaneurysm. (d) RICA injection from a catheter angiogram 2 weeks after admission shows enlargement of the pseudoaneurysm in the supraclinoid RICA (*black arrow*). (e) RICA injection from a catheter angiogram 1 week later now demonstrates a carotid-cavernous fistula arising from the RICA (*black arrow*). In the studies at 2 weeks (d) and 3 (e) weeks after injury, the right anterior cerebral artery no longer filled from the RICA.

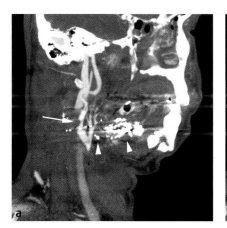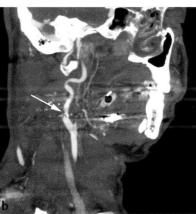

Fig. 8.4 Gunshot wound (GSW) to the neck. (a,b) These are two oblique maximum-intensity projection images through the right common internal carotid artery (ICA) bifurcation. Bullet fragments were present (*arrowheads*), as well as an injury to the proximal right ICA (*arrows*). This appears equivalent to a Biffl type II injury, although the Biffl classification was created in the setting of blunt, and not penetrating, trauma. The more proximal common carotid artery is patent but not present on these slices.

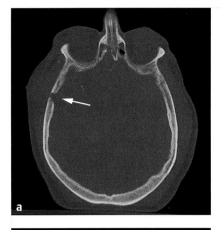
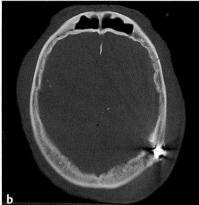
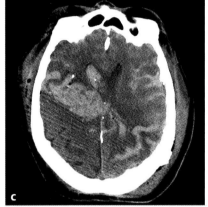

Fig. 8.5 Self-inflicted gunshot wound with 0.22-caliber bullet: (a) Computed tomography with bone kernel shows typical beveling of the entrance wound in the right temporal bone (*arrow*) and (b) the retained bullet fragment at the contralateral parietal cranium. (c) The bullet tract crosses the midline in the midcoronal plane with intraventricular hemorrhage. Patients with injury of this extent and pattern of intracranial involvement have little chance of survival.

8.3 Gunshot Wounds to the Head

In the trauma literature, GSWs to the head are frequently separated into civilian and military injuries. One of the major reasons for this is their significantly different ballistics and mortality rates. Penetrating brain injuries in the military setting are also frequently collections of all penetrating missiles, artillery shrapnel, bullets, and such, and these injuries have lower mortality rates. In one case series of 964 patients involved in the Iran-Iraq War of the 1980s, overall mortality was just 14% (133 patients).[17] Multiple series from urban settings in the United States have very different results. These have demonstrated that most civilian GSW to the head are fatal and never reach trauma centers for evaluation or care,[18] and many that do reach trauma centers are not survivable. In one series of 250 cases of GSW to the head from Maryland, 71% died at the scene, and the total mortality was 89%.[7] Of the patients who reach trauma centers, most have a Glasgow Coma Scale score of 8 or lower,[7] limiting physical examination and increasing the relative importance of diagnostic imaging.

8.3.1 Ballistics

Bullets entering the scalp frequently devitalize the adjacent soft tissue. If the gun barrel is very near the scalp, propellant gas may be demonstrated in layers of the scalp near the entrance wound. Despite the heat of a fired bullet, the wounds are frequently contaminated by skin, hair, fabric, and superficial flora. Prophylactic antibiosis is the standard of care. The offending

bacteria in subsequent intracranial infections have been frequently identified as contaminating skin flora.[7]

Cranial fracture and fragmentation are highly variable. Small-bore entrance fractures can be seen as well as large stellate fracture patterns involving much of the cranial hemisphere. If the bullet exits the cranium, the exit wounds tend to be larger than the entrance wounds. The beveled edge of the cranium frequently indicates the direction of bullet passage. That is, the wider opening of the bevel at the inner table of the skull facing the intracranial compartment is suggestive of the entrance wound (▶ Fig. 8.5).[6]

Numerous investigations of the bullet and brain parenchyma interaction have been made using both gelatin and animal models. These suggest that a bullet's behavior creates a large radial force as it passes through brain parenchyma with a high-pressure wave at the front of the bullet, which contributes to a pressure differential on the order of 1000 atm. With sufficient kinetic energy (equals one-half the mass multiplied by the velocity squared), the force radiating from the bullet tract can create a transient cavity and vacuum in the wake of the bullet that pulls loose hair, soft tissue, bone fragments, and other contaminants into the cavity. Transient reverberation of the tissue adjacent to the bullet tract is also present as kinetic energy dissipates.[19] With the radial dissipation of energy, it is important to assess parenchyma distant to the bullet tract for possible contusion or other injury. Additionally, experimental GSW in cats demonstrated respiratory depression and bradycardia even when the bullet tract was more than 2 cm from the brainstem and while using low-velocity bullets.[5] Most handguns generate

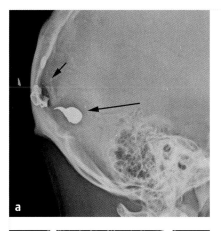

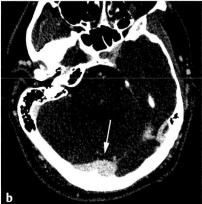

Fig. 8.6 Gunshot wound with minimal penetration: (a) The metal jacket of the bullet (*short black arrow*) was separated from the lead core of the bullet *(long black arrow)*, which went on to penetrate the occipital cortex. This was best demonstrated by this follow-up radiograph (for posterior skin breakdown). (b) The dural venous sinuses, including the confluence (*white arrow*), were intact on computed tomography venogram (CTV) performed at the time of the initial injury. (c) CTV was moderately limited by streak artifact from the bullet, a common problem when evaluating penetrating gunshot injuries.

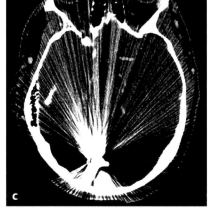

only "low" muzzle velocity,[6] much less than the 700 to 1000 m per second of a typical rifle.[7] Such velocity demonstrates minimal transient cavitation in the bullet tract and much less vacuum phenomenon.[19]

Bullet construction is worthy of brief consideration (▶ Fig. 8.6). The Hague Convention of 1899 prohibits the use in international warfare of bullets that easily expand or flatten in the human body, and this has been generally adhered to since then; thus, standard military full-metal-jacket bullets tend to pass through tissue with minimal deformation. Hunting ammunition, on the other hand, is theoretically designed to minimize the suffering of the animal by causing death as quickly as possible. As such, hunting and other civilian ammunition rounds usually deform significantly, with rapid dispersion of their energy in a broad cone within the tissue, unlike the relatively narrow distribution by military rounds. The best examples are hollow-point bullets that essentially deform or "puddle" after limited passage through soft tissue. These are used by some police forces to minimize the likelihood that bystanders might be struck by bullets penetrating through the intended target. As a result of the differences in construction, police and civilian ammunition rounds, unlike military rounds, rarely contain ferromagnetic material. Unfortunately, there is frequently enough uncertainty that an MR examination remains an inappropriate risk. As such, MR is very rarely used after GSW to the head with retained fragments,[5] particularly as symptomatic spontaneous fragment migration has been described without any MR exposure.[20,21]

Shotgun shells can be made with multiple small pellets—also known as "shot"—or with a large single slug of missile material.

In the setting of pellets or shot, the shot is separated from the propellant by a layer of wadding that acts as a piston to accelerate all of the shot on firing. The pellets disperse with distance in a cone pattern to become independent low-velocity projectiles. Notably, the wadding tends to be relatively radiolucent, but this is rarely a diagnostic issue, as described by Jandial and colleagues[19]; wadding can reach the patient only at close range, and such events are almost always fatal in any case. Rarely, in the setting of a near-miss event where only a few of the shotgun pellets reach the patient, wadding can be seen at the patient's skin, although this is generally evident on physical examination.[19]

8.3.2 Prognosis

Many findings have demonstrated prognostic value. As one might expect, prognosis is worse with involvement of multiple lobes rather than one. Other factors include passage of the bullet across midline, violation of one or both lateral ventricles, and whether the injury was self-inflicted (i.e., a GSW to the head in a suicide attempt has a worse prognosis).[6] Additional predictors of poor outcome are herniation and intraventricular hemorrhage (▶ Fig. 8.7).[7,22]

Aarabi and colleagues[7] summarize the accumulated literature well; see ▶ Table 8.1 for bullet tract findings and associated mortality rates.

The central brain frequently involved with such catastrophic cases has been referred to as the zona fatalis and demonstrates similar mortality (nearing 100%) in both civilian and military GSW to the head. The zona fatalis has been defined as the 4 cm

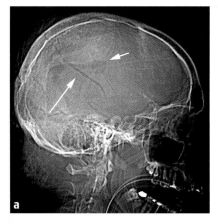

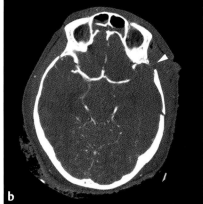

Fig. 8.7 Self-inflicted gunshot wound to the left frontotemporal skull. (a) There is a radiating skull fracture (*long arrow*) and the contralateral parietal exit site (*short arrow*) is visible on the lateral scout image. (b) A computed tomographic arteriogram maximal-intensity projection (MIP) image at the level of the entrance site (*arrowhead*) shows preserved M1 and A1 flow bilaterally. MIP images allowed for tracing of the distal right middle cerebral artery branches, which revealed (c) active extravasation (*arrow*) at the exit wound from one of these extruded right middle cerebral artery branches.

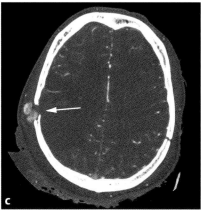

Table 8.1 Mortality rates by bullet pathway.

Brain Tract Involved	Mortality (%)
Any lobar injury	48
Unilateral with multiple lobes	72
Crossing midline	77
Crossing the midcoronal plane	84
Crossing both midline and midcoronal plane	96

above the dorsum sella involving the ventricles, the hypothalamus, and the thalamus.[23,24] Special comment should be made about any bullet tract that violates the inferior cranial dura. In particular, bullet passage near the paranasal sinuses, mastoid air spaces, orbits, and the skull base all increase the risk for subsequent CSF leak. As previously discussed, such injuries are associated with increased risk of infection despite the prophylactic antibiosis that is standard of care. Many of these may require operative debridement and watertight closure of the dura.[7]

The extent of operative debridement after GSW to the head is controversial. Lack of improved outcome with aggressive debridement of the missile tract has been reported. However, debridement of superficial nonviable tissue and closure of the dura are frequent goals.[19] There are also reports of neurologic sequelae from retained lead and copper from bullets.[25] Identifying large fragments of in-driven bone and bullet fragments are appropriate for surgical planning and on follow-up imaging.

Attention on follow-up imaging to such fragments is also important as migration of missiles has been reported with serious neurologic sequelae.[20,21]

8.3.3 Late Complications

Infection after GSW to the head has been seen in essentially every anatomic space violated by a missile: meningitis, abscess, ventriculitis, and so forth.[5] The rates of infection and abscess have decreased with the use of prophylactic antibiosis[6,7] but are not eliminated. The infection rate varies by series, but rates from 2 to 8% have been reported.[26,27] As previously mentioned, post-traumatic CSF leak increases the rate of infection to as high as 31%, although broad-spectrum prophylactic antibiotics were not yet standard of care in that series (▶ Fig. 8.8).[11]

Penetrating gunshot GSWs to the head have been associated with varying rates of traumatic intracranial aneurysm development. Depending on the population being studied and the pretest risk assessment, rates have been noted between 3 and 40% in different series. Traumatic AV fistulae are less frequent and naturally require angiographic characterization to assess for possible intervention.[7] As with all possible vascular compromise, infarction and subsequent evolution may be seen on follow-up examinations.

Seizures are known secondary complications to penetrating brain injury. In the military setting, epilepsy has been demonstrated in 32% of a series from the Iran-Iraq War involving 489 patients (median follow-up of 23 months). In addition to antibiotic prophylaxis, antiepileptic prophylaxis is used for such

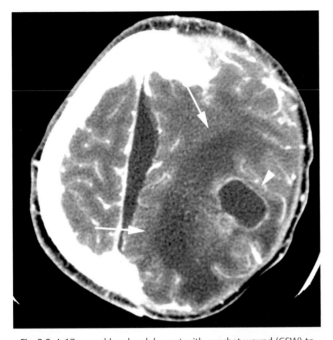

Fig. 8.8 A 17-year-old male adolescent with gunshot wound (GSW) to head from a drive-by shooting: 15 days after surgical decompression, the patient had altered mental status and fever. Axial contrast-enhanced computed tomography through the centrum semiovale shows diffuse vasogenic edema (*arrows*) and ring enhancement (*arrowhead*) in the left posterior frontal lobe. Although there is a large differential for ring enhancing lesions, in this young patient with a GSW, infection is more likely than any other causes. Operative debridement and culture confirmed the diagnosis.

injuries in the acute setting. Unfortunately, this may not change the rate of epilepsy development in the long term.[6,28]

Follow-up imaging should assess for any retained fragments and possible migration. Such migration is frequently associated with adjacent fluid (intraventricular CSF, abscess, or hemorrhage). This migration can manifest with neurologic deterioration clinically and can contribute to obstructive hydrocephalus.[5,20,21] In the military setting, removal of an intracranial fragment has been suggested if there is demonstrated migration or abscess formation or if the fragment abuts a major vessel (▶ Fig. 8.9). Additionally, the presence of porous material (not bone or bullet fragment) in continuity with the CSF has been suggested as an indication for operative extraction.[24]

As previously mentioned, CSF leak may develop, particularly with skull-base injuries, which can be evaluated with CT cisternography or radionuclide cisternography. Shindo's series of 43 patients with GSW involving temporal bones reported a CSF-leak rate of 14%.[10] Another series of 79 civilians with GSW to the head demonstrated eight patients (10%) with subsequent CSF leak.[29]

8.4 Penetrating Injury by Wood

Penetrating injury by wood deserves independent consideration, as several published reports have demonstrated penetrating wood that has been missed by typical head CT evaluations.[15,30,31] Subsequent morbidity from such events has included meningitis, abscess, and vascular injury. One of the primary difficulties is relatively low density of wood compared

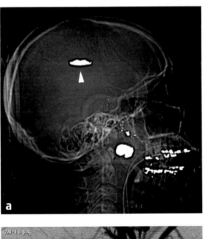
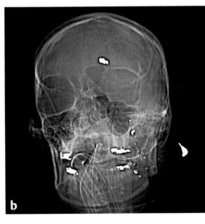
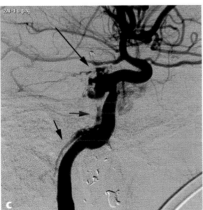
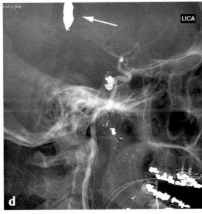

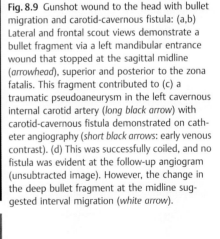

Fig. 8.9 Gunshot wound to the head with bullet migration and carotid-cavernous fistula: (a,b) Lateral and frontal scout views demonstrate a bullet fragment via a left mandibular entrance wound that stopped at the sagittal midline (*arrowhead*), superior and posterior to the zona fatalis. This fragment contributed to (c) a traumatic pseudoaneurysm in the left cavernous internal carotid artery (*long black arrow*) with carotid-cavernous fistula demonstrated on catheter angiography (*short black arrows*: early venous contrast). (d) This was successfully coiled, and no fistula was evident at the follow-up angiogram (unsubtracted image). However, the change in the deep bullet fragment at the midline suggested interval migration (*white arrow*).

9 Skull-Base Trauma

Shivani Gupta and Kathleen R. Fink

9.1 Introduction

Skull-base trauma is an important cause of long-term neurologic sequelae, permanent disability, and death. Because of the complex anatomy at the skull base, the initial injury can result in various complications, ranging from cranial nerve deficits to devastating vascular injury.[1] Recent advances in medical imaging have allowed for increased detection of subtle injuries in a rapid, noninvasive manner.

Fractures of the skull are reported in 3.5 to 24% of patients with head injury.[2] Of patients with facial trauma, the overall frequency of skull-base trauma is 25%.[3] In patients with trauma to the upper cervical spine, 23% will also have a fracture of the skull base.[4] Hence, the presence of spinal or maxillofacial trauma predicts a higher likelihood of a skull-base fracture.

Computed tomography (CT) is the mainstay imaging modality in the initial assessment of patients with suspected skull-base trauma. Imaging of the skull base requires high-resolution axial images with coronal and sagittal reformats. The need for additional imaging is determined by the clinical scenario and the presence of injury. This may include a CT angiogram of the head and neck or magnetic resonance imaging (MRI) of the craniocervical junction to look for associated complications. MRI may also detect associated injuries, for example, spinal trauma or subtle intracranial injuries that are poorly delineated by CT, including diffuse axonal injury, brainstem trauma, and small cortical contusions. MRI is also useful for evaluation of long-term post-traumatic sequelae such as cranial nerve injury.

Conventional angiography plays a limited role in the immediate assessment of skull-base trauma, but it may be helpful after initial imaging has been obtained to evaluate for traumatic vascular injury, especially if computed tomographic angiography (CTA) is limited or equivocal. Vascular complications, such as an arteriovenous fistula, are often best evaluated on conventional angiography with the potential for immediate endovascular intervention. Skull x-rays play a limited role in evaluation for trauma at the skull base.[5] Underlying brain parenchymal injury or vascular injury is not evaluated on skull x-rays, and the presence or absence of a skull fracture does not adequately predict concomitant injuries.

9.2 Imaging Technique

For the diagnosis of skull-base trauma, CT is the mainstay modality. In addition to a routine head CT (5-mm axial slices), high-resolution images through the skull base are needed to evaluate skull-base injury (1- to 3-mm axial slices). Coronal reformations are helpful to further evaluate 1 to 2-mm subtle fracture lines and are especially helpful in evaluating the superior orbital roof and petrous bone. If there is clinical suggestion of a temporal bone fracture or suspicious findings on standard CT (such as mastoid fluid in the setting of trauma), dedicated images through the temporal bone in thin sections (1- to 2-mm-thick axial slices with coronal and sagittal reformations) with a reduced field of view using bone reconstruction algorithms are necessary. Contrast is not necessary for evaluation of osseous trauma.

Often, CTA is obtained after noncontrast imaging to evaluate for vascular injury. The use of both coronal and sagittal reformations is important, as subtle injury can be missed in one imaging plane but better appreciated on another.

9.3 Clinical Presentation

Depending on the underlying injury, patients may exhibit various signs on physical examination. Some clinical signs suggest the location of the skull fracture. Fractures of the anterior skull base may initially manifest as rhinorrhea, raccoon eyes (periorbital ecchymosis), anosmia, and visual changes. Fractures of the middle skull base, particularly those involving the petrous temporal bones, can manifest as hemotympanum (blood in the middle ear), blood in the external auditory canal, vestibular changes, Battle's sign (retroauricular hematoma), facial paralysis, CSF otorrhea, or strabismus. Fractures of the clivus and posterior skull base may present as craniocervical dissociation or brainstem dysfunction. Involvement of any aspect of the skull base can result in a cranial nerve deficit or vascular injury (especially of the petrous and cavernous portions of the internal carotid artery).

In cases of depressed skull fractures, a palpable abnormality may be felt at the site of the depressed fracture fragment. In open skull fractures involving the skin, there will be a visible soft tissue laceration.

9.4 Normal Anatomy

9.4.1 Cranial Fossae

The skull base anatomy is notably complex, comprising the ethmoid, sphenoid, frontal, temporal, and occipital bones.[6] These bones each have a complex shape, and it is often easier to consider them together based on overall structure. One way to consider the skull base is as a cradle for the intracranial components. This cradle can be divided also into three regions: the anterior, middle, and posterior cranial fossae. This terminology is helpful to describe the location of an extra-axial hematoma, for example:

- **Anterior cranial fossa**: Bounded anteriorly by the inner table of the frontal sinus, posteriorly by the anterior clinoid processes and the planum sphenoidale, and laterally by the frontal bone.
- **Middle cranial fossa**: Bounded anteriorly by the anterior clinoid processes and posterior margin of the lesser wing of the sphenoid; posteriorly by the superior margin of the petrous temporal bone and dorsum sellae of the sphenoid bone; and laterally by the squamous temporal bone, parietal bone, and greater wing of the sphenoid.
- **Posterior cranial fossa**: Composed mainly of the occipital bone; bounded anteriorly by the dorsum sellae and clivus,

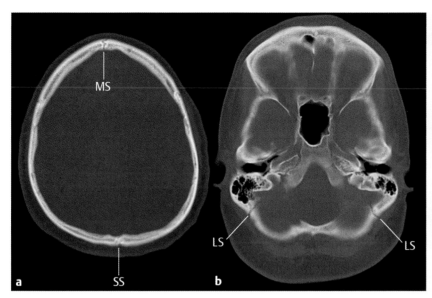

Fig. 9.1 Cranial sutures. Axial computed tomography of the skull (a) showing the metopic suture (MS), sagittal suture (SS), and (b), the lambdoid suture (LS).

and laterally by the posterior aspect of the petrous temporal bone and the lateral aspect of the occipital bone. Some classification systems separate the clivus as the central skull base, as is done in this chapter.

Because fractures do not respect the anatomic borders of the cranial fossa, another way to consider the skull base when evaluating the results of trauma, particularly skull-base fractures, is to divide the skull base into four parts: the anterior, middle, central, and posterior skull base. Although fractures may involve more than one of these areas, traumatic injury can be categorized based on which of these four areas is primarily affected.

9.4.2 Anterior Skull Base

The anterior skull base consists of the crista galli, cribriform plate, fovea ethmoidalis (the roof of the ethmoid sinus), and orbital roofs.[7] The cribriform plate is an important aspect of the anterior skull base, as it is the most inferiorly positioned aspect of the floor of the anterior skull base, and is not covered by dura. Thus, fractures of the cribriform plate may lead to development of a cerebrospinal fluid (CSF) leak. Immediately adjacent to the anterior skull base are the upper paranasal sinuses (sphenoid sinus, posterior walls of the frontal sinus, and roof of the ethmoid sinus).

9.4.3 Middle Skull Base

The middle skull base consists of the sella turcica and the floor of the middle cranial fossa. Major foramina within the middle skull base are the superior orbital fissure, foramen ovale, foramen rotundum, foramen spinosum, foramen lacerum, and the pterygoid (vidian) canal.

9.4.4 Central Skull Base

The central skull base consists of the clivus, which is formed by the basisphenoid and basiocciput.

9.4.5 Posterior Skull Base

The posterior skull base consists of the occiput and bilateral petrous ridges. Major foramina of the posterior skull base include the foramen magnum, hypoglossal canal, jugular foramen, carotid canal, and internal auditory canal.

9.5 Normal Fissures and Sutures

Cranial sutures consist of fibrous bands of tissue uniting the skull bones together.[8] They are important sites of bone growth. Knowledge of the various sutures and their appearance on CT imaging is vital to avoid mistaking these normal structures for a nondisplaced fracture. Important sutures to consider include the following (▶ Fig. 9.1):

- Metopic suture: Interfrontal suture between the two frontal bones that usually fuses in childhood
- Sagittal suture: Between the parietal bones
- Coronal sutures (paired): Between the two frontal and two parietal bones
- Lambdoid sutures (paired): Between the occipital and parietal bones
- Squamosal sutures (paired): Between the parietal, temporal and sphenoid bones
- Sphenosquamous suture: Between the posterolateral margin of the greater wing of the sphenoid and the anterior border of the squamous temporal bone
- Occiptomastoid suture: Between the lateral aspect of the occipital bone and the superior mastoid part of the temporal bone

Cranial fissures are also an important aspect of skull base anatomy and may be mistaken for skull fractures. These include the petrosphenoidal and petro-occipital fissures.

Skull-base trauma can involve the skull-base foramina (▶ Fig. 9.2). Patients can initially show various cranial nerve palsies. Knowledge of the various foramina and their location and contents is important to predict cranial nerve injury (▶ Table 9.1).

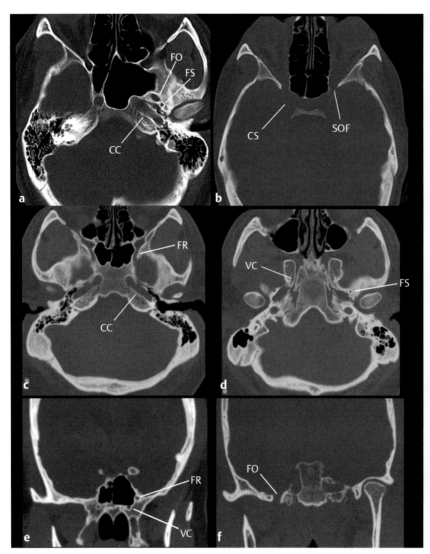

Fig. 9.2 Skull base foramina on computed tomography (CT). Axial CT images (a–d) and coronal reformat (e,f) demonstrate the foramen ovale (FO), foramen spinosum (FS), carotid canal (CC), superior orbital fissure (SOF) cavernous sinus (CS), foramen rotundum (FR), vidian canal (VC)

Table 9.1 Skull-base foramina and their contents

Foramen	Contents
Optic canal	Cranial nerve (CN) II (optic) Ophthalmic artery
Superior orbital fissure	CN III, IV, V1, VI (oculomotor, trochlear, ophthalmic and abducens) Superior ophthalmic vein
Foramen rotundum	CN V2 (maxillary)
Foramen ovale	CN V3 (mandibular) Lesser petrosal nerve
Foramen spinosum	Middle meningeal artery
Vidian canal	Greater superficial and deep petrosal nerves (vidian nerve)
Jugular foramen	CN IX, X, XI (glossopharyngeal, vagus, spinal accessory, sympathetic nerve)
Internal acoustic meatus	CN VII, VIII (facial, vestibulocochlear)
Hypoglossal canal	CN XII (hypoglossal)
Foramen magnum	Brainstem Vertebral arteries

In pediatric patients, the appearance of developing bones and unfused cranial sutures may be confused with a fracture, and knowledge of these normal age-related variations is crucial to avoid misdiagnosis. Most of the skull-base forms by endochondral ossification.[9] Ossification begins in the occipital bones and continues anteriorly.[10] Evaluating symmetry often aids in determining whether a finding is a true fracture versus normal ossification of the cartilaginous skull base.

The skull base of an infant contains many synchondroses (▶ Fig. 9.3). The major synchondroses are the intersphenoid, spheno-occipital, frontosphenoidal, and posterior occipital. Accessory synchondroses are also possible along cranial sutures. In addition, the newborn and young infant skull contains fontanelles (anterior, posterior, and lateral).

In the evaluation of skull-base trauma, it is important to recognize the spheno-occipital synchondrosis, located at the junction of the sphenoid and occipital bones. It usually fuses by age 18 years.[11] Closure occurs from above, and a thin sclerotic scar often persists into adulthood. Incomplete closure of the spheno-occipital synchondrosis is possible and is a site of weakness with a higher predisposition to fracture.

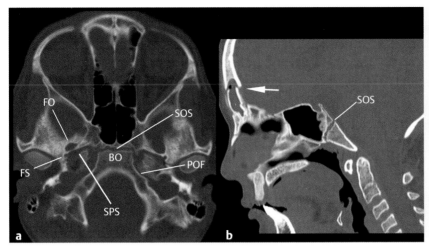

Fig. 9.3 Pediatric skull. Axial computed tomography of the skull base (a) with sagittal reformat (b) in a child with frontal sinus fractures (*arrow*) demonstrates the spheno-occipital synchondrosis (SOS), basiocciput (BO), petrooccipital fissure (POF), foramen ovale (FO), foramen spinosum (FS), and the sphenopetrosal synchondrosis (SPS).

9.6 Fractures of the Anterior Skull Base

Fractures of the anterior skull base are often associated with maxillofacial trauma. Fractures may involve the cribriform plate, fovea ethmoidalis (▶ Fig. 9.4), sphenoid sinus (▶ Fig. 9.5), and the orbital plate of the frontal bone or the walls of the frontal sinuses (▶ Fig. 9.6). Frontal sinus fractures are described more fully in Chapter 10, Maxillofacial Trauma, of this book. Evaluation for associated orbital injury, either intraconal, extraconal, or involving the globe, is key, as is detecting involvement of the optic canal. Orbital injuries are more fully described in Chapter 11, Traumatic Orbital Injury.

9.6.1 Classification

Reporting fractures of the anterior skull base is best done in a descriptive manner, describing the specific bones involved and extent of injury. In the neurosurgical literature, Sakas et al have described a classification system that is helpful in understanding the various types of injuries that may affect the anterior skull base. Although fractures of the anterior skull base are not usually classified radiographically by this system, it provides a framework on which to consider anterior skull-base fractures. Four fracture types are described:[12]

- Type I: Cribriform fracture. This fracture extends through the cribriform plate but does not involve the ethmoid or frontal sinuses.
- Type II: Frontoethmoidal fracture. This fracture extends through the walls of the ethmoid or medial walls of the frontal sinus and involves the medial portion of the anterior skull base.
- Type III: Lateral frontal fracture. This fracture extends through the lateral aspect of the frontal sinus through the superomedial aspect of the orbit.
- Type IV: Complex fracture. This type of fracture describes a complex injury involving any of the injuries classified in types I through III (▶ Fig. 9.7).

9.6.2 Associated Injuries

When evaluating anterior skull-base fractures, always consider what secondary injuries may be present. For example, exten-

sion of a fracture into the petrous carotid canal necessitates evaluation of the carotid artery for injury (▶ Fig. 9.5). Fractures extending into the orbit require careful assessment of orbital complications (▶ Fig. 9.6). Certain anterior skull-base fractures, particularly those of the cribriform plate and fovea ethmoidalis, are associated with CSF leaks (▶ Fig. 9.4). Fractures involving both the inner and outer table of the frontal sinus may result in a CSF leak. Additionally, inner-table fractures may require surgical evaluation and treatment resulting from communication between the paranasal sinuses and the intracranial compartment, with a potential for intracranial infection, intracranial hemorrhage, and delayed mucocele formation. This topic is discussed further in Chapter 10, Maxillofacial Trauma. With significant fractures, even without direct petrous carotid canal involvement, vascular injury is an important entity to exclude (▶ Fig. 9.8).

9.6.3 Treatment

Treatment of fractures of the anterior cranial fossa depends on the extent of injury. Emergent surgery may be indicated for open or significantly depressed fracture, foreign bodies, or to decompress the optic canal.[13] Dural repair may be needed to avoid or close a post-traumatic CSF leak and to prevent intracranial infection. CSF leaks sometimes close without direct repair after ventricular drainage, such as with a lumboperitoneal shunt. Vascular injuries may require endovascular or surgical care. Cosmesis is an important consideration in long-term management.

9.7 Fractures of the Central Skull Base

9.7.1 Clival Fractures

Detection of clival fractures has increased with the use of CT and improved image resolution. These fractures are often associated with other craniofacial trauma. Neurologic prognosis in patients with clival fractures is poor, and the mortality rate is high, up to 24%.[14] Fracture of the clivus indicates a severe mechanism of injury, and clinical outcome is correlated to the patient's initial Glasgow Coma Scale score and associated injuries.[15]

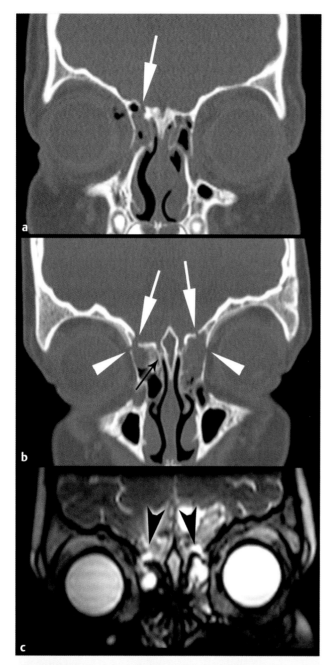

Fig. 9.4 Fractures of the fovea ethmoidalis. Coronal computed tomography (CT) (a) shows a fracture through the roof of the right ethmoid sinus (fovea ethmoidalis, *white arrow*) associated with a right orbital roof fracture (not shown). Coronal CT in a different patient (b) shows bilateral fractures of the fovea ethmoidalis (*white arrows*) associated with fractures of the medial orbital walls (*white arrowheads*). Note that the cribiform plate is spared (*black arrow*). High-resolution T2-weighted image (c) demonstrates cerebrospinal fluid (CSF) leaks (*black arrowheads*), manifested as T2 hyperintense CSF on either side of the fracture lines.

Classification

Clival fractures can be classified into three types, depending on the orientation:

- Longitudinal fractures extend from the sphenoid body to the foramen magnum in the anteroposterior direction.

- Transverse fractures extend from right to left (usually one carotid canal to the other).
- Oblique fractures extend at an angle through the clivus, traversing the lateral aspect of the dorsum sellae toward the contralateral petroclival fissure (▶ Fig. 9.9).

Associated Injuries

Fractures of the clivus are associated with significant morbidity and mortality owing to the proximity of important neurovascular structures. Longitudinal fractures have the highest rate of mortality from associated injuries. Vascular injuries, including dissection and pseudoaneurysm, may affect the vertebrobasilar system (longitudinal fractures) or carotid circulation (transverse fractures), with a reported incidence of up to 46%.[16] A traumatic carotid-cavernous fistula may develop acutely or in a delayed fashion. Although rare, longitudinal fractures of the clivus can result in incarceration of the basilar artery.[17]

Additional injuries associated with clivus fractures include pituitary dysfunction, injury to the brainstem, CSF leaks, and cranial nerve deficits. The sixth cranial nerves in particular are susceptible to injury, as they are fixed by their course through Dorello's canal in the clivus. Cranial nerves III, IV, V, and VII may also be injured in association with clivus fractures because of their close proximity.

Treatment

Fractures of the clivus are often associated with other injuries and are associated with various complications. Treatment is best achieved via a multidisciplinary approach that initially targets life-threatening complications such as vascular injury.

9.8 Fractures of the Posterior Skull Base

9.8.1 Fractures of the Occipital Bone

Fractures of the occipital bone can be nondisplaced, displaced, or comminuted; they can also be classified as closed or open (▶ Fig. 9.10). A ring fracture of the skull base is a specific type of occipital skull fracture that is particularly associated with motorcycle accidents.[18] The fracture is orientated in the transverse plane and encircles the foramen magnum. This injury is important because it can result in severe vascular and parenchymal injury.

Associated Injuries

Some fractures of the occipital bone are isolated injuries. Others are associated with other osseous trauma, including occipital condyle fractures, cervical spine fractures, and central skull-base trauma. Careful evaluation for an underlying extra-axial hematoma is key. If the fracture is near a venous sinus, dural venous sinus thrombosis or injury must be excluded (▶ Fig. 9.11).

Extra-axial hematomas may result in compression of an adjacent dural venous sinus. CT venography is helpful to exclude extrinsic dural venous sinus compression and direct venous injury. Magnetic resonance venography may also be considered if

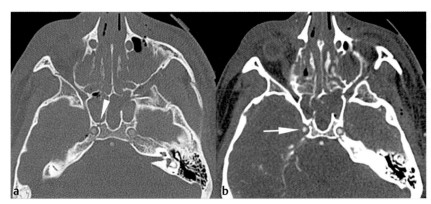

Fig. 9.5 Fractures of the sphenoid sinus. (a) Axial computed tomography (CT) shows a fracture through the posterior wall of the right sphenoid sinus extending through the anterior wall of the adjacent carotid canal (*arrowhead*). Additional maxillofacial injuries are present. CT angiography at the same level (b) demonstrates slight narrowing of the right internal carotid artery compared with the left (*arrow*), consistent with a Denver grade I injury.

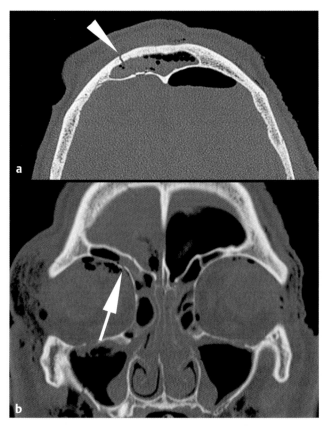

Fig. 9.6 Fractures of the anterior skull base with orbital involvement. (a) Axial computed tomography demonstrates fractures of the inner and outer table of the frontal sinus (*arrowhead*) with pneumocephalus. Coronal reformat (b) shows extension into the right orbital roof (*arrow*), in addition to other sinus fractures and extensive subcutaneous and orbital emphysema.

the patient is clinically stable to undergo MRI scan. Parenchymal and extra-axial hemorrhages may result in sufficient mass effect to cause tonsillar herniation or upward tentorial herniation. If associated brainstem compression is severe, decompressive surgery may be required. Additionally, if there is significant mass effect on the fourth ventricle, hydrocephalus may develop.

Contrecoup frontotemporal injury accounts for significant mortality and morbidity associated with fractures of the occipital bone (▶ Fig. 9.12). Careful attention to areas of potential contrecoup injury is required to find subtle injuries, including contrecoup parenchymal hematomas and extra-axial

hemorrhages. Sites of involvement include the medial subfrontal and anterior temporal locations.

Treatment

Nondisplaced linear fractures without associated injuries are treated conservatively. Open or depressed injuries often require surgical intervention with antibiotic prophylaxis.

9.8.2 Fractures of the Occipital Condyles

Occipital condyle fractures (OCFs) are usually the result of high-energy blunt trauma.[19] Patients often have other concomitant injuries, including traumatic brain injury and soft tissue injury at the craniocervical junction. Accurate diagnosis of OCFs is important to decrease morbidity and improve outcomes. CT is the imaging modality of choice, with sagittal and coronal reconstructions to optimally evaluate the occipital condyles.[20] In some cases, an MRI of the craniocervical junction can be useful to evaluate for additional cord or ligamentous injury.[21]

Classification

The Anderson and Montesano[22] classification system is the most widely used classification system for OCFs, and it takes into consideration both the mechanism of injury and injury morphology. In this classification system, OCFs are classified into three types (▶ Fig. 9.13):

- Type I: Comminuted and impacted fracture, with or without displacement, which occurs as a result of axial loading
- Type II: Skull-base fracture that extends into the occipital condyle(s), which occurs after direct impact to the skull
- Type III: Avulsion fracture of the occipital condyle that occurs after forced rotation and lateral bending

The type III fracture can be associated with disruption of the craniocervical ligaments resulting in craniocervical dissociation. The avulsed fragment is usually displaced medially.

Associated Injuries

OCFs are commonly associated with other injuries sustained in high-energy trauma affecting both cranial and extracranial compartments. Intracranial injuries (including intracranial

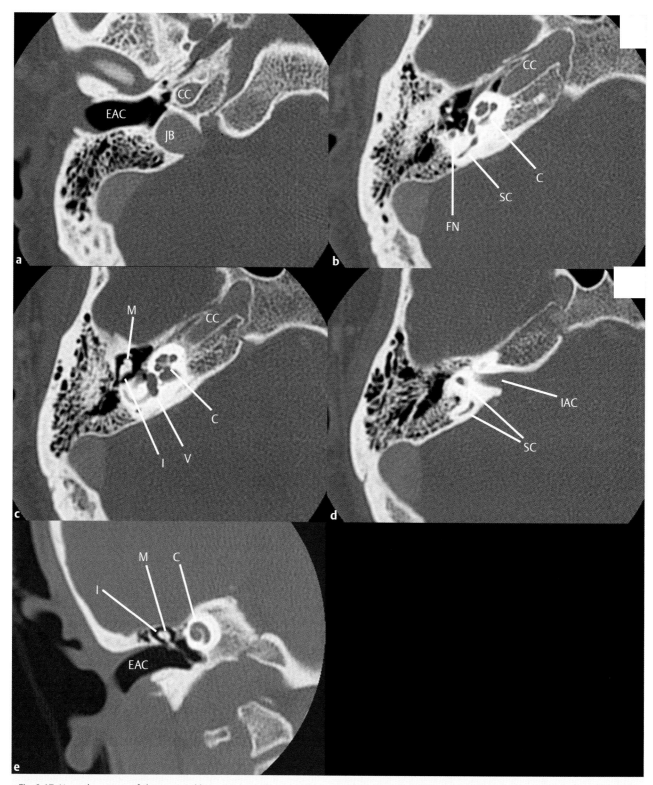

Fig. 9.17 Normal anatomy of the temporal bone. High-resolution axial (a–d) and coronal (e) computed tomography demonstrates normal temporal bone structures: carotid canal (CC), jugular bulb (JB), external auditory canal (EAC), internal auditory canal (IAC), cochlea (C), semicircular canals (SC), vestibule (V), facial nerve canal (FN), malleus (M) and incus (I).

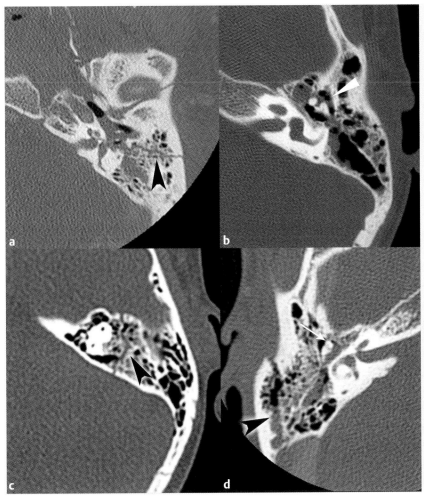

Fig. 9.18 Fractures of the petrous temporal bone. Longitudinal temporal bone fracture (a) (*arrowhead*) involving glenoid fossa, and, in a different patient, associated with disruption of the ossicular chain (b). Note widening of the incudomalleolar joint (*arrowhead*). Transverse petrous temporal bone fractures (c,d) (*arrowheads*) in two different patients that spared the otic capsules and ossicular chains. Note the normal arrangement of the incus and malleus in an "ice cream cone" configuration (d) (*white arrow*).

Treatment

Treatment of petrous temporal bone fractures is targeted at the complications associated with the fracture. For example, sensorineural hearing loss may require cochlear implantation.[39] Patients with facial nerve paralysis can be treated medically (with corticosteroids) or surgically. Other complications are addressed on an individual basis.

9.10 Trauma to Cranial Sutures and Fissures

Diastasis of cranial sutures can be as common as skull-base fractures; often these injuries occur in conjunction with skull fractures. In adults, the most common suture to be affected is the lambdoid suture (▶ Fig. 9.23). Studies have suggested criteria for lambdoid suture diastasis, including width greater than 1.5 mm or a difference in width between the right and left sides of 1 mm or greater.[40] The importance of diastasis of cranial sutures lies in their association with other injuries, particularly an epidural hematoma. Other important considerations include injury to an adjacent dural venous sinus.

9.11 Complications and Associated Injury

Complications of skull-base fractures depend on the location, morphology, and severity of the underlying traumatic injury. As discussed previously, each type of fracture is prone to specific complications related to the surrounding anatomy. Fractures at the skull base, independent of whether specifically involving the anterior, middle, or posterior skull base, can also have additional potential complications or concomitant injuries.

9.11.1 Arterial Injury

Trauma to the intracranial arterial circulation may occur with skull-base fractures. Arterial trauma includes thrombosis, occlusion, dissection, post-traumatic aneurysms, incarceration or arteriovenous fistulas.[41] The internal carotid artery, especially its petrous and cavernous segments, is the most commonly affected vessel (▶ Fig. 9.24). Involvement of the petrous segment places patients at risk for cerebrovascular ischemia. Cerebrovascular injuries are classified by the Denver Grading System[42] and are discussed in depth in Chapter 7, Blunt Cerebrovascular Injury. CTA

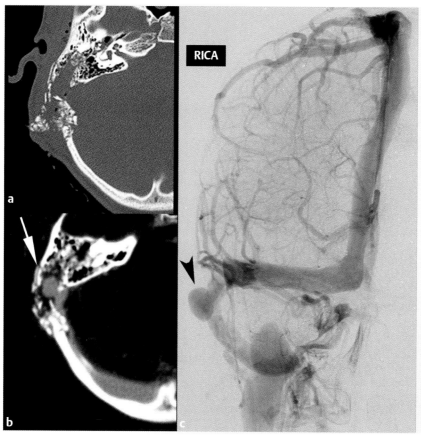

Fig. 9.19 Pseudoaneurysm of the transverse sinus secondary to a temporal bone fracture. Axial high-resolution multidetector computed tomographic (CT) image of the right temporal bone (a) demonstrates a comminuted fracture. Axial maximum-intensity projection (MIP) from CT angiography (b) shows an abnormal vascular structure protruding through the fracture defect and communicating with the right transverse sinus (*arrow*). Anteroposterior venous phase angiographic image from right internal carotid artery (RICA) injection (c) confirms a pseudoaneurysm of the right transverse sinus (*arrowhead*).

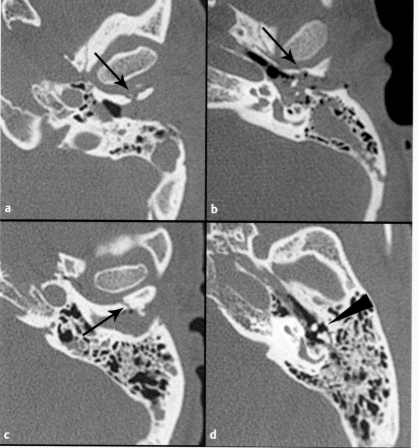

Fig. 9.20 Involvement of the external auditory canal (EAC) with fractures of the temporal bone. (a) Axial computed tomography image in a patient with a mixed left temporal bone fracture extending through the anterior wall of the EAC (*arrow*). (b) Involvement of both the anterior and posterior walls of the EAC in association with a longitudinal temporal bone fracture. In a different patient, a fracture through the anterior wall of the EAC (c) (*arrow*) was associated with incudomalleolar separation (d) (*arrowhead*).

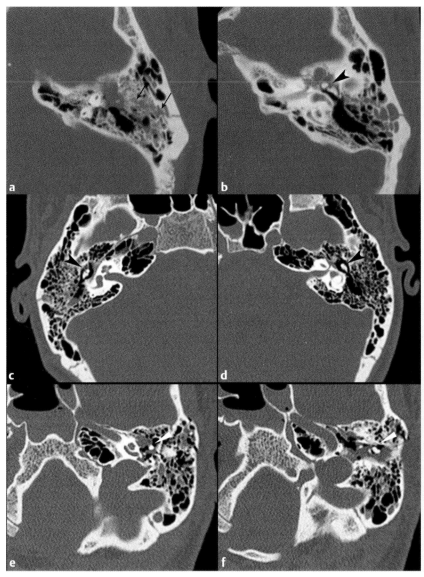

Fig. 9.21 Ossicular injury secondary to temporal bone fractures. Axial computed tomographic images show a longitudinal temporal bone fracture (*arrows*) (a) with associated incudomalleolar dislocation (*arrowhead*) (b). Subtle right ossicular dislocation in a different patient (c) (*arrowhead*), evident only as a slight widening of the incudomalleolar joint compared with the normal left side (d) (*arrowhead*). Third patient with obvious ossicular chain disruption (e,f) with an absence of the normal "ice cream cone" appearance (e) (*arrowhead*) and with ossicles evident in the external auditory canal (f) (*arrowhead*).

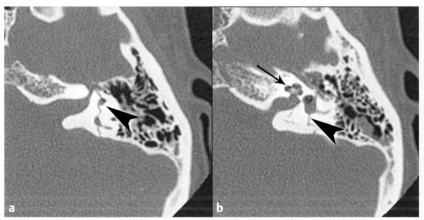

Fig. 9.22 Otic capsule involvement with temporal bone fracture. (a) Axial computed tomography demonstrates a transverse petrous temporal bone fracture that extends through the semicircular canals (*arrowhead*). (b) Fracture line extends through the vestibule (*arrowhead*) with gas evident in the cochlea and vestibule (pneumolabyrinth, *arrow*).

is sensitive for the diagnosis of cerebrovascular injury, although conventional angiography is sometimes necessary.[43]

The mainstay of therapy for traumatic vascular occlusion is medical management in the form of anticoagulation.[44] Other supportive measures, such as blood pressure augmentation, may also help with recovery. Traumatic aneurysms can be true, mixed, or false. Traumatic aneurysms usually involve the internal carotid artery but can also affect other intracranial vessels. Surgical or endovascular treatment is often necessary, as these types of aneurysms do not typically regress.

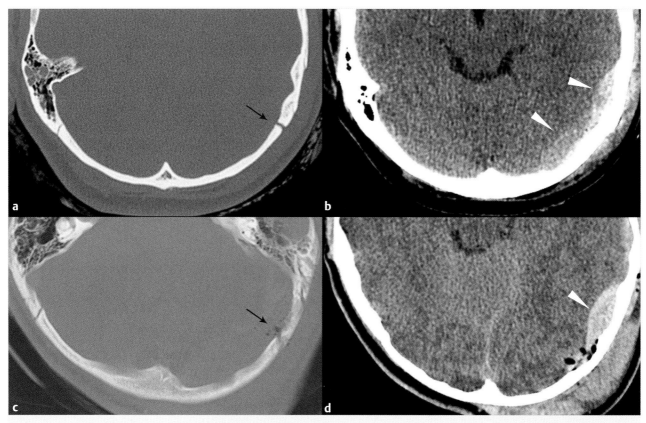

Fig. 9.23 Traumatic diastasis of a cranial suture. (a) Axial computed tomography demonstrates traumatic diastasis of the left lambdoid suture (*arrow*) with an associated epidural hematoma (b) (*arrowhead*). Similar findings are seen in a different patient (c,d).

9.11.2 Cerebrospinal Fluid Leak

The dura closely apposes the skull base and is vulnerable to injury in the presence of a skull-base fracture. Dural tears may result in a CSF leak and increase the risk for intracranial infection. Dural tears allow communication between the basal subarachnoid space and the paranasal sinuses, middle ear cavity, and mastoid air cells. Patients may develop meningitis, encephalitis, or a cerebral abscess, regardless of whether they present with rhinorrhea. Pneumococcus is the most commonly found organism in patients with meningitis in the presence of a CSF fistula.[45] CSF leaks usually occur within 48 hours after the initial injury. The "double-ring sign" describes a bedside test for CSF leak, in which the bloody nasal discharge is blotted with a paper tower. CSF diffusion occurs more rapidly than that of blood, so if a CSF leak is present, a larger clear ring will become evident around the central bloody area on the paper towel. Other confirmatory tests for CSF in bloody or nonbloody fluid include testing for the presence of beta-2-transferrin, which is found exclusively in CSF and perilymph.

Imaging may assist in the diagnosis of a CSF leak. Radionuclide cisternography is a sensitive means to detect CSF rhinorrhea. Pledgets are placed in the nose. After injection of radiotracer into the thecal sac by lumbar puncture, the pledgets are tested for radiotracer. If present, CSF leak is confirmed. Contrast-enhanced CT cisternography, in which contrast is injected into the thecal sac via lumbar puncture followed by high-resolution CT of the area of concern, may be used to localize the leak

(▶ Fig. 9.25). MRI can also be used, especially high-resolution T2-weighted imaging (▶ Fig. 9.4).

Management of CSF leaks includes conservative and surgical approaches.[46] Most CSF leaks resolve spontaneously, and a trial of conservative management is usually indicated before more aggressive treatments, such as external CSF drainage or direct leak repair, are performed. The use of prophylactic antibiotics is controversial, as several studies have shown that prophylactic antibiotics do not decrease the risk of meningitis. Important indications for surgery include a persistent leak, development of meningitis, and persistent or worsening pneumocephalus.

9.11.3 Traumatic Carotid-Cavernous Fistula

A carotid-cavernous (CC) fistula is an abnormal communication between the cavernous segment of the internal carotid artery and the cavernous sinus. It can occur secondary to skull-base trauma, whether involving the anterior, middle, or posterior cranial fossae.[47] Patients may initially have reduced vision, exophthalmos, headache, or a cranial nerve deficit. On CT or MRI, imaging findings include proptosis, orbital edema, enlargement of the extraocular muscles, and dilatation of the superior ophthalmic vein and cavernous sinus. MRI may also demonstrate abnormal flow voids within the cavernous sinus. Conventional angiography is the mainstay of diagnosis. On injection of the internal carotid artery, there is rapid filling of the

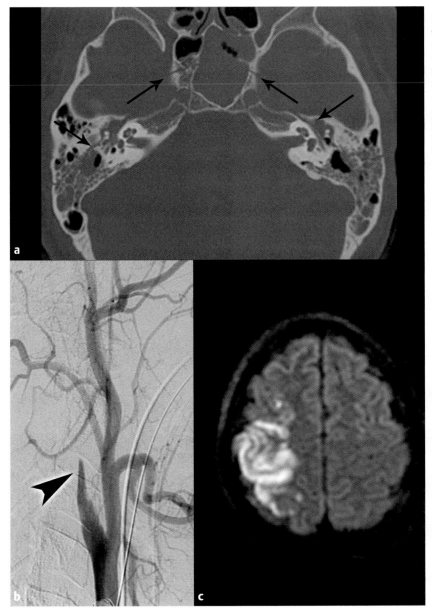

Fig. 9.24 Blunt cerebrovascular injury associated with skull base fracture. Axial computed tomography (a) shows several skull-base fractures, including fractures of the sphenoid and petrous temporal bones bilaterally (*arrows*). (b) Digital subtraction angiography, lateral view, right common carotid artery injection, demonstrates dissection of the internal carotid artery just distal to its origin. Diffusion-weighted magnetic resonance image (c) shows an acute infarction in the right middle cerebral artery territory.

cavernous sinus and ophthalmic veins, which are dilated (▶ Fig. 9.26). Treatment options include embolization or surgery. Long-term sequelae include vision loss and ischemic ocular necrosis.

9.11.4 Intracranial Hemorrhage

Patients with trauma at the skull base often have associated intracranial hemorrhage, including epidural and subdural hematomas, subarachnoid hemorrhage, and hemorrhagic contusions (▶ Fig. 9.27). Patients who have a posterior fossa subdural hematoma often have associated fractures of the posterior skull base or occipital condyles.[48] If there is significant posterior fossa mass effect, emergent decompressive surgery may be required. Although CT is the imaging modality of choice, MRI can be helpful, especially when evaluating for smaller contusions or diffuse axonal injury.

9.11.5 Spinal Trauma

Depending on the mechanism of injury, imaging of the spine may be indicated to evaluate for associated spinal trauma. Imaging modalities include x-rays, CT, or MRI, or a combination of these modalities. Trauma at the craniocervical junction is often associated with fractures of the skull base, and MRI is helpful to exclude ligamentous and soft tissue injury.

9.11.6 Maxillofacial Trauma

Skull-base trauma is often found in conjunction with maxillofacial trauma, particularly fractures involving the floor of the anterior cranial fossa. High-resolution axial imaging through the maxillofacial bones is an important adjunct to imaging of the skull base, particularly in the setting of high-energy trauma.

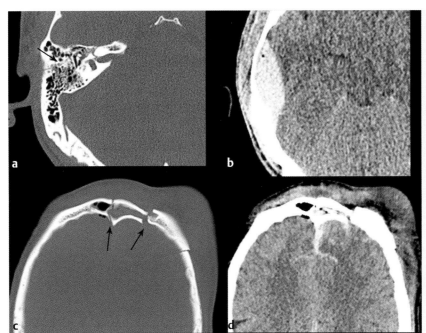

Fig. 9.27 Intracranial hemorrhage associated with skull-base fractures. Axial computed tomographic images demonstrate (a) a nondisplaced longitudinal fracture through the right petrous temporal bone (*arrow*) with an associated epidural hematoma (b). In a different patient, comminuted and displaced fractures through the inner and outer table of the frontal sinus (c) (*arrows*) are associated with subarachnoid hemorrhage, as well as hemorrhage within the frontal sinus (d).

tube placement is possible and has been reported.[57] Hence, enteric tube placement should be via the orogastric route.

9.12 Pearls

- Fractures of the anterior cranial fossa are often associated with maxillofacial trauma, and close evaluation of the facial structures is required. Post-traumatic CSF leak, particularly with fractures of the cribriform plate and fovea ethmoidalis, should be considered.
- Clivus fractures are highly associated with severe concomitant injuries, including vascular injury and parenchymal trauma.
- Occipital condyle fractures are the result of high-energy trauma and are classified into three types. MRI may be used to evaluate the craniocervical junction and cervical spinal cord.
- Temporal bone fractures are classified into longitudinal, transverse, and mixed types and are best identified on axial images. Assess adjacent structures, including the otic capsule, facial nerve, carotid canal, and ossicular chain for injury.
- Sellar fractures are often radiologically occult and can result in an endocrinopathy.
- Traumatic diastasis of the cranial sutures can manifest with complications similar to those of other skull base fractures. In adults, the most common suture to be affected is the lambdoid suture.

References

[1] Muñoz-Sánchez MA, Murillo-Cabezas F, Cayuela-Domínguez A, Rincón-Ferrari MD, Amaya-Villar R, León-Carrión J. Skull fracture, with or without clinical signs, in mTBI is an independent risk marker for neurosurgically relevant intracranial lesion: a cohort study. Brain Inj 2009; 23: 39–44

[2] Slupchynskyj OS, Berkower AS, Byrne DW, Cayten CG. Association of skull base and facial fractures. Laryngoscope 1992; 102: 1247–1250

[3] Mulligan RP, Friedman JA, Mahabir RC. A nationwide review of the associations among cervical spine injuries, head injuries, and facial fractures. J Trauma 2010; 68: 587–592

[4] Iida H, Tachibana S, Kitahara T, Horiike S, Ohwada T, Fujii K. Association of head trauma with cervical spine injury, spinal cord injury, or both. J Trauma 1999; 46: 450–452

[5] Lloyd DA, Carty H, Patterson M, Butcher CK, Roe D. Predictive value of skull radiography for intracranial injury in children with blunt head injury. Lancet 1997; 349: 821–824

[6] Laine FJ, Nadel L, Braun IFCT. CT and MR imaging of the central skull base. Part 1: Techniques, embryologic development, and anatomy. Radiographics 1990; 10: 591–602

[7] Parmar H, Gujar S, Shah G, Mukherji SK. Imaging of the anterior skull base. Neuroimaging Clin N Am 2009; 19: 427–439

[8] Opperman LA. Cranial sutures as intramembranous bone growth sites. Dev Dyn 2000; 219: 472–485

[9] Nemzek WR, Brodie HA, Hecht ST, Chong BW, Babcook CJ, Seibert JAMR. MR, CT, and plain film imaging of the developing skull base in fetal specimens. AJNR Am J Neuroradiol 2000; 21: 1699–1706

[10] Mann SS, Naidich TP, Towbin RB, Doundoulakis SH. Imaging of postnatal maturation of the skull base. Neuroimaging Clin N Am 2000; 10: 1–21, vii.

[11] Bassed RB, Briggs C, Drummer OH. Analysis of time of closure of the spheno-occipital synchondrosis using computed tomography. Forensic Sci Int 2010; 200: 161–164

[12] Sakas DE, Beale DJ, Ameen AA et al. Compound anterior cranial base fractures: classification using computerized tomography scanning as a basis for selection of patients for dural repair. J Neurosurg 1998; 88: 471–477

[13] Asano T, Ohno K, Takada Y, Suzuki R, Hirakawa K, Monma S. Fractures of the floor of the anterior cranial fossa. J Trauma 1995; 39: 702–706

[14] Ochalski PG, Spiro RM, Fabio A, Kassam AB, Okonkwo DO. Fractures of the clivus: a contemporary series in the computed tomography era. Neurosurgery 2009; 65: 1063–1069

[15] Menkü A, Koç RK, Tucer B, Durak AC, Akdemir H. Clivus fractures: clinical presentations and courses. Neurosurg Rev. 2004; 27: 194–198

[16] Ochalski PG, Spiro RM, Fabio A, Kassam AB, Okonkwo DO. Fractures of the clivus: a contemporary series in the computed tomography era. Neurosurgery 2009; 65: 1063–1069

[17] Taguchi Y, Matsuzawa M, Morishima H, Ono H, Oshima K, Hayakawa M. Incarceration of the basilar artery in a longitudinal fracture of the clivus: case report and literature review. J Trauma 2000; 48: 1148–1152

[18] Young HA, Schmidek HH. Complications accompanying occipital skull fracture. J Trauma 1982; 22: 914–920

[19] Alcelik I, Manik KS, Sian PS, Khoshneviszadeh SE. Occipital condylar fractures. Review of the literature and case report. Neurologist 2012; 18: 152–154

[20] Raila FA, Aitken AT, Vickers GN. Computed tomography and three-dimensional reconstruction in the evaluation of occipital condyle fracture. Skeletal Radiol 1993; 22: 269–271

[21] Hanson JA, Deliganis AV, Baxter AB et al. Radiologic and clinical spectrum of occipital condyle fractures: retrospective review of 107 consecutive fractures in 95 patients. AJR Am J Roentgenol 2002; 178: 1261–1268

[22] Anderson PA, Montesano PX. Morphology and treatment of occipital condyle fractures. Spine 1988; 13: 731–736

[23] Leone A, Cerase A, Colosimo C, Lauro L, Puca A, Marano P. Occipital condylar fractures: a review. Radiology 2000; 216: 635–644

[24] Young WF, Rosenwasser RH, Getch C, Jallo J. Diagnosis and management of occipital condyle fractures. Neurosurgery 1994; 34: 257–261

[25] Dublin AB, Poirier VC. Fracture of the sella turcica. AJR Am J Roentgenol 1976; 127: 969–972

[26] Kusanagi H, Kogure K, Teramoto A. Pituitary insufficiency after penetrating injury to the sella turcica. J Nippon Med Sch 2000; 67: 130–133

[27] Brodie HA, Thompson TC. Management of complications from 820 temporal bone fractures. Am J Otol 1997; 18: 188–197

[28] Little SC, Kesser BW. Radiographic classification of temporal bone fractures: clinical predictability using a new system. Arch Otolaryngol Head Neck Surg 2006; 132: 1300–1304

[29] Gurdjian ES, Lissner HR. Deformations of the skull in head injury studied by the stresscoat technique, quantitative determinations. Surg Gynecol Obstet 1946; 83: 219–233

[30] Swartz JD. Trauma. In: Swartz JD, Harnsberger HR, eds. Imaging of the Temporal Bone. 3rd ed. New York, NY: Thieme, 1997:318–344.

[31] Ghorayeb BY, Yeakley JW. Temporal bone fractures: longitudinal or oblique? The case for oblique temporal bone fractures. Laryngoscope 1992; 102: 129–134

[32] McHugh HE. The surgical treatment of facial paralysis and traumatic conductive deafness in fractures of the temporal bone. Ann Otol Rhinol Laryngol 1959; 68: 855–889

[33] Lambert PR, Brackmann DE. Facial paralysis in longitudinal temporal bone fractures: a review of 26 cases. Laryngoscope 1984; 94: 1022–1026

[34] Resnick DK, Subach BR, Marion DW. The significance of carotid canal involvement in basilar cranial fracture. Neurosurgery 1997; 40: 1177–1181

[35] Meriot P, Veillon F, Garcia JF et al. CT appearances of ossicular injuries. Radiographics. 1997; 17: 1445–1454

[36] Swartz JD. Temporal bone trauma. In: Som PM, Curtin HD, eds. Head and Neck Imaging. 3rd ed. St Louis, Mo: Mosby, 1995:1425–1431.

[37] Kollias SS. Temporal bone trauma. In: Lemmerling M, Kollias SS, eds. Radiology of the Petrous Bone. Berlin, Germany: Springer, 2003:49–58.

[38] Brodie HA, Thompson TC. Management of complications from 820 temporal bone fractures. Am J Otol 1997; 18: 188–197

[39] Hagr A. Cochlear implantation in fractured inner ears. J Otolaryngol Head Neck Surg 2011; 40: 281–287

[40] Grossart KW, Samuel E. Traumatic diastasis of cranial sutures. Clin Radiol 1961; 12: 164–170

[41] Feiz-Erfan I, Horn EM, Theodore N et al. Incidence and pattern of direct blunt neurovascular injury associated with trauma to the skull base. J Neurosurg 2007; 107: 364–369

[42] Biffl WL, Moore EE, Offner PJ, Burch JM. Blunt carotid and vertebral arterial injuries. World J Surg 2001; 25: 1036–1043

[43] Bub LD, Hollingworth W, Jarvik JG, Hallam DK. Screening for blunt cerebrovascular injury: evaluating the accuracy of multidetector computed tomographic angiography. J Trauma 2005; 59: 691–697

[44] Miller PR, Fabian TC, Bee TK et al. Blunt cerebrovascular injuries: diagnosis and treatment. J Trauma 2001; 51: 279–286

[45] Briggs M. Traumatic pneumocephalus. Br J Surg 1974; 61: 307–312

[46] Bell RB, Dierks EJ, Homer L, Potter BE. Management of cerebrospinal fluid leak associated with craniomaxillofacial trauma. J Oral Maxillofac Surg 2004; 62: 676–684

[47] Liang W, Xiaofeng Y, Weiguo L, Wusi Q, Gang S, Xuesheng Z. Traumatic carotid cavernous fistula accompanying basilar skull fracture: a study on the incidence of traumatic carotid cavernous fistula in the patients with basilar skull fracture and the prognostic analysis about traumatic carotid cavernous fistula. J Trauma. 2007; 63: 1014–1020

[48] Takeuchi S, Takasato Y, Wada K et al. Traumatic posterior fossa subdural hematomas. J Trauma Acute Care Surg 2012; 72: 480–486

[49] Lehn AC, Lettieri J, Grimley R. A case of bilateral lower cranial nerve palsies after base of skull trauma with complex management issues: case report and review of the literature. Neurologist. 2012; 18: 152–154

[50] Kapila A, Chakeres DW. Clivus fracture: CT demonstration. J Comput Assist Tomogr 1985; 9: 1142–1144

[51] Katsuno M, Yokota H, Yamamoto Y, Teramoto A. Bilateral traumatic abducens nerve palsy associated with skull base fracture—case report. Neurol Med Chir (Tokyo) 2007; 47: 307–309

[52] Hato N, Nota J, Hakuba N, Gyo K, Yanagihara N. Facial nerve decompression surgery in patients with temporal bone trauma: analysis of 66 cases. J Trauma 2011; 71: 1789–1793

[53] Sanuş GZ, Tanriöver N, Tanriverdi T, Uzan M, Akar Z. Late decompression in patients with acute facial nerve paralysis after temporal bone fracture. Turk Neurosurg 2007; 17: 7–12

[54] de P Djientcheu V, Njamnshi AK, Ongolo-Zogo P et al. Growing skull fractures. Childs Nerv Syst 2006; 22: 721–725

[55] Ciurea AV, Gorgan MR, Tascu A, Sandu AM, Rizea RE. Traumatic brain injury in infants and toddlers, 0–3 years old. J Med Life 2011; 4: 234–243

[56] Holsti M, Kadish HA, Sill BL, Firth SD, Nelson DS. Pediatric closed head injuries treated in an observation unit. Pediatr Emerg Care. 2005; 21: 639–644

[57] Fremstad JD, Martin SH. Lethal complication from insertion of nasogastric tube after severe basilar skull fracture. J Trauma 1978; 18: 820–822

10 Maxillofacial Trauma

Jayson L. Benjert, Kathleen R. Fink, and Yoshimi Anzai

10.1 Introduction

Maxillofacial trauma represents a significant cause of morbidity and financial cost in the United States. More than three million people sustain maxillofacial injuries each year,[1] and many of these injuries require hospital admission. In 2007, the cost of treatment of facial fractures in U.S. emergency departments was nearly one billion dollars.[2]

Imaging plays an important role in the management of patients with maxillofacial trauma. Proper imaging allows for the rapid diagnosis of craniofacial fractures and associated injuries. Cross-sectional imaging, particularly the use of three-dimensional (3D) reconstructions, has become vital to surgical planning. Intraoperative computed tomography (CT) has increasingly been used to provide essential anatomic information directly at the point of care. This chapter discusses the causes of maxillofacial injuries, the major patterns of facial fractures, and current imaging practices concerning maxillofacial trauma.

10.2 Epidemiology

Maxillofacial trauma accounts for a major use of health care resources in the United States, with an average hospitalization of 6 days and a mean cost of $60,000 per patient.[2] Motor-vehicle collisions and assault cause most maxillofacial trauma. In industrialized nations, assault accounts for an increasing proportion of maxillofacial trauma, with increasing numbers of cases reported in some countries.[3] Motor-vehicle collisions are also an increasing cause of such fractures in developing countries.[3] The cause of maxillofacial fractures also may vary within a country from region to region, with interpersonal violence more frequent in urban areas and motor-vehicle collisions and falls more common in rural areas.[4] Falls, sports, and work-related injuries round out the most common causes of maxillofacial trauma, with falls accounting for most maxillofacial injuries in the older population.[5]

The typical patient with maxillofacial trauma is a man in the third decade of life. Maxillofacial trauma affects men more than women, with male-to-female ratios reported as high as 11:1, but more commonly found in the range of two to four men affected for every woman affected.[6–8] Alcohol use plays a significant factor in maxillofacial injury, with some reports finding as many as 87% of maxillofacial trauma cases to involve alcohol.[9]

The increased use of seat belts and air bags in automobiles has decreased the incidence of facial fractures and lacerations resulting from motor-vehicle collisions.[10] An analysis of the effect of safety devices on the incidence of facial trauma found that 59% of patients with facial fractures resulting from motor-vehicle collisions did not use any safety device.[11] Further, the lack of use of air bags or seat belts during motor-vehicle collision increased the incidence of facial fractures.[11]

10.3 Normal Anatomy

The facial bones and supporting musculature and tissues provide both function and form. The facial bones provide important protection for the brain and eyes. They house the structures necessary for sight, smell, and taste. The facial skeleton provides the framework for the vital functions of ventilation, mastication, and phonation. Lastly, the face is the portal to the outside world and is the organ of social interaction. In patients with congenital or post-traumatic facial deformity, appearance is rated as the fifth most important function of the face after breathing, vision, speech, and eating.[12]

The buttress system of the face is helpful in conceptualizing facial anatomy and is essential in planning surgical reconstruction. The facial buttresses are composed of regions of relatively thickened bone that support the physiologic functions of the face, such as mastication.[13] They also provide targets of sufficient thickness to accommodate surgical fixation hardware.

There are four pairs of vertically oriented buttresses (► Fig. 10.1):
- Nasomaxillary or medial maxillary buttress runs from the anterior maxillary alveolar process superiorly along the frontal process of the maxilla to the region of the glabella.
- The zygomaticomaxillary or lateral maxillary buttress extends from the lateral maxillary alveolar process over the

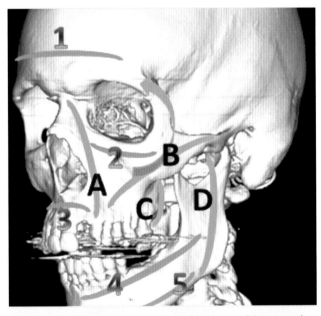

Fig. 10.1 Facial buttress anatomy. Vertical buttresses: (A) Nasomaxillary or medial maxillary buttress, (B) zygomaticomaxillary or lateral maxillary buttress, (C) pterygomaxillary or posterior maxillary buttress, (D) vertical mandibular buttress. Horizontal buttresses: (1) frontal bar, (2) upper transverse maxillary buttress, (3) lower transverse maxillary buttress, (4) upper transverse mandibular buttress, (5) lower transverse mandibular buttress.

zygoma and includes the lateral orbital wall. This buttress bifurcates at the zygoma and travels posteriorly along the zygomatic arch.

- Pterygomaxillary or posterior maxillary buttress is located at the posterior maxillary alveolar process and extends along the posterior wall of the maxillary sinus to the base of the pterygoids. This buttress is not surgically accessible.
- Vertical mandibular buttress courses along the vertical ramus of the mandible to the mandibular condyle and skull base at the glenoid fossa of the temporomandibular joint.

The bony nasal septum also represents a weak vertical buttress present centrally. There are five horizontal buttresses of the face (▶ Fig. 10.1):

- The frontal bar extends along the thickened frontal bone of the inferior forehead at the supraorbital ridges between the frontozygomatic sutures.
- Upper transverse maxillary buttress travels along the infraorbital rims and includes the insertion site of medial canthal tendon in the medial orbit, an important structure for naso-orbito-ethmoid (NOE) fracture evaluation, described below.
- The lower transverse maxillary buttress is located centrally at the palatoalveolar complex and extends laterally and posteriorly along the maxilla.
- The upper and lower transverse mandibular buttresses are the lower-most buttresses. The upper mandibular buttress extends from the central portion of the mandible along the dentoalveolar arch. The lower mandibular buttress travels along the most inferior aspect of the mandible.

10.4 Imaging

CT is the modality of choice for evaluating maxillofacial trauma. CT has supplanted conventional radiography for this purpose, given CT's speed of data acquisition, wide availability, and high sensitivity and specificity.[14] In cases of severe trauma, CT examinations of the head and cervical spine are often performed concurrently. The use of a 64- or 128-slice multidetector row CT scanner allows for the maxillofacial CT to be reformatted from the source images obtained for head and cervical spine CT, thereby eliminating unnecessary radiation exposure and time.

Current multidetector CT scanners provide isometric voxel size with excellent spatial resolution of reformatted and 3D images. The CT protocol for evaluation of maxillofacial trauma should include axial images no more than 1 mm thick from the top of the frontal sinuses to the bottom of the mandible. Coronal and sagittal reformats can then be reconstructed at 0.5- to 1-mm intervals. The use of 3D reconstructions in maxillofacial trauma has steadily increased as multidetector row CT technology has advanced.

The 3D images allow easy visualization of the degree of fracture comminution and displacement, aid in localizing displaced fracture fragments, and allow evaluation of complex facial fractures in multiple planes.[15] 3D images are helpful for planning fracture fixation and operative reconstruction by surgeons[16,17] and provide an overall "big picture" as to the extent of facial injuries.

The reported sensitivity of CT in the detection of facial fractures ranges from 45 to 97%, with specificity of near 100%. The wide range of reported sensitivity is likely due to the difficulty of visualizing some fractures in a single plane, such as identifying an orbital floor fracture using only axial images. Coronal reformats in addition to axial source images are particularly helpful in facilitating fracture detection, thus improving sensitivity. In fact, one study found that using a combination of axial images, multiplanar reconstructions, and 3D volume-rendered reformats was more accurate than using either axial images alone or axial images with multiplanar reconstructions.[15] Evaluation of all three sets of images yielded a sensitivity of 95.8% and specificity of 99% for maxillofacial fractures.[15]

Surgeons are increasingly requesting intraoperative CT to assess the adequacy of facial fracture reduction and fixation during surgery, which allows for immediate revision and reduces the need for future revision procedures.[18] Additionally, early complications such as graft malposition can be identified.

Although clearly displaced or comminuted fractures are readily detectible by CT, nondisplaced fractures can be more difficult to identify, and some fractures are occult. In these cases, recognizing the presence of soft tissue injury or secondary signs of injury may be the only way to detect these fractures. Soft tissue swelling, subcutaneous stranding, and hematoma identify the site where blunt injury occurred. Subcutaneous emphysema within the masticator space, malar region, or orbits, along with pneumocephalus, may indicate a fracture involving the paranasal sinus walls. Hemorrhagic effusions with the paranasal sinuses, manifested as hypderdense layering fluid, should always prompt a thorough search for fractures.

10.5 Facial Fractures

10.5.1 Nasal Fractures

The nasal bones are the most commonly fractured facial bones.[19] Nasal fractures are commonly caused by motor-vehicle collisions, assaults, and sports-related injuries.[20] The bony components of the nose include the nasal process of the frontal bone, the frontal processes of the maxilla, the ethmoid, the vomer, and the nasal bones (▶ Fig. 10.2). The distal portions of the nasal bones are susceptible to fracture because of the broadness and thinness of the bone in this region.

The signs and symptoms of nasal fractures include tenderness to palpation, palpable deformity, malposition, ecchymosis, epistaxis, and cerebrospinal fluid (CSF) rhinorrhea. Some authors suggest that imaging is not required for suspected simple nasal fractures because management is influenced chiefly by clinical rather than imaging findings.[21] Clinical suspicion for other facial fractures or any concerning physical examination finding, such as copious epistaxis or rhinorrhea, dictates the need for CT evaluation.

Nasal fractures are classified clinically by severity (▶ Table 10.1). Type I injury refers to soft tissue injury without underlying damage to the bony structures of the nose. Type IIa injury is defined as a simple unilateral nondisplaced nasal bone fracture, and type IIb injury is simple bilateral nondisplaced fractures. Type III injury refers to simple displaced fractures. Type IV injury denotes a closed comminuted fracture. Type V

Many classification schemes have been designed for zygomaticomaxillary fractures.[28] Zingg et al[29] developed a fairly simple classification system (▶ Table 10.2), in which type A fracture refers to incomplete zygomatic fractures in which

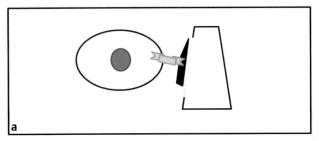

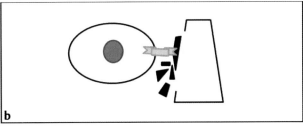

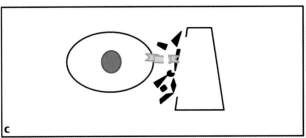

Fig. 10.5 Markowitz-Manson classification of naso-orbito-ethmoid (NOE) fractures. Iris of the eye shown in blue. Medial canthal tendon denoted in green; fracture fragments in black. (a) Type I demonstrates large central fragment. (b) Type II refers to comminuted central fragment with fragments external to medial canthal tendon insertion. (c) Type III refers to marked comminution of central fragment and disruption of medial canthal tendon.

only one of the zygomatic pillars is fractured. Subtypes include isolated zygomatic arch fractures (A1), lateral orbital wall fractures (A2), or infraorbital rim fractures (A3). There is no displacement of the zygomatic complex because the remaining pillars are intact. Type B fracture describes the classic "tripod" fracture wherein all four pillars are fractured and displacement may occur. Again, this is more correctly referred to as a tetrapod fracture. Type C fractures involve the same structures as type B fractures but demonstrate greater comminution.

Type B fractures are the most common (▶ Fig. 10.8; ▶ Fig. 10.9).[29] Surgical fixation and reconstruction are generally performed as soon as possible, usually within 2 weeks of injury.[30] ZMC fractures associated with other facial fractures, comminuted fractures, malocclusion, or infraorbital nerve sensory disturbances are more likely to be treated surgically.[31]

10.5.4 Central Midface Fractures

Most central midface fractures fall within the Le Fort (pterygofacial) category of fractures. The classification system of these fractures was developed by Rene Le Fort in 1901[32] and is based on observations that blunt trauma results in specific fracture patterns along three lines of inherent weakness of the facial bones. CT is the imaging modality of choice for evaluating central midface fractures because it allows good delineation of fracture patterns within the complex anatomy of the midface. Axial and coronal thin-section images are the standard. 3D CT also plays a role in operative planning.

A key feature of Le Fort fracture is involvement of the pterygoid bones, and the presence of a pterygoid plate fracture almost always indicates a Le Fort fracture. Pterygoid plate fractures sometimes occur from a direct blow, such as with a lateral pterygoid plate fracture in association with a mandibular fracture. Such cases do not fall within the Le Fort series of fractures. Rhea and Novelline[33] discussed a method for simplifying the evaluation of Le Fort fracture patterns by CT by looking for the presence of specific defining fracture components for each fracture type.

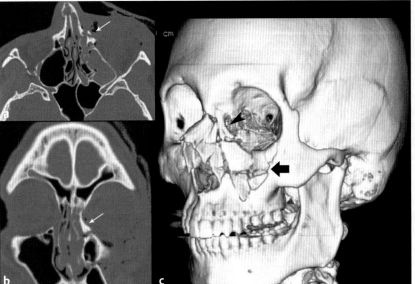

Fig. 10.6 Type I naso-orbito-ethmoid (NOE) fracture. Axial computed tomography (CT) (a) showing fracture involving medial canthal tendon attachment site (arrow). Coronal CT (b) demonstrates large single central fragment (arrow). Three-dimensional reformat CT (c) better demonstrates large central fragment (arrowhead) consistent with type I NOE fracture. Comminuted depressed fracture of the left anterior maxillary sinus wall and inferior orbital rim are also present (black arrow).

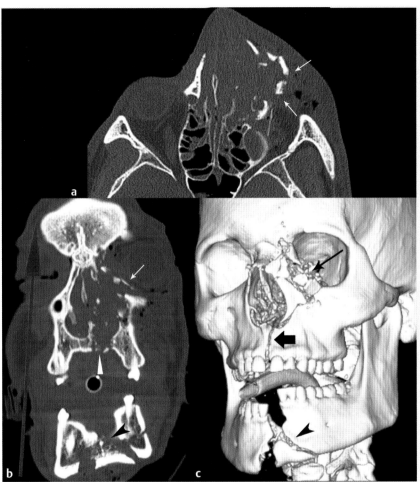

Fig. 10.7 Self-inflicted gunshot wound with type III naso-orbito-ethmoid (NOE) fracture. Axial computed tomography (CT) (a) shows comminuted and severely laterally displaced left NOE fracture (*arrows*). Injury to the medial canthal tendon is inferred from the comminution and displacement of fragments. Coronal reformat (b) shows additional fractures of the left nasal wall, medial orbital wall, infraorbital rim (*arrow*), hard palate (*white arrowhead*), and mandible (*black arrowhead*). Bullet trajectory is suggested by the pattern of fractures (*red arrow*). Volume-rendered reformat (c) shows comminution and displacement of the NOE fracture (*black arrow*), anterior maxillary fracture extending superiorly to infraorbital foramen (*thick black arrow*), and comminuted, displaced symphyseal fracture of the mandible (*arrowhead*).

Table 10.2 Zygomatic Fracture Classification

Classification	Description
Type A	Incomplete zygomatic fracture
A1	Isolated zygomatic arch fracture
A2	Lateral orbital wall fracture
A3	Infraorbital rim fracture
Type B	Complete zygomatic fracture (tetrapod fracture), single fragment
Type C	Multifragment zygomatic fracture (type B + greater comminution)

Adapted from Zingg M, Laedrach K, Chen J, et al. Classification and treatment of zygomatic fractures: a review of 1,025 cases. J Oral Maxillofac Surg. 1992;50(8):778–790.

The Le Fort I fracture consists of a horizontal fracture through the maxilla (▶ Fig. 10.10) and results in the separation of the hard palate from the skull, resulting in a floating palate. This fracture involves the anterolateral margin of the nasal fossa and traverses the inferior aspects of the medial and lateral maxillary buttresses. The key fracture component to diagnose Le Fort I injury is a fracture through the anterolateral nasal fossa.[33]

The Le Fort II fracture is sometimes referred to as a pyramidal fracture because of the triangular shape of the fracture fragment, with the maxillary teeth at the base and nasal arch at the tip. The Le Fort II fracture (▶ Fig. 10.11) involves the pterygoid plates, posterior and lateral walls of the maxillary sinuses, inferior orbital rim, and medial orbital wall. The fracture terminates near the nasofrontal suture. Fracture of the inferior orbital rim is unique to this fracture pattern and aids in proper classification.[33] The maxilla and nose are separated from the skull in Le Fort II injuries and move as a unit in relation to the remainder of the face.

The Le Fort III fractures result in "facial dissociation," with the maxillary teeth, nose, and zygomatic bones freely mobile with respect to the remainder of the skull. A Le Fort III fracture (▶ Fig. 10.11) includes fractures of the pterygoid plates, superior aspect of the posterior maxillary wall, lateral orbital wall, zygomatic arch, greater wing of the sphenoid at the posterior aspect of the orbit, and medial orbital wall. The fracture of the zygomatic arch is unique to this fracture pattern,[33] aiding in correct categorization, although isolated zygomatic arch fractures without involvement of the other Le Fort III injuries may be present with Le Fort I and II fracture types.

Le Fort fractures often occur in combination with other fractures of the orbit, nose, and zygoma. The different types of Le Fort fractures may occur concurrently in severe trauma; that is, one may sustain LeFort I, II, and III fractures on the same side of

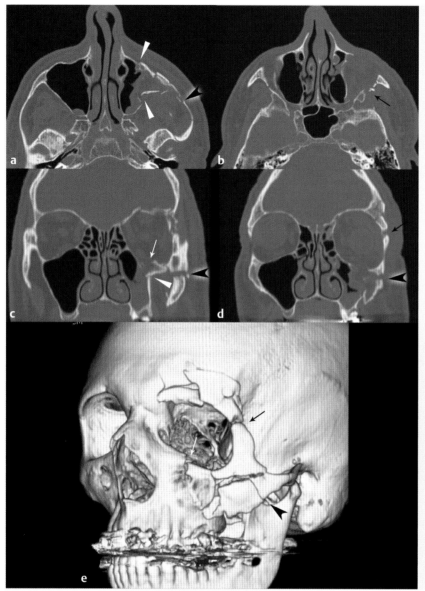

Fig. 10.8 Left zygomaticomaxillary complex (ZMC) fracture. Axial (a,b), coronal (c,d) and volume-rendered reformat (e) computed tomography demonstrating components of left ZMC fracture. Multiple fractures of left zygomatic arch (*black arrowheads*), anterior and lateral maxillary sinus wall (*white arrowheads*). Fracture of the left lateral orbital wall (*black arrow*), and orbital floor (*white arrow*).

the face (▶ Fig. 10.11). Additionally, a patient may sustain different types of Le Fort fractures on either side of the face (▶ Fig. 10.11).

Treatment of Le Fort fractures is surgical. The goals of treatment are to restore occlusion, facial height, and facial projection. Important considerations for treatment include the degree of comminution of the facial buttresses, as this may necessitate bone grafting for adequate reconstruction.[34]

10.5.5 Mandibular Fractures

The mandible is one of the most commonly fractured bones in the face owing to its anatomic prominence, mobility, and relatively lack of bony support. Fractures may affect any part of the mandible and are described by location.[35] Symphyseal fractures traverse the mandibular symphysis, which is the space between the roots of the central incisors. Parasymphseal fractures are lateral to the central incisors but medial to the lateral roots of the canine teeth. Mandibular body fractures occur between the lateral roots of the canine teeth and the second molar (4 mm

anterior to the mandibular foramen in edentulous patients). Mandibular angle fractures occur posteriorly to body fractures, but they do not involve the vertically oriented mandibular ramus. The mandibular ramus gives off two processes, the condylar process and the coronoid process. The mandibular condyle consists of the condylar head and neck.

The most common locations of mandibular fracture are the mandibular condyle (36%), followed by the body (21%) and angle (20%).[36] Mandibular angle fractures occur more frequently in assaults.[37] Fractures are multiple in 50 to 60% of cases,[38] and the observation of one fracture through the mandible should prompt a thorough search for the second fracture.

Important considerations when describing mandibular fractures include involvement of the mandibular foramen, alveolar canal, or mental foramen because of the possibility of injury to the inferior alveolar nerve. Involvement of the alveolar ridge, including the involved teeth sockets, should be described. Careful examination for fractures or subluxation of the teeth is important for the surgeon to assess the need for tooth repair or extraction.

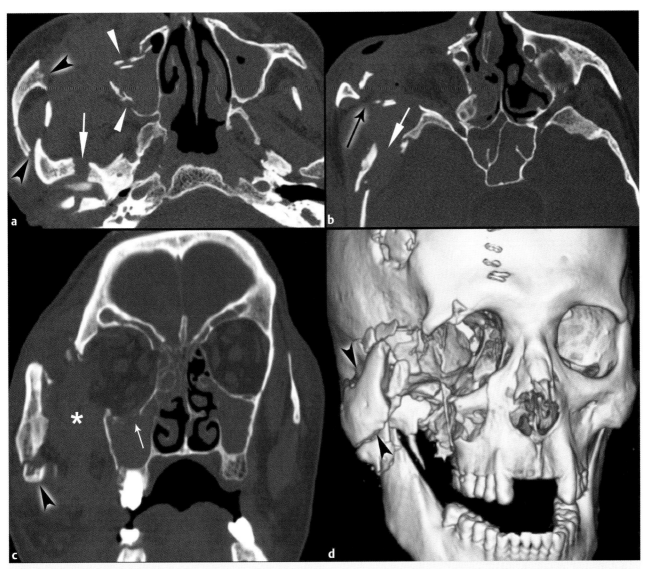

Fig. 10.9 Laterally displaced right zygomaticomaxillary complex (ZMC) fracture. Axial computed tomography (CT) (a) demonstrates laterally displaced fractures of the right zygoma and zygomatic arch (*black arrowheads*), comminuted fractures of the walls of the right maxillary sinus (*white arrowheads*), and (b) comminuted fracture of the lateral orbital wall (*black arrow*). Fracture disrupts the glenoid fossa of the right temporomandibular junction (*white arrow*) (a) and extends into the right greater wing of sphenoid bone and squamous temporal bone (*white arrow*) (b). (c) Coronal reformat depicts the lateral displacement of the right zygoma and lateral orbital wall (*black arrowhead*) with hematoma of the masseter muscle (*). Note the orbital floor component to the fracture (*white arrow*). Three-dimensional volume-rendered reformat (d) demonstrates displaced fracture fragment composed of the zygoma and lateral orbital wall (*black arrowheads*).

Like fractures elsewhere, mandibular fractures can be described as simple or comminuted and open or closed. Open fractures may communicate externally through a skin laceration or internally through the socket of a tooth. Mandibular fractures may also be defined as favorable or unfavorable, depending on whether or not the fracture fragments are displaced by muscular pull; favorable fractures are not displaced. Examples of unfavorable fractures include symphyseal and parasymphyseal fractures subject to downward pull by the suprahyoid musculature (▶ Fig. 10.12); mandibular angle fractures displaced horizontally by muscles of mastication, and high condylar fractures subject to medial displacement by the lateral pterygoid muscles (▶ Fig. 10.13).

For the evaluation of mandibular trauma, CT has replaced Panorex and other mandibular radiographs. CT allows for rapid identification of mandibular fractures along with evaluation of other facial fractures and associated injuries. 3D reconstructions are useful in treatment planning. CT is reported to be up to 100% sensitive for identifying mandibular fractures, whereas Panorex is only 86% sensitive.[39] In addition, obtaining Panorex radiographs may not be feasible in someone with multisystem trauma or severe maxillofacial trauma because the images are obtained in the upright sitting position.

Mandibular fractures are treated conservatively, by closed reduction, or by open reduction and internal fixation. Most symphyseal and parasymphyseal fractures, displaced fractures of

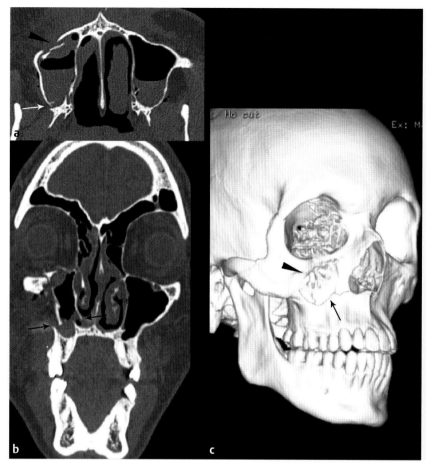

Fig. 10.10 Right hemi Le Fort I fracture. Axial computed tomography (a) shows fracture through the base of the right pterygoid (*white arrow*) and comminuted fracture of the right anterior maxillary sinus wall (*black arrowhead*). Coronal reformat (b) demonstrates fractures at the inferior aspects of the medial and lateral maxillary buttresses (*black arrows*). Three-dimensional volume-rendered reformat (c) better delineates the horizontal fracture line through the maxilla characteristic of the Le Fort I fracture (*black arrow*). Depressed, comminuted fracture of the anterior wall of the maxillary sinus redemonstrated (*black arrowhead*).

the angle and body, and some condylar fractures[36] are treated by open reduction. Infection, particularly in the setting of open fractures, is the most common complication. Malocclusion and sensory disturbances of the inferior alveolar nerve may also occur.[40]

10.5.6 Frontal Sinus Fractures

Fractures of the frontal sinus account for 5 to 15% of facial fractures and are typically caused by high-energy trauma.[41] Frontal sinus fractures may involve the anterior (outer) table, posterior (inner) table, or both. Penetrating trauma may result in fractures completely traversing the fronal sinuses, involving injuries to the skin, anterior and posterior tables, dura, and possibly frontal lobes. Frontal sinus fractures most commonly involve both the anterior and posterior tables (▶ Fig. 10.14), with this pattern accounting for approximately two thirds of frontal sinus fractures.[42] Fractures of the anterior table have important aesthetic consequences for the appearance of the forehead and supraorbital ridge. The posterior table is important because of the intimate association with the adjacent underlying dura. The status of the inferior frontal recess and frontal sinus ostia (nasofrontal recess) is key when evaluating frontal sinus fractures because obstruction of the outflow tract has important clinical implications, described as follows.

Fractures can be simple, displaced, comminuted, and depressed (▶ Fig. 10.15). Up to 56 to 87% of patients with frontal sinus fractures have associated craniofacial injuries,[34,42,43] and CT is the imaging modality of choice in evaluating these

fractures. CT also allows for the evaluation of other facial fractures and identification of associated intracranial injuries such as cerebral contusions, dural injury, and extra-axial hemorrhage. Thin-slice axial and coronal images are typically obtained. Sagittal reconstructions allow improved evaluation of the frontal sinus outflow tract and nasofrontal recess, an hourglass-shaped structure comprising the frontal sinus infundibulum, ostia, and recess.[44]

Treatment of frontal sinus fractures is determined by the involved structures and the degree of displacement. Nondisplaced anterior table fractures are usually treated conservatively with observation. The presence of a small CSF leak does not preclude conservative treatment, as most small leaks will resolve with conservative management in 7 to 10 days.[45] Comminuted or depressed anterior table fractures can result in significant facial deformity and require surgical reduction and fixation.

If the inferior frontal recess or frontal sinus ostia is obstructed, the frontal sinus will become nonfunctional (▶ Fig. 10.16), with attendant risks of complications, including mucocele formation. If frontal sinus outflow obstruction is recognized at the time of injury, the frontal sinus may be obliterated, with surgical removal of the frontal sinus mucosa and blockage of the outflow tract (nasofrontal duct). Cranialization of the frontal sinuses, defined as removal of the posterior wall of the frontal sinus, sinus mucosa, and obstruction of the frontal sinus outflow tract, is reserved for severe posterior table fractures and persistent CSF leaks.[46]

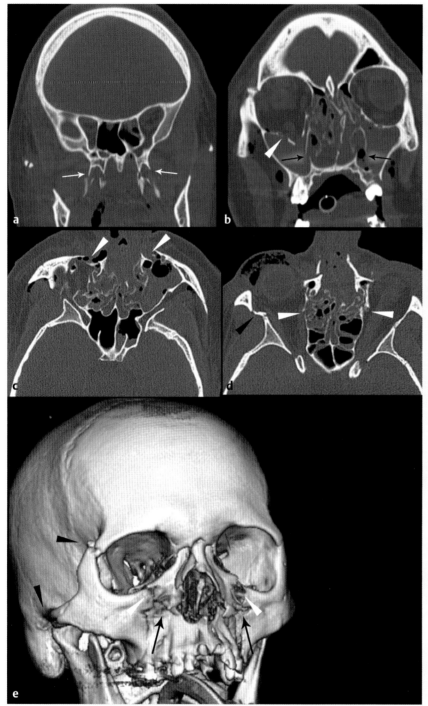

Fig. 10.11 Bilateral Le Fort I and II fractures and right Le Fort III fracture. Coronal computed tomography (CT) reformat (a,b) and axial CT (c,d) demonstrates bilateral pterygoid plate fractures (*white arrows*), indicating Le Fort fracture pattern. In this case, there are fractures through the medial maxillary buttress (*black arrows*), right orbital floor (*white arrowhead*) (b), bilateral infraorbital rims (*white arrowheads*) (c), right lateral orbital wall (*black arrowhead*) (d), and bilateral medial orbital walls (*white arrowheads*) (d). Three-dimensional (3D) CT volume-rendered reformat nicely demonstrates the three fracture patterns, including Le Fort I fracture involving the anterior maxilla and anterolateral nasal fossae (*black arrows*), Le Fort II fracture involving bilateral infraorbital rims (*white arrowheads*), and right Le Fort III fracture, including the zygomatic arch and lateral orbital wall components (*black arrowheads*). 3D reconstruction also demonstrates depressed "smash type" injury to the central midface.

Delayed complications of frontal sinus fractures may occur after facial trauma. One of the most common complications of frontal sinus fractures is mucocele formation, which can result from untreated obstruction of the frontal sinus outflow tract. A mucocele can also form if frontal sinus mucosa is left behind following frontal sinus fracture surgery. CSF leak, another delayed complication of frontal sinus fracture, may be transient or persist. Persistent CSF leaks require surgical treatment and may lead to the development of meningitis or empyema. Antibiotic prophylaxis is recommended in these patients. Chronic frontal sinus pain is another complication of frontal sinus fracture. It is difficult to predict which patients will develop chronic sinus pain, but multiple fractures seem to be an associated factor.[47]

10.6 Associated Injuries

Approximately 25% of patients with maxillofacial fractures will have associated injuries,[48] which will depend on the mechanism of trauma. Trauma of sufficient force to fracture the bones of the face is likely to involve other areas of the body and result in additional areas of injury. Motor-vehicle collisions are a major cause of systemic injury. In one study, 70% of patients with

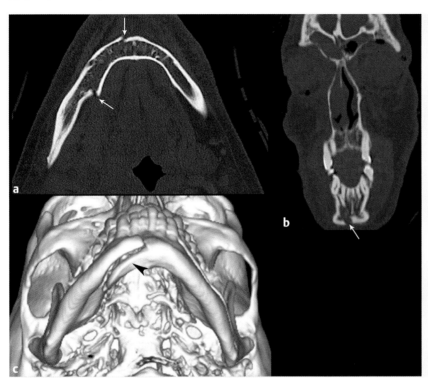

Fig. 10.12 Obliquely orientated right parasymphyseal fracture of the mandible. Axial computed tomography (CT) (a) demonstrates oblique orientation of mandibular fracture (*white arrows*). Coronal reformat (b) in this case clearly localizes the fracture to the right parasymphyseal region of the mandible (*white arrow*). Three-dimensional CT (c) is helpful in demonstrating the degree of displacement (*black arrowhead*).

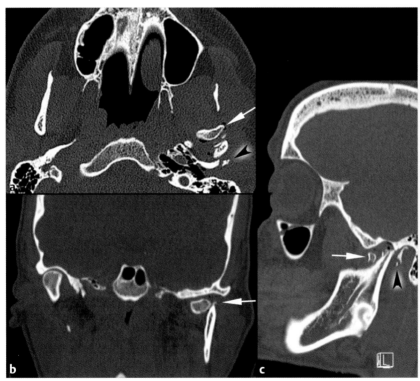

Fig. 10.13 Left subcondylar fracture of the mandible. Axial computed tomography (CT) (a) demonstrates fracture of the left mandible with anterior subluxation of condylar fragment (*white arrow*). Note the fracture of the anterior wall of the bony external auditory canal (EAC) (*black arrowhead*) with hemorrhage in the EAC. Coronal (b) and sagittal (c) reformats show subluxation of the condylar fragment medially (*white arrow*) (b) and anteriorly (*white arrow*) (c). Fracture of the anterior wall of the bony EAC redemonstrated on sagittal reformat (*arrowhead*) (c).

facial fractures from motor-vehicle crashes sustained concomitant injuries.[49]

Traumatic brain injury is an important associated finding in patients with maxillofacial fractures, with a reported incidence of 5.4 to 85%.[50–52] The wide variation of reported head injury rates may be due to differences in selection criteria. One study reported cerebral trauma to be the most commonly associated injury in patients with facial fractures, with cerebral hematoma the most common manifestation, occurring in 44% of patients with facial fractures.[53] Thus, careful analysis of the intracranial structures is warranted in patients found to have facial fractures. If needed, 5-mm axial images in standard algorithm may be reconstructed from the maxillofacial CT to best evaluate the brain and extra-axial spaces.

There is a well-known association between maxillofacial trauma and cervical spine injury, with one report finding an

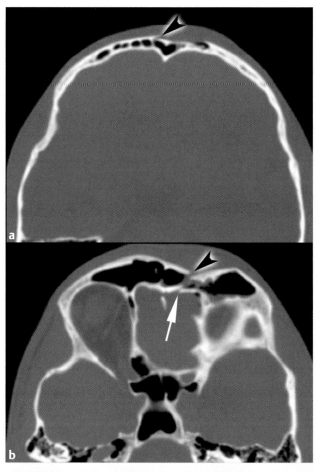

Fig. 10.14 Frontal sinus fractures. (a) Axial computed tomography demonstrates depressed fracture of the anterior (outer) table of the frontal sinus (*arrowhead*) with minimally depressed fracture of the posterior (inner) table (*white arrow*) (b).

incidence of 6.28% of combined cervical spine and maxillofacial fractures.[54] Because of this association, patients with maxillofacial fractures should be placed in cervical spine precautions until injury is excluded either clinically or radiographically.

Acute visual loss is a devastating complication of facial fractures, particularly those that affect the orbit and orbital apex, such as Le Fort III and ZMC fractures. The reported incidence of visual loss and blindness secondary to facial fractures is 1.7%.[55] Ocular and orbital injury is discussed further in Chapter 11, Traumatic Orbital Injury.

10.7 Pearls

- Maxillofacial trauma is a substantial source of morbidity and financial cost in the United States. Motor-vehicle collisions and assaults are the two most common causes of maxillofacial trauma; alcohol is frequently involved, and facial fractures are more common in men aged 20 to 40 years.
- Thin-slice CT with multiplanar reformats, particularly in the coronal plane, is the recommended modality to assess for facial fractures. Reviewing a combination of thin-slice axial images, multiplanar reformats, and 3D CT improves accuracy of detection of these fractures. 3D CT images are useful for presurgical planning, assessing the degree of comminution, localizing displaced fracture fragments, and evaluating complex multiplanar fractures.
- Secondary signs of trauma, such as subcutaneous hematoma, hemorrhagic paranasal sinus effusion, subcutaneous gas, and pneumocephalus, should guide the search for subtle maxillofacial fractures.
- Understanding the concept of facial buttresses is helpful in assessing the fracture pattern and the structures that are involved. Facial buttresses are also vital to facial stabilization and surgical reconstruction.

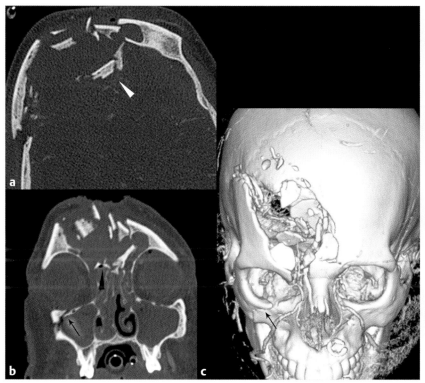

Fig. 10.15 Severely comminuted and depressed fractures of the frontal sinuses. Axial computed tomography (a) demonstrates markedly comminuted and depressed frontal sinus and frontal bone fractures. Fracture fragments intrude deeply into the brain parenchyma (*arrowhead*). Coronal reformat (b) redemonstrates severe frontal sinus fractures and shows involvement of the ethmoid roof (*arrowhead*) and infraorbital rim (*black arrow*). Three-dimensional volume-rendered reformat (c) demonstrates the extent of comminution and displacement of the frontal sinus and frontal bone fracture. Right infraorbital fracture (*black arrow*) extends into the right zygoma.

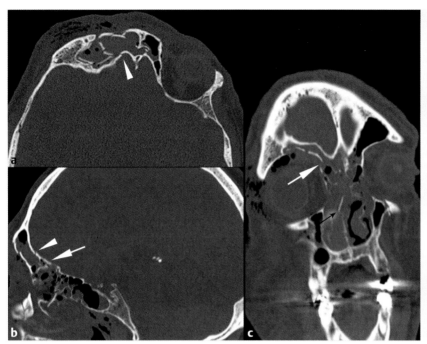

Fig. 10.16 Frontal sinus fracture with nasofrontal duct obstruction. Axial computed tomography (a) demonstrates comminuted and depressed fractures of the anterior table of the right frontal sinus with nondisplaced fracture of the posterior table (*arrowhead*). Note the fracture fragments within the sinus. Sagittal reformat (b) redemonstrates the frontal sinus fractures (*arrowhead*) with obstruction of the inferior frontal recess/nasofrontal duct by a fracture fragment (*arrow*). Coronal reformat (c) shows orbital roof fracture, with incursion of fracture fragments into the inferior frontal sinus (*white arrow*). Note also nasal septal fracture (*black arrow*).

• The forces responsible for maxillofacial trauma can cause severe injury to other parts of the body. Radiologists should be vigilant for associated injuries in patients with facial fractures, particularly head and cervical spine trauma.

References

[1] Roden KS, Tong W, Surrusco M, Shockley WW, Van Aalst JA, Hultman CS. Changing characteristics of facial fractures treated at a regional, level 1 trauma center, from 2005 to 2010: an assessment of patient demographics, referral patterns, etiology of injury, anatomic location, and clinical outcomes. Ann Plast Surg 2012; 68: 461–466

[2] Allareddy V, Allareddy V, Nalliah RP. Epidemiology of facial fracture injuries. J Oral Maxillofac Surg 2011; 69: 2613–2618

[3] Kostakis G, Stathopoulos P, Dais P, et al. An epidemiologic analysis of 1,142 maxillofacial fractures and concomitant injuries. Oral Surg Oral Med Oral Pathol Oral Radiol. 2012;114.

[4] Smith H, Peek-Asa C, Nesheim D, Nish A, Normandin P, Sahr S. Etiology, diagnosis, and characteristics of facial fracture at a midwestern level I trauma center. J Trauma Nurs. 2012; 19: 57–65

[5] Al-Qamachi LH, Laverick S, Jones DC. A clinico-demographic analysis of maxillofacial trauma in the elderly. Gerodontology 2012; 29: e147–e149

[6] Hwang K, You SH. Analysis of facial bone fractures: An 11-year study of 2,094 patients. Indian J Plast Surg . 2010; 43: 42–48

[7] Kapoor P, Kalra N. A retrospective analysis of maxillofacial injuries in patients reporting to a tertiary care hospital in East Delhi. Int J Crit Illn Inj Sci. 2012; 2: 6–10

[8] Naveen Shankar A, Naveen , Shankar V, Hegd , N , Sharma , Prasad R. The pattern of the maxillofacial fractures: a multicentre retrospective study. J Craniomaxillofac Surg 2012;

[9] Lee KH. Interpersonal violence and facial fractures. J Oral Maxillofac Surg. 2009; 67: 1878–1883

[10] Murphy RX Jr Birmingham KL, Okunski WJ, Wasser T. The influence of airbag and restraining devices on the patterns of facial trauma in motor vehicle collisions. Plast Reconstr Surg 2000; 105: 516–520

[11] Stacey DH, Doyle JF, Gutowski KA. Safety device use affects the incidence patterns of facial trauma in motor vehicle collisions: an analysis of the National Trauma Database from 2000 to 2004. Plast Reconstr Surg 2008; 121: 2057–2064

[12] Borah GL, Rankin MK. Appearance is a function of the face. Plast Reconstr Surg. 2010; 125: 873–878

[13] Linnau KF, Stanley RB Jr Hallam DK, Gross JA, Mann FA. Imaging of high-energy midfacial trauma: what the surgeon needs to know. Eur J Radiol 2003; 48: 17–32

[14] Tanrikulu R, Erol B. Comparison of computed tomography with conventional radiography for midfacial fractures. Dentomaxillofac Radiol. 2001; 30: 141–146

[15] Dos Santos DT, Costa e Silva AP, Vannier MW, Cavalcanti MG. Validity of multislice computerized tomography for diagnosis of maxillofacial fractures using an independent workstation. Oral Surg Oral Med Oral Pathol Oral Radiol Endod 2004; 98: 715–720

[16] Mayer JS, Wainwright DJ, Yeakley JW, Lee KF, Harris JH, Jr, Kulkarni M. The role of three-dimensional computed tomography in the management of maxillofacial trauma. J Trauma 1988; 28: 1043–1053

[17] Saigal K, Winokur RS, Finden S, Taub D, Pribitkin E. Use of three-dimensional computerized tomography reconstruction in complex facial trauma. Facial Plast Surg 2005; 21: 214–220

[18] Rabie A, Ibrahim AM, Lee BT, Lin SJ. Use of intraoperative computed tomography in complex facial fracture reduction and fixation. J Craniofac Surg 2011; 22: 1466–1467

[19] Hussain K, Wijetunge DB, Grubnic S, Jackson IT. A comprehensive analysis of craniofacial trauma. J Trauma 1994; 36: 34–47

[20] Renner GJ. Management of nasal fractures. Otolaryngol Clin North Am 1991; 24: 195–213

[21] Logan M, O'Driscoll K, Masterson J. The utility of nasal bone radiographs in nasal trauma. Clin Radiol 1994; 49: 192–194

[22] Higuera S, Lee EI, Cole P, Hollier LH, Jr, Stal S. Nasal trauma and the deviated nose. Plast Reconstr Surg 2007; 120 Suppl 2: 64S–75S

[23] Markowitz BL, Manson PN, Sargent L et al. Management of the medial canthal tendon in nasoethmoid orbital fractures: the importance of the central fragment in classification and treatment. Plast Reconstr Surg 1991; 87: 843–853

[24] Paskert JP, Manson PN. The bimanual examination for assessing instability in naso-orbitoethmoidal injuries. Plast Reconstr Surg 1989; 83: 165–167

[25] Daly BD, Russell JL, Davidson MJ, Lamb JT. Thin section computed tomography in the evaluation of naso-ethmoidal trauma. Clin Radiol 1990; 41: 272–275

[26] Remmler D, Denny A, Gosain A, Subichin S. Role of three-dimensional computed tomography in the assessment of nasoorbitoethmoidal fractures. Ann Plast Surg 2000; 44: 553–563

[27] Gerlock AJ, Sinn DP. Anatomic, clinical, surgical, and radiographic correlation of the zygomatic complex fracture. AJR Am J Roentgenol 1977; 128: 235–238

[28] Jackson IT. Classification and treatment of orbitozygomatic and orbitoethmoid fractures: the place of bone grafting and plate fixation. Clin Plast Surg 1989; 16: 77–91

[29] Zingg M, Laedrach K, Chen J et al. Classification and treatment of zygomatic fractures: a review of 1,025 cases. J Oral Maxillofac Surg 1992; 50: 778–790

[30] Kelley P, Hopper R, Gruss J. Evaluation and treatment of zygomatic fractures. Plast Reconstr Surg 2007; 120 Suppl 2: 5S–15S

[31] Olate S, Lima SM Jr Sawazaki R, Moreira RW, de Moraes M. Variables related to surgical and nonsurgical treatment of zygomatic complex fracture. J Craniofac Surg 2011; 22: 1200–1202

[32] Tessier P. The classic reprint: experimental study of fractures of the upper jaw. I and II. René Le Fort, M.D. Plast Reconstr Surg 1972; 50: 497–506

[33] Rhea JT, Novelline RA. How to simplify the CT diagnosis of Le Fort fractures. AJR Am J Roentgenol 2005; 184: 1700–1705

[34] Fraioli RE, Branstetter BF, IV, Deleyiannis FW. Facial fractures: beyond Le Fort. Otolaryngol Clin North Am 2008; 41: 51–76, vi.

[35] Follmar KE, Baccarani A, Das RR, Erdmann D, Marcus JR, Mukundan S. A clinically applicable reporting system for the diagnosis of facial fractures. Int J Oral Maxillofac Surg 2007; 36: 593–600

[36] Stacey DH, Doyle JF, Mount DL, Snyder MC, Gutowski KA. Management of mandible fractures. Plast Reconstr Surg 2006; 117: 48e–60e

[37] van den Bergh B, van Es C, Forouzanfar T. Analysis of mandibular fractures. J Craniofac Surg 2011; 22: 1631–1634

[38] Rhea JT, Rao PM, Novelline RA. Helical CT and three-dimensional CT of facial and orbital injury. Radiol Clin North Am 1999; 37: 489–513

[39] Wilson IF, Lokeh A, Benjamin CI et al. Prospective comparison of panoramic tomography (zonography) and helical computed tomography in the diagnosis and operative management of mandibular fractures. Plast Reconstr Surg 2001; 107: 1369–1375

[40] Shankar DP, Manodh P, Devadoss P, Thomas TK. Mandibular fracture scoring system: for prediction of complications. Oral Maxillofac Surg. 2012;16 (4):355–360.

[41] Yavuzer R, Sari A, Kelly CP et al. Management of frontal sinus fractures. Plast Reconstr Surg 2005; 115: 79e–95e

[42] Strong EB, Pahlavan N, Saito D. Frontal sinus fractures: a 28-year retrospective review. Otolaryngol Head Neck Surg 2006; 135: 774–779

[43] Wallis A, Donald PJ. Frontal sinus fractures: a review of 72 cases. Laryngoscope 1988; 98: 593–598

[44] Jain SA, Manchio JV, Weinzweig J. Role of the sagittal view of computed tomography in evaluation of the nasofrontal ducts in frontal sinus fractures. J Craniofac Surg 2010; 21: 1670–1673

[45] Tedaldi M, Ramieri V, Foresta E, Cascone P, Iannetti G. Experience in the management of frontal sinus fractures. J Craniofac Surg 2010; 21: 208–210

[46] Echo A, Troy JS, Hollier LH, Jr. Frontal sinus fractures. Semin Plast Surg. 2010; 24: 375–382

[47] Metzinger SE, Metzinger RC. Complications of frontal sinus fractures. Craniomaxillofac Trauma Reconstr 2009; 2: 27–34

[48] Thorén H, Snäll J, Salo J et al. Occurrence and types of associated injuries in patients with fractures of the facial bones. J Oral Maxillofac Surg 2010; 68: 805–810

[49] Follmar KE, Debruijn M, Baccarani A et al. Concomitant injuries in patients with panfacial fractures. J Trauma 2007; 63: 831–835

[50] Lim LH, Lam LK, Moore MH, Trott JA, David DJ. Associated injuries in facial fractures: review of 839 patients. Br J Plast Surg 1993; 46: 635–638

[51] Luce EA, Tubb TD, Moore AM. Review of 1,000 major facial fractures and associated injuries. Plast Reconstr Surg 1979; 63: 26–30

[52] Sinclair D, Schwartz M, Gruss J, McLellan B. A retrospective review of the relationship between facial fractures, head injuries, and cervical spine injuries. J Emerg Med 1988; 6: 109–112

[53] Alvi A, Doherty T, Lewen G. Facial fractures and concomitant injuries in trauma patients. Laryngoscope 2003; 113: 102–106

[54] Jamal BT, Diecidue R, Qutob A, Cohen M. The pattern of combined maxillofacial and cervical spine fractures. J Oral Maxillofac Surg 2009; 67: 559–562

[55] Magarakis M, Mundinger GS, Kelamis JA, Dorafshar AH, Bojovic B, Rodriguez ED. Ocular injury, visual impairment, and blindness associated with facial fractures: a systematic literature review. Plast Reconstr Surg 2012; 129: 227–233

11 Traumatic Orbital and Occular Injury

Roberta W. Dalley and Sarah J. Foster

11.1 Introduction

Bony orbital and ocular trauma is common in the setting of head trauma. Double vision, a partial loss of vision, or a complete loss of vision in one or both eyes may occur. Facial disfigurement by fractures, lacerations, or loss of an eye may require facial reconstruction or even an ocular prosthesis. High-quality, precise, and complete ocular and orbital imaging is crucial to assessment of the degree of injury to the orbit, as well as to plan surgical approaches for emergency treatment or subsequent reconstruction.

11.2 Ocular and Orbital Soft Tissue Anatomy

An understanding of ocular anatomy is critical to appreciating how trauma can affect distinct parts of the orbit and globe. The globe has an anterior segment containing aqueous humor and a posterior segment containing more viscous vitreous humor (▶ Fig. 11.1). The anterior segment is further divided into an anterior and posterior chamber separated by the iris. The lens is situated posterior to the iris and is held in suspension by zonular radial fibers of the ciliary body. The globe has three layers: an outer fibrous sclera, a middle vascular choroid, and an innermost neural layer (the retina). The sclera is continuous anteriorly with the conjunctiva, and the choroidal layer attaches to the ora serrate at the level of the ciliary body anteriorly. The ocular muscles are in the conal space and are surrounded by a fibrous layer called the tenons capsule. The muscles attach to the globe via their respective tendons and pierce the sclera at their points of attachment. The optic nerve sheath contains the optic nerve, veins, and lymphatics. The sheath itself is a dural reflection. The central retinal artery lies outside the sheath.

11.3 Orbital Imaging Modalities

11.3.1 Volume Computed Tomography

Computed tomography (CT) is the primary modality for assessing orbital soft tissue and bony injury in the emergency setting. CT scanning of the orbits is very quick, which significantly reduces motion artifacts. The following discussion assumes a volume CT technique using a multidetector scanner when referring to CT. Volume CT also allows multiplanar reformations in any desired plane. It can distinguish a variety of soft tissue orbital injuries, including foreign bodies, gas, edema, hemorrhage, and ocular injures. CT is also useful for assessing bone thickness, fracture, and displacements, as well as intracranial complications. The major concern with orbital CT is the radiation dose to the ocular lens. Current-generation CT scanners are able to decrease the radiation dose by at least 50% compared with earlier CT scanner generations. In addition, using volume scanning to reconstruct coronal and sagittal reformations eliminates the need for direct coronal scans, which in combination with axial scans, doubles the radiation dose to the lens. A further disadvantage of direct coronal orbital imaging was that it was often significantly degraded by dental metallic streak artifact. CT angiography also can be performed rapidly to assess adjacent vascular injury of the internal carotid (ICA) and external carotid artery (ECA) branches.

11.3.2 Magnetic Resonance Imaging

Magnetic resonance imaging (MRI) of the orbit is less frequently used than CT is in the setting of traumatic injury. MRI of the orbit requires more time and a cooperative patient who can hold his or her eyes relatively still. In acute orbital trauma, any suspicion of a potential foreign body in the orbit needs initial evaluation by CT to exclude a metal foreign body. If no foreign body is suspected or if a metal foreign body has been excluded by CT, then MRI may have a limited role in evaluating orbital soft tissue injury and any associated intracranial complications of the trauma.

Ultrasound

Radiologists in the United States do not commonly use ultrasound for orbital trauma, but ophthalmologists may use it in their office to quickly locate an intraocular foreign body, retinal detachment, or choroidal detachment. This testing is particularly useful if direct visualization via ophthalmoscopic examination is obscured by intraocular hemorrhage. Ultrasound of the orbit is highly sensitive and specific for globe injury and is easy to implement in the emergency department setting. Ultrasound, however, must not be used in the setting of known or

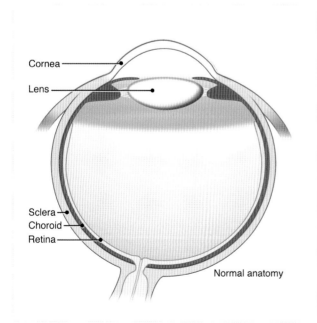

Fig. 11.1 Illustration showing the layers and structures of the normal globe.

Cornea
Lens
Sclera
Choroid
Retina
Normal anatomy

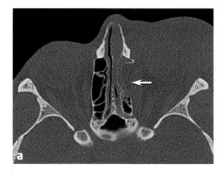

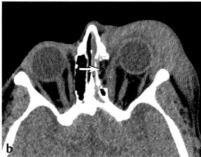

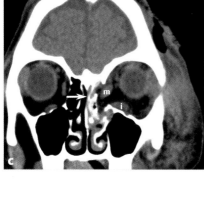

Fig. 11.2 Medial orbital blowout fracture. (a) Axial bone and (b) axial and (c) coronal computed tomography soft tissue images demonstrate an acute medial orbital blowout fracture (*arrow*) of the left orbit, with medial herniation of the medial rectus muscle into the ethmoid sinus fracture. Moderate periorbital soft tissue swelling is present. Note the distortion and swelling of both the left medial (m) and inferior (i) rectus muscles on the coronal view.

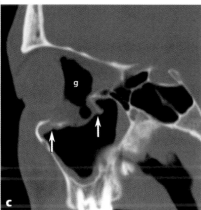

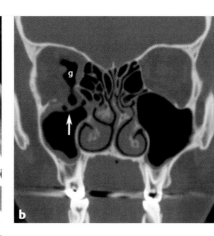

Fig. 11.3 Orbital floor blowout fracture. (a) Axial computed tomographic view showing right globe proptosis and retro-ocular gas (g). (b) Coronal bone image shows depressed right orbital floor fracture with orbital fat and retro-ocular gas herniating (*vertical arrow*) into the defect. (c) Sagittal view demonstrates the anterior and posterior extent (*vertical arrows*) of the depressed floor fracture.

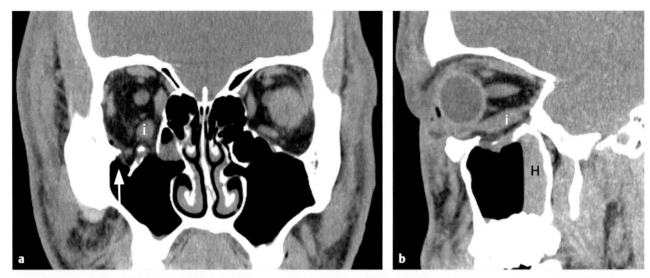

Fig. 11.4 Inferior extraocular muscle distortion. (a) Coronal and (b) sagittal computed tomographic views showing only fat herniating into the depressed orbital floor defect (*arrow*) but associated edema and distortion of the inferior rectus muscle (*i*) without downward herniation. Note the hemorrhagic air-fluid level (*H*) in the maxillary sinus on the sagittal view.

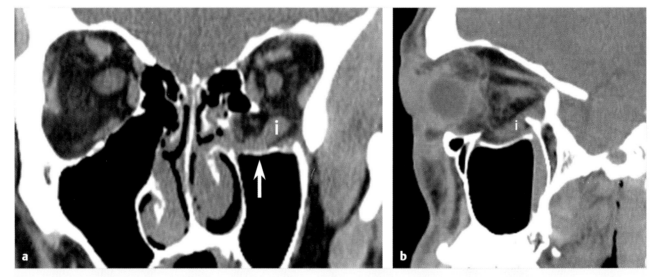

Fig. 11.5 Inferior extraocular muscle distortion. (a) Coronal and (b) sagittal soft tissue computed tomographic images of the acute left orbit depressed floor fracture (*arrow*) with both fat and inferior rectus muscle (*i*) herniation into the defect. Although the inferior rectus muscle is displaced, it is not entrapped by bone.

suspected globe rupture because it could potentially aggravate the injury.

11.4 Fractures of the Bony Orbit

Fractures can involve any of the bones that border the bony orbit. These bones include frontal, zygomatic, lacrimal, ethmoid, and sphenoid bones. Orbital fractures may be isolated (e.g., blowout fracture, orbital rim fracture) or part of a more complex maxillofacial or skull-base fracture (e.g., zygomaticomaxillary fracture, Le Fort II or III fracture, naso-orbito-ethmoid fracture, orbital apex fracture, and sphenoid wing fracture). A combination of several patterns of fracture may

coexist. Classification of fractures involving the orbit is a means of simplifying the description of the injury.

11.4.1 Blowout Fracture

An orbital blowout fracture refers to two kinds of fractures that can occur through the weakest portions of the orbit: (1) medial orbital wall with the thin weak lamina papyracea of the ethmoid bone (▶ Fig. 11.2); and (2) orbital floor with the linear weak infraorbital canal (▶ Fig. 11.3). These fractures do not involve the orbital rim and are usually a result of blunt trauma from an object larger than the orbital rim, such as a fist or softball. The most common complications of this fracture are dysfunction of the medial rectus in a medial wall fracture or dysfunction of the inferior rectus with an orbital floor fracture (▶ Fig. 11.4; ▶ Fig. 11.5). The extraocular muscles may be edematous or have an intramuscular hematoma.

In addition, displacement or entrapment may occur through the bony defect (▶ Fig. 11.6; ▶ Fig. 11.7). Subperiosteal hematoma is either not present or is a minor component of this injury. Subperiosteal abscess is a rare complication of blowout fracture (▶ Fig. 11.8). Anesthesia of the maxillary division of cranial nerve V may occur if the fracture involves V2 in the infraorbital canal. Surgical repair with an implant reinforcing the floor or wall is often recommended in the first week or two after injury to prevent fibrosis and scarring from causing permanent muscular dysfunction (▶ Fig. 11.9).

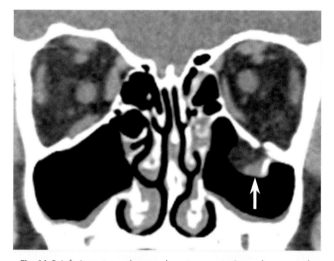

Fig. 11.6 Inferior extraocular muscle entrapment. Coronal computed tomographic view shows acute left orbital blowout fracture with both fat and inferior rectus muscle (*vertical arrow*) entrapped below the orbital floor.

11.4.2 Orbital Roof Fracture

Fractures of the orbital roof are usually seen in combination with extension of linear frontal bone fractures or with complex cranial-facial fractures, including Le Fort III, naso-orbito-ethmoidal (NOE), skull-base fractures extending into the anterior skull base. A supraorbital subperiosteal hematoma is commonly seen (▶ Fig. 11.10; ▶ Fig. 11.11), which often causes acute ocular proptosis. These are usually treated noninvasively unless a bone fragment is rotated or displaced with impingement on the superior muscle complex or optic nerve.

11.4.3 Blow-In Fracture

A blow-in fracture is an uncommon subtype of orbital roof fracture. A high-velocity projectile penetrating the skull and passing through the brain causes a blow-in fracture. The shock wave from the projectile causes a caudal or downward directed force on the floor of the anterior cranial fossa, resulting in comminuted, inferiorly displaced fractures through one or both orbital roofs (▶ Fig. 11.12).

11.4.4 Zygomaticomaxillary Fracture

This relatively common facial fracture has gone by several names: tripod fracture, trimalar fracture, and now zygomaticomaxillary (ZMC) fracture. These fractures are usually caused by blunt-force injury to the malar eminence of the body of the zygoma. The fractures essentially pass through or near the zygoma's sutures with adjacent bones, including the frontozygomatic, zygomatico-maxillary, and the zygomatico-temporal sutures. A ZMC fracture may be nondisplaced or have both a displacement and rotary component. By definition, the fractures involve the lateral and inferior orbital rim, orbital floor, and lateral orbital wall (▶ Fig. 11.13). Anesthesia from the orbital floor fracture crossing the infraorbital canal may injure V2, the maxillary division of cranial nerve V. Subperiosteal hematomas or intrasinus hemorrhage may also occur with this injury.

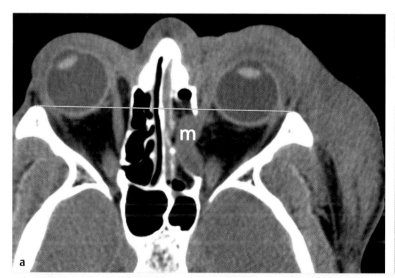
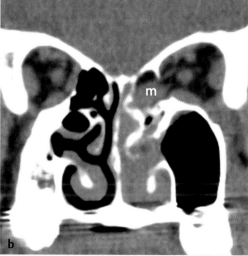

Fig. 11.7 Medial extraocular muscle entrapment. (a) Axial and (b) coronal computed tomographic images demonstrate complete herniation and entrapment of the swollen medial rectus muscle (*m*) into the acute medial orbital wall defect with associated enophthalmos.

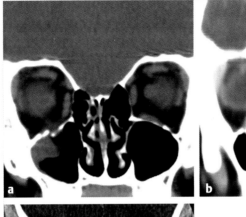

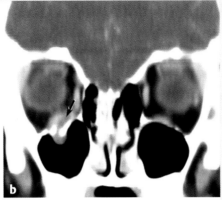

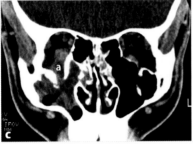

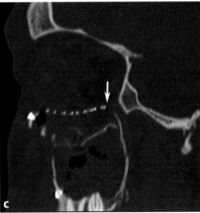

Fig. 11.8 Abscess complicating blowout fracture. (a) Coronal computed tomographic (CT) images showing an acute right orbital floor fracture. (b) Coronal CT in the same patient 3 weeks later returning with proptosis and pain showing a new subperiosteal abscess (*arrow*) between the inferior rectus and the orbital floor. (c) A different patient returned to the emergency department after being punched in the right eye a week earlier, now experiencing redness and swelling of the right orbit. Note the subperiosteal abscess (a) elevating the inferior rectus muscle and the associated maxillary sinus inflammation.

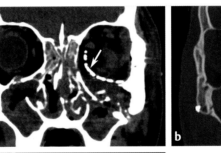

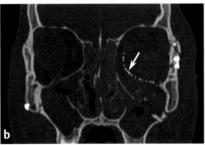

Fig. 11.9 Postoperative repair blowout fracture. (a) Coronal soft tissue and (b) bone computed tomographic images show a large depressed left medial and inferior orbital floor defect repaired with the placement of a curved mesh implant (*arrow*) underneath the inferior rectus muscle to approximate the normal position of the new orbital floor. (c) Sagittal image indicates the anterior-posterior extent (*arrow*) of the implant.

Displaced fractures are usually treated with surgical fixation along the lateral or infraorbital rim.

11.4.5 Le Fort II and Le Fort III Fractures

Le Fort fractures are seen with high-velocity or high-impact energy blunt trauma, most commonly with a victim in a high-speed motor-vehicle collision. Le Fort injuries are usually bilateral and involve the pterygoid plates and the nasal septum. Orbital involvement is seen only in Le Fort II and Le Fort III

fractures. A Le Fort II fracture passes through the infraorbital rim and medial orbit (▸ Fig. 11.14a,b). It may injure V2 if it passes through the infraorbital canal or foramen. A Le Fort III fracture passes through the frontozygomatic suture, lateral orbital wall, orbital floor, and medial orbit (▸ Fig. 11.14c–f). V2 injury may be seen with this injury as well. Intraorbital soft tissue and subperiosteal hematomas are common. Ocular injury may be present. Displaced Le Fort fractures are usually treated operatively with plates.

11.4.6 Naso-Orbito-Ethmoid

A naso-orbito-ethmoid (NOE) fracture may be more accurately described as a naso-ethmoid-frontal fracture pattern. This fracture is most commonly caused by a blunt-force injury to the central midface, nose, and frontal bones (▶ Fig. 11.15a,b). It tends to fracture the medial buttresses but spares the lateral buttresses of the face. This injury drives the anterior portion of the ethmoid bone and/ or glabella of the frontal bone posteriorly or the glabella of the frontal bone posteriorly, telescoping the impacted bones into the deeper midface. Hypertelorism with widening of the interpupillary distance is common and is caused by the lateral expansion of the collapsed anterior ethmoid complex (▶ Fig. 11.15c–f). Involvement of the nasolacrimal duct may cause epiphora as a result of obstruction of lacrimal drainage. Ocular and retro-ocular soft tissue injury is often present. Displaced naso-ethmoid-frontal fractures are usually treated operatively with plates.

11.4.7 Medial Buttress Fracture

A medial buttress fracture can be thought of as a unilateral subtype of the naso-orbito-ethmoid. This medial buttress comprises the medial maxilla, frontal process of the maxilla, and nasal bone. This fracture often has its superior extent at the frontal-maxillary suture at the glabella (▶ Fig. 11.16). Like the NOE fracture, the medial buttress fracture can obstruct the nasolacrimal duct and cause epiphora.

11.4.8 Orbital Apex Fracture and Optic Canal Fracture

Fractures of the anterior skull base and central skull base may include the orbital apex. These fractures may include the sagittal plane posterior extension of the frontal bone and NOE

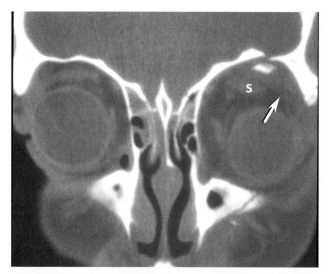

Fig. 11.10 Orbital roof fracture. Coronal computed tomographic image showing an inferiorly displaced orbital roof fracture fragment with an associated subperiosteal hematoma (*arrow*) displacing the superior muscle complex (s) and globe inferiorly.

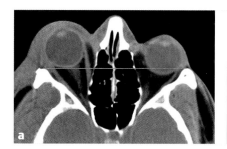
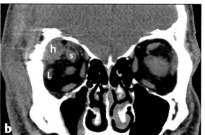

Fig. 11.11 Postoperative subperiosteal hematoma. (a) Axial computed tomography shows proptosis of the right globe. (b) Coronal image demonstrates postoperative superolateral right subperiosteal hematoma (*h*) from a pterional craniotomy, which is causing an intraorbital mass effect and displacing the superior (*s*) muscle complex and lateral (*L*) rectus muscle.

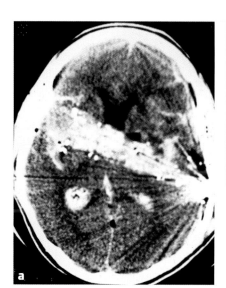
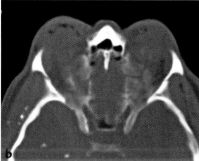

Fig. 11.12 Orbital blow-in fracture. (a) Axial head computed tomography shows a gunshot wound traversing the frontal lobes and basal ganglia with a high density hemorrhagic tract. (b) Axial bone windows show bilateral comminuted orbital roof fractures depressed down into the obits by the shock wave of the bullet traversing the brain.

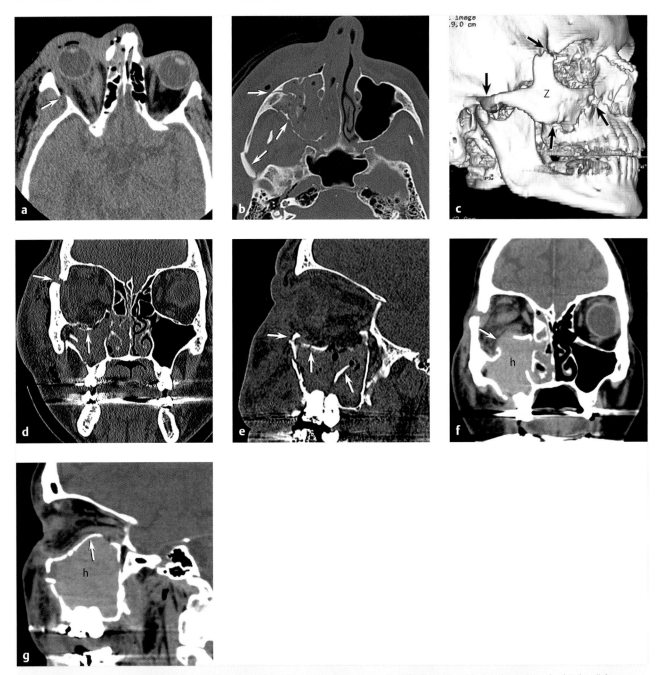

Fig. 11.13 Zygomaticomaxillary complex (ZMC) fracture. (a) Axial computed tomography (CT) through midorbit shows lateral orbital wall fracture (*arrow*) and retro-ocular hemorrhage. (b) Axial CT through maxillary sinus shows zygomatic arch and maxillary wall fractures (*arrows*). (c) Three-dimensional CT reformations showing ZMC fractures (*arrows*) with free zygomatic (Z) bone fragment. (d) Coronal and (e) sagittal images demonstrating a depressed orbital floor, infraorbital rim, and frontozygomatic suture fractures (*arrows*) with hemorrhage in the maxillary sinus. (f) Coronal and (g) sagittal repeat CT 4 hours later showing increased maxillary sinus bleeding (*h*) with unusual reversal of the orbital floor fracture now herniating up into the orbit (*arrow*) causing new proptosis.

fractures, coronal plane fractures extending from one or both longitudinal temporal fractures that extend into the sphenoid bone, and complex fractures of the greater sphenoid wing. Fracture fragments and orbital apex hematoma may compromise the optic nerve (► Fig. 11.17a,b).

An optic canal fracture is a subtype of the orbital apex fracture, which specifically involves the body of the sphenoid bone at the confluence of the lesser sphenoid wing and anterior clinoid process, which form the margins of the optic canal. With the optic nerve and ophthalmic artery passing through the optic canal, displaced fragments and shearing forces may injure the tightly confined optic nerve resulting in visual loss (► Fig. 11.17c,d,e).

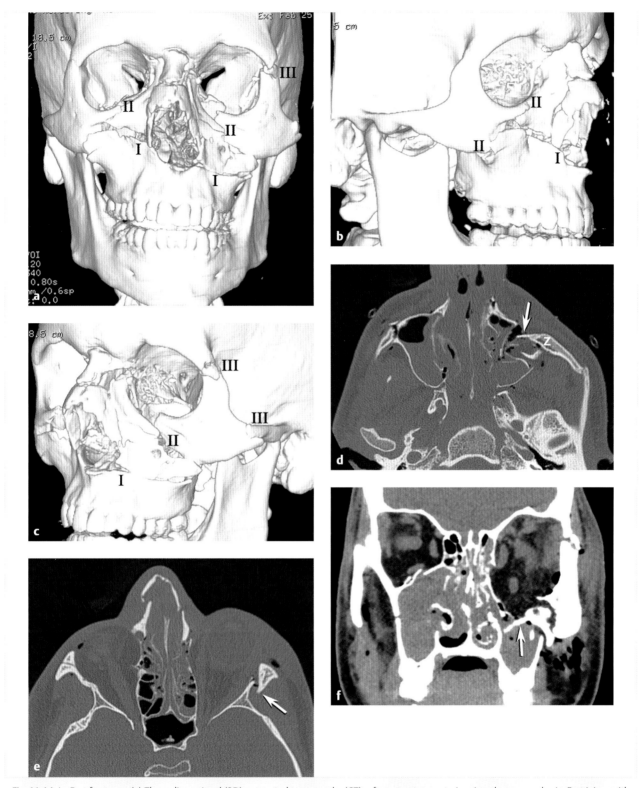

Fig. 11.14 Le Fort fractures. (a) Three-dimensional (3D) computed tomography (CT) reformat anteroposterior view shows complex Le Fort injury with bilateral Le Fort I, right Le Fort II, and left Le Fort III fractures. (b) 3D CT reformat right oblique view shows that this Le Fort II fracture involves the right infraorbital rim, anterior-lateral maxilla, and nasal arch, sparing the zygomatic arch and frontozygomatic suture. (c) 3D CT reformat left oblique view shows Le Fort III fracture through infraorbital rim, nasal arch, frontozygomatic suture, and zygomatic arch resulting in a free zygomatic fragment. (d) Axial CT shows medial and posterior rotation (*arrow*) of free zygomatic fragment (*z*) in left complex Le Fort I and III fracture. (e) Axial CT demonstrates Le Fort III fracture on the left with lateral orbital wall (*arrow*) and nasal arch and bilateral anterior ethmoid fractures. Le Fort II on right spares lateral orbital wall. (f) Coronal CT shows left orbital floor displaced fracture (*arrow*) as a component of the left Le Fort III injury.

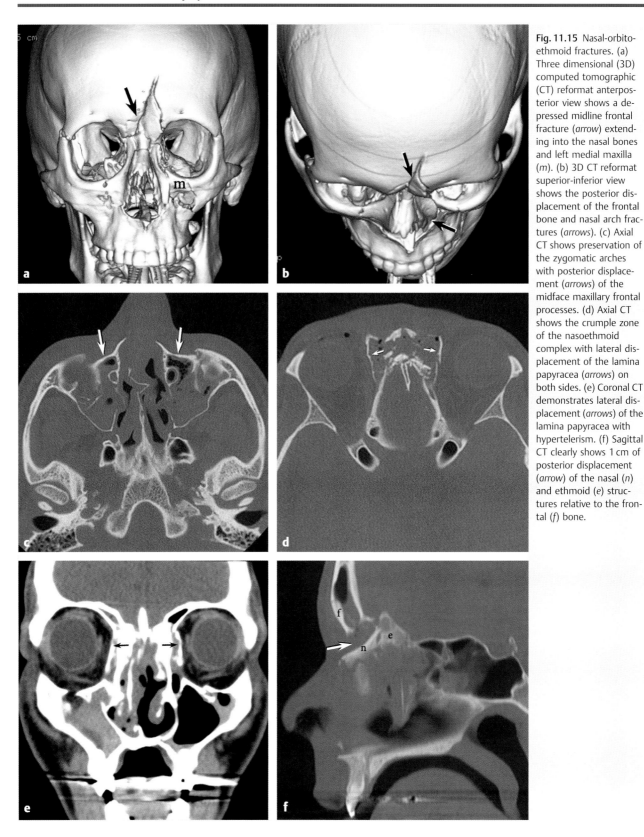

Fig. 11.15 Nasal-orbito-ethmoid fractures. (a) Three dimensional (3D) computed tomographic (CT) reformat anterposterior view shows a depressed midline frontal fracture (*arrow*) extending into the nasal bones and left medial maxilla (*m*). (b) 3D CT reformat superior-inferior view shows the posterior displacement of the frontal bone and nasal arch fractures (*arrows*). (c) Axial CT shows preservation of the zygomatic arches with posterior displacement (*arrows*) of the midface maxillary frontal processes. (d) Axial CT shows the crumple zone of the nasoethmoid complex with lateral displacement of the lamina papyracea (*arrows*) on both sides. (e) Coronal CT demonstrates lateral displacement (*arrows*) of the lamina papyracea with hypertelerism. (f) Sagittal CT clearly shows 1 cm of posterior displacement (*arrow*) of the nasal (*n*) and ethmoid (*e*) structures relative to the frontal (*f*) bone.

11.5 Injury to the Orbital Soft Tissues

The soft tissues of the orbit may be injured in both blunt and penetrating facial trauma. Assessment of the optic pathway for injury or foreign body is critical and should include the eye and optic nerve. Hematoma and edema may affect the preseptal soft tissues, retro-ocular fat, and subperiosteal space. These tissues can be readily assessed using volume CT techniques.

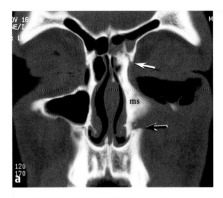

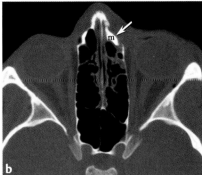

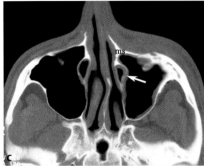

Fig. 11.16 Medial buttress fracture. (a) Coronal computed tomography (CT) shows medial rotation of the left medial maxilla (*ms*, medial strut) at the nasofrontal suture (*white arrow*) superiorly and the anterior maxilla fracture zone (*black arrow*) inferiorly. Subcutaneous emphysema in the left lower eyelid. (b) Axial CT shows posteromedial displacement (*arrow*) of the frontal process of maxilla (*m*) superiorly. (c) Axial CT demonstrates medial rotation of the medial strut (*ms*) and compression of the nasolacrimal duct (*arrow*) inferiorly.

11.5.1 Mass Effect

Acute mass effect in the orbit may manifest as compression of one side of the globe, axial proptosis, or off-axis displacement of the globe. Orbital soft tissue mass effect is more commonly unilateral, but it can be bilateral.

Proptosis can be assessed by the globe position relative to the orbital rim. At the midglobe level on an axial CT slice, the interzygomatic line (a line drawn from one frontozygomatic suture or lateral orbital rim to the contralateral lateral orbital rim) will normally show about a third of the posterior globe behind the interzygomatic line (▶ Fig. 11.18a). The inner-to-outer canthal line is often more challenging to use because the medial bony landmark of the frontal process of the maxilla is often harder to define (▶ Fig. 11.18b). In a normal orbit, about half of the globe should lie posterior to this line. Relative proptosis can then be measured, especially if only one eye or orbit is injured. Difficulty occurs in ZMC, Le Fort III, and NOE fractures, which disrupt and displace bony landmarks, making the drawing of these lines problematic.

Globe tenting is another measure of acute orbital tension associated with axial globe proptosis. As the globe is pushed anteriorly, the optic nerve begins to straighten and stretch, tethering the posterior globe margin at the optic nerve head, causing a conical deformation of the posterior globe (▶ Fig. 11.18c). When an angle is measured subtending the tethered posterior globe margin at the optic nerve head, an angle less than 120 degrees (▶ Fig. 11.18d,e) may correlate with a high incidence of afferent pupillary defect.[1] Urgent decompression of the proptosis and globe tenting are needed to preserve vision.

Enophthalmos, or a sunken globe position, may be noted when the orbital fractures effectively increase the bony orbital volume compared with the pretrauma volume, such as in large displaced medial and inferior blowout fractures (▶ Fig. 11.19) or laterally displaced ZMC fractures.

11.5.2 Blunt Orbital Trauma

Blunt Globe Trauma

Ocular injury in the setting of major trauma arriving in emergency departments ranges in the literature between 2 and 3%. More than half of cases are secondary to motor-vehicle accidents. The term *blunt trauma* refers to all nonpenetrating injuries to the orbit; these injuries represent more than 95% of the causes of ocular injury according to studies in the literature; penetrating injuries are in the minority as mechanisms of injury.[2] (Penetrating injuries are discussed in a separate section to follow). The aim of ocular imaging in the setting of trauma is to address the specific injury to help in management decisions that may save threatened visual loss and determine prognosis.

The risk of ocular injury is significantly greater in the setting of fracture of the seven bones that constitute the walls of the orbit. Fractures of the walls of the orbit have decreased by 50% with the advent of seat-belt laws. Blunt ocular injuries result from either direct laceration or impingement by a periorbital fracture or by the transmission of shear forces or increased intraocular pressures by the trauma itself or resultant hematoma.

The most common injuries seen in blunt trauma of the orbit include lens dislocation or subluxation, corneal abrasions, anterior chamber hematomas, posterior segment vitreous hemorrhage, retinal or choroidal detachments, optic nerve injury, extraocular muscle injury or entrapment, and carotid-cavernous fistula. Periorbital facial fractures are covered separately.

Corneal Tear

A tear in the cornea will result in decreased volume of the anterior chamber (▶ Fig. 11.20). This loss of volume is a secondary sign of the underlying corneal injury, and the tear itself is not directly seen on CT. Careful assessment of the lens is required,

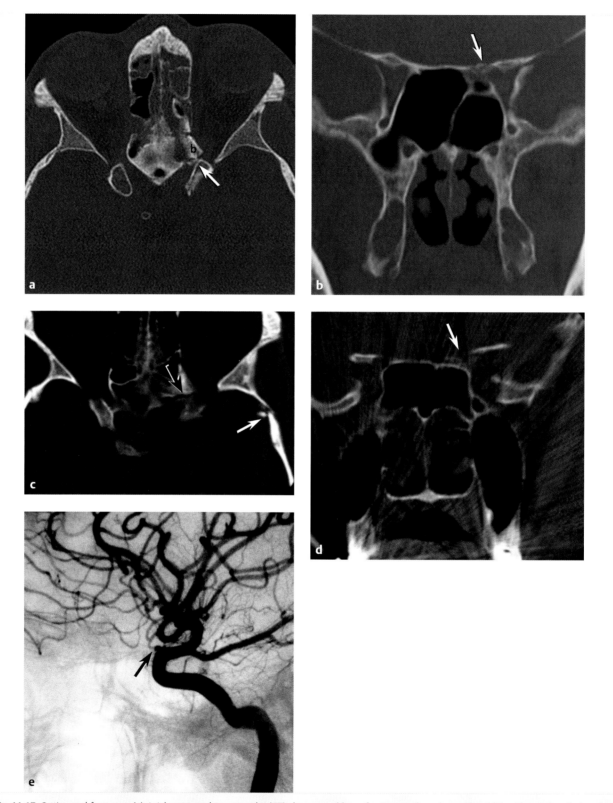

Fig. 11.17 Optic canal fractures. (a) Axial computed tomography (CT) shows an oblique fracture at the sphenoethmoid junction and a displaced fracture fragment (*b*) in the left optic canal (*arrow*). (b) Coronal CT same patient with fracture through the sphenoid lesser wing and medial-superior wall (*arrow*) of the left optic canal. (c) Axial CT in a different patient with complete visual loss in the left eye after a motor-vehicle collision; CT shows fractures laterally through the left greater sphenoid wing (*white arrow*) extending medially into the lesser sphenoid wing (*black arrow*) structures of the anterior clinoid and left optic canal. (d) Coronal CT demonstrates disruption of the left anterior clinoid and bone fragments (*arrow*) in the left optic canal. (e) Lateral left internal carotid artery angiogram shows complete cutoff of the left ophthalmic artery (*arrow*).

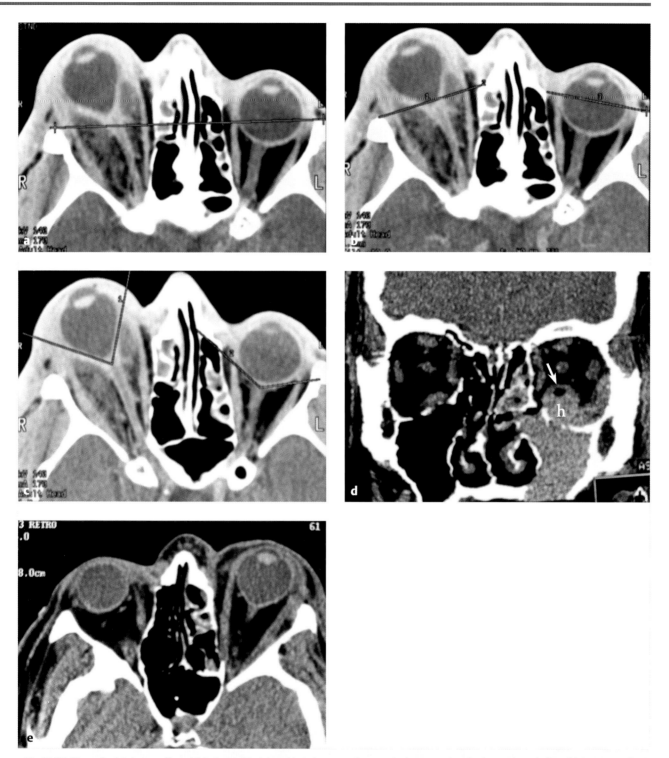

Fig. 11.18 Signs of orbital mass effect. (a) Patient with right orbital abscess and proptosis demonstrating the interzygomatic line. (b) Demonstration of the inner-to-outer canthal lines. (c) Globe tenting on the right with a posterior globe angle of 85 degrees compared with a normal left posterior globe angle of 135 degrees. (d) Coronal computed tomography (CT) shows a different patient with an inferior blowout fracture with subperiosteal hematoma (*h*) elevating the inferior rectus muscle (*arrow*). (e) Axial CT from the same patient demonstrates proptosis and moderate acute globe tenting.

however, because an anterior subluxation of the lens will also decrease the depth of the anterior chamber mimicking a corneal injury.

Globe Rupture

The globe can rupture in the absence of penetrating trauma. Shear injury with laceration of the sclera can result in rupture, as can direct impact causing a transient peak of high intraocular pressure (▶ Fig. 11.21). The globe will appear distorted and of small volume (▶ Fig. 11.22a,b). The classic appearance is the "flat-tire sign"[3] or "drooping lily" sign (▶ Fig. 11.22c,d). A subperiosteal hematoma may result in mass effect and proptosis with stretching of the optic nerve. The long-term sequela of chronic globe rupture is a shrunken calcified globe termed *phthisis bulbi* (▶ Fig. 11.23), in which the lens, vitreous, or sclera may calcify.

Anterior Chamber Hematoma

Blood products in the anterior chamber result from tearing of the small arteries within the ciliary body. The anterior chamber will have attenuation higher than the contralateral normal side

(▶ Fig. 11.24) and will have variable T1 and T2 signal on MRI, depending on the degradation state of the hemoglobin.

Lens Injury

When the orbit sustains an impact of force anteriorly, such as from a fist, dashboard, or bat, the globe is compressed in the anteroposterior dimension and is deformed outwardly. The outward pressures can disrupt the zonular fibers partially or completely, leading to lens subluxation or dislocation (▶ Fig. 11.25a). The iris usually inhibits an anterior lens dislocation; therefore, a posterior subluxation or dislocation is the most common finding.[4] Rupture of the lens capsule is unusual without a penetrating injury (▶ Fig. 11.25b,c). In the setting of complete lens dislocations, the lens is usually found lying in the dependent area of the vitreous in the posterior chamber (▶ Fig. 11.26a,b,c). Bilateral lens detachment is unusual in the trauma setting and should alert the clinician to the possibility of an underlying connective tissue disorder, such as Marfan syndrome (▶ Fig. 11.26d,e).[3]

Posterior Segment Hematoma

Hemorrhage into the vitreous will result in increased density in this compartment on CT (▶ Fig. 11.27a). On magnetic resonance

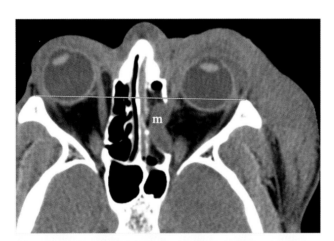

Fig. 11.19 Acute enophthalmos. Axial computed tomography shows acute soft tissue left periorbital swelling and large medial orbital wall fracture. The medial rectus muscle (*m*) is entrapped in the medial defect with enophthalmos of the left globe relative to the normal right side.

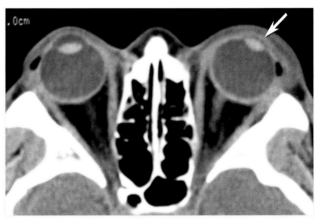

Fig. 11.20 Corneal tear. Axial computed tomography in a patient with a corneal laceration reveals collapse of the left anterior chamber (*arrow*), without intraocular hemorrhage.

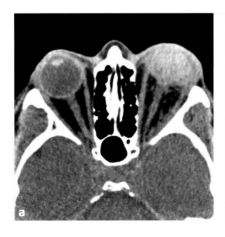

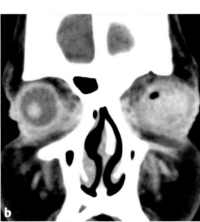

Fig. 11.21 Globe rupture and vitreal hemorrhage. (a) Axial computed tomography (CT) of patient with blunt trauma to the left globe reveals diminished anteroposterior diameter of the hemorrhage-filled globe. (b) Coronal CT in the same patient shows both hemorrhage and air in the partially collapsed left globe.

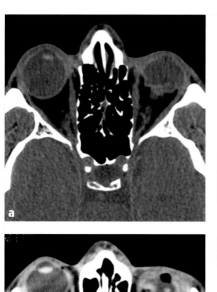

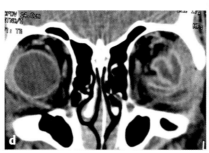

Fig. 11.22 Globe rupture with vitreal extrusion. (a) Axial and (b) coronal computed tomographic (CT) scans show the deflation of the posterior left globe with multiple folds. Also note the left lens is absent due to extrusion. (c) Axial and (d) coronal CT in a different patient shows the "flat tire" or "drooping lily" sign of near total collapse, with extrusion of the lens and vitreous.

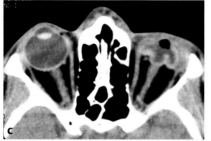

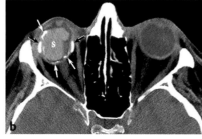

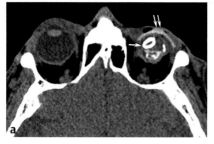

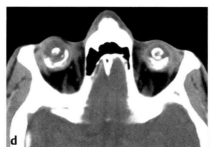

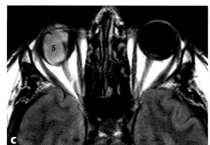

Fig. 11.23 Phthisis bulbi. (a) Axial computed tomography (CT) shows old left eye trauma with a shrunken globe with calcification of the lens (*arrow*) and vitreous. A cosmetic glass prosthesis (*double arrow*) covers the left eye. (b) Axial CT and (c) axial magnetic resonance show the calcified posterior and lateral sclera (*white arrows*) of small right globe, which has had a prior vitrectomy with silicone oil (*s*) and a scleral banding (*black arrows*). (d) Axial CT in a child with mental disability reveals bilateral shrunken globes with calcification of the lenses and vitreal structures caused by repetitive self-injury.

(MR), the normal vitreous is T2 bright, but not as bright as cerebrospinal fluid; however, methemoglobin will be T1 bright on CT (▶ Fig. 11.27b,c). It is important to note that silicone oil positioned between the vitreous and the retina as a treatment for retinal detachment can mimic a vitreous hemorrhage (▶ Fig. 11.27d). Careful history and comparison to previous examinations can thus be helpful.[3]

Choroidal Detachment

When the choroid separates from the sclera, usually secondary to hemorrhage in this space, the configuration is distinct and needs to be distinguished from a retinal detachment. The shape is similar to the appearance of an intracranial biconvex epidural collection. This shape occurs as a result of the choroidal attachment sites at the vortex veins and the ora serrata (▶ Fig. 11.28a). The choroidal membranes' appearance is similar to the stitching on a baseball (▶ Fig. 11.28b). Acute choroidal detachments have tense hemorrhage-filled membranes that bow internally into the vitreous (▶ Fig. 11.28c,d,e). With time, chronic choroidal detachments may deflate and lose tension with undulating membranes (▶ Fig. 11.28f).[5,6]

Retinal Detachment

Shear injury or laceration can result in retinal detachment. The appearance on CT is of an inverted triangle with the apex of the triangle or a "gull-wing" appearance, creating a V-shape at the optic nerve head (▸ Fig. 11.29a,b). This appearance is due to the retina's strong attachments at the level of the optic nerve posteriorly and at the ora serrata anteriorly (▸ Fig. 11.29c–f). A similar appearance can also be detected with MR (▸ Fig. 11.29b,c).[6,7]

Optic Nerve Injury

The optic nerve can be injured by direct laceration, mass effect, or ischemia secondary to devascularization. Fracture is the most common cause of optic nerve injury, with 63% of cases secondary to fracture as stated in the literature (▸ Fig. 11.30a–d). Conversely, 2% of patients with periorbital fractures will have optic nerve damage.[8] A fracture at the orbital apex can impinge on the optic nerve and have devastating consequences to vision unless recognized and surgically corrected (▸ Fig. 11.30e). These fractures can be very subtle, so careful scrutiny of this area using multiplanar CT reformats is important. The optic nerve can be affected by mass effect from a

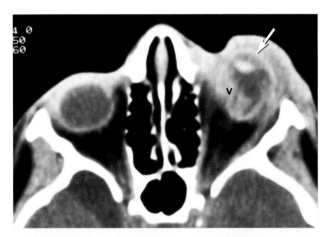

Fig. 11.24 Anterior chamber hematoma. Axial computed tomography in a patient stabbed in the eye with scissors shows both high-density hemorrhage anterior to the lens in the anterior chamber (*arrow*), as well as posterior vitreal (*v*) blood with globe rupture.

subperiosteal hematoma, as stated previously. Shear injury with disruption of the vascular supply to the optic nerve can result in ischemia. Rapid vision loss without an identifiable fracture or mass on CT can raise this possibility. MRI will demonstrate high T2 signal within the nerve indicative of edema in this setting.[9] Some studies have demonstrated the utility of diffusion tensor imaging to assess disruption of the optic nerve tract. Altered fractional anisotropy may be used to evaluate the severity of optic nerve fiber disruption.[10]

Extraocular Muscle Tear

The extraocular muscles have tendon attachments of the globe, which pierce the sclera. Avulsion can lead to a scleral tear, with vitreous extrusion resulting in loss of volume in the posterior chamber and mild enophthalmos. Most commonly, the muscle belly will partially or completely tear, as it is weaker than the tendon insertion (▸ Fig. 11.31).

Periorbital Hematoma

Preseptal hematoma rarely causes ocular problems except to make clinical assessment of the eye difficult, and it may reflect the severity of trauma to the area. Subperiosteal hematomas can displace the extraocular muscles and cause proptosis (▸ Fig. 11.32); hematoma within the extraocular muscles will cause them to expand (▸ Fig. 11.4a). Hematoma near the orbital apex is a critical finding because mass effect on the optic nerve can lead to vision loss and may require decompression.

Orbital Compartment Syndrome

Normal intraocular pressure (IOP) is between 3 and 6 mm Hg. When the IOP exceeds the pressure of the vasa nervorum, the optic nerve is at risk of ischemia. Ischemia to the nerve for more than 60 to 100 minutes has been shown to result in irreversible vision loss. If the IOP exceeds that of the central retinal artery, the retina itself becomes at risk of ischemia. Lack of lymphatics in the orbit compounds the inability for the orbit to decom-

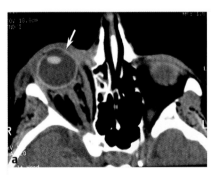

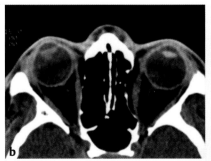

Fig. 11.25 Lens injury. (a) Axial computed tomography (CT) shows partial dislocation of the nasal attachment (*arrow*) of the right lens from blunt trauma. (b) Axial and (c) coronal CT in a different patient show disruption of the posterior margin of the right lens capsule and decreased lens density caused by edema from a penetrating metal foreign body. Note the old left medial wall blowout fracture.

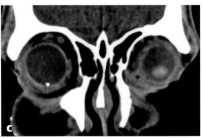

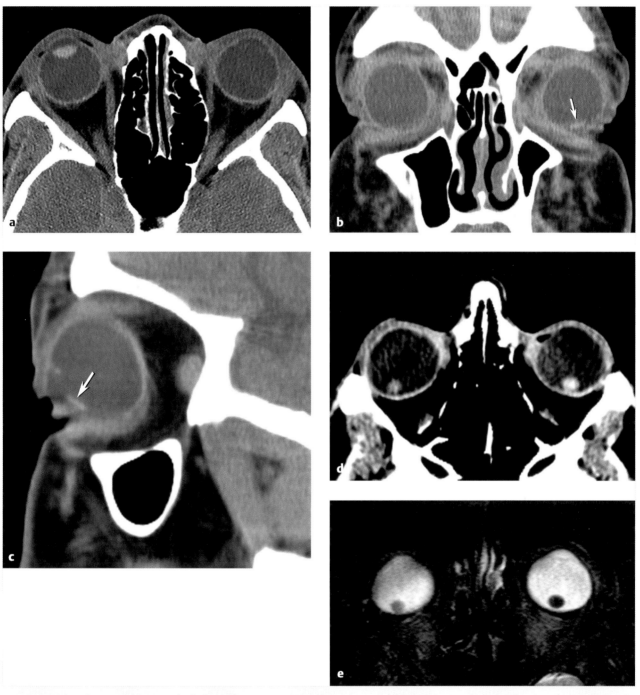

Fig. 11.26 (a) Axial computed tomography (CT) in a blunt trauma patient shows absence of the plastic intraocular lens replacement from its expected position. (b) Coronal and (c) sagittal reformatted views demonstrate inferior and anterior location of the dislocated intraocular lens replacement. (d) Axial CT and (d) axial short-inversion imaging recovery magnetic resonance show bilateral far posterior dislocations of the native lenses.

press. The only other mechanism of orbital decompression is via the draining veins, such as the superior ophthalmic vein. The cause of the increased IOP can be a large intraocular hematoma or tension pneumo-orbita (▶ Fig. 11.33). The anteroposterior dimension of the globe on imaging will be increased and the globe may become proptotic. Globe tenting with afferent pupillary defect may develop as the proptosis increases.

Carotid-Cavernous Fistula

Traumatic laceration of the cavernous segment of the ICA can result in a fistulous communication with the cavernous sinus. As a result of increased pressure on the venous side, there is resultant reflux flow with engorgement of the cavernous sinus and superior ophthalmic vein. The periorbital fat will demonstrate stranding, and the globe can be proptotic. Clinically, the

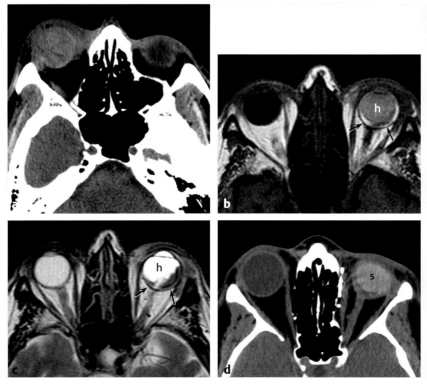

Fig. 11.27 Vitreal hematoma. (a) Axial computed tomography (CT) in a psychotic patient who attempted to pluck out his own right eye, resulting in globe rupture and vitreal hemorrhage. (b) Axial T1 W and (c) axial T2 W of a trauma patient with left vitreal bleed (*h*), which is higher signal than normal vitreous on both T1 W and T2 W sequences. A retinal detachment (*arrows*) is also present. (d) Axial CT in a third patient shows high-density vitreal silicone oil (*s*) from a vitrectomy in the left eye that mimics the density of acute hemorrhage.

patient will have chemosis resulting from arterialization of the conjunctiva and may have reduced visual acuity. The fistula is best demonstrated on CT angiography or with formal angiography (▶ Fig. 11.34). Treatment is embolization. Isolated enlargement of the superior ophthalmic vein can mimic a carotid-cavernous fistula. The patient will not be symptomatic in this setting, and there will be a lack of venous congestion with stranding of the periorbital fat and an absence of proptosis in these cases. The isolated enlargement of the vein can be idiopathic or the result of varix or cavernous thrombosis.[3]

Chronic Post-traumatic Fat Atrophy

A rare complication of chronic orbital soft tissue injury is a paradoxical atrophy of the retro-ocular fat causing a chronic enophthalmos (▶ Fig. 11.35a,b). This complication manifests on CT as decreased orbital fat with a somewhat infiltrated appearance of the residual retro-ocular fat (▶ Fig. 11.35c,d).

Chronic Post-traumatic Neuroma

Injury to the cranial nerves can rarely result in a post-traumatic neuroma (▶ Fig. 11.36). Post-traumatic neuromas generally show less enhancement than do schwannomas or neurofibromas.

Penetrating Orbital Trauma

Penetrating injury is defined by the passage of a foreign object through the periorbital soft tissues, globe, retro-ocular soft tissues, or bones constituting the orbit. The penetrating objects may be metallic, such as bullets, shrapnel, metal filings, pellets, knives, skewers, screw drivers, screws, nails, and such. Common nonmetallic orbital foreign bodies include glass, wooden sticks, pencils, pens, and plastic objects. The penetrating object may transiently pass through the orbit, or it may be retained within or adjacent to the orbit. Volume CT is the modality of choice for locating the foreign body or bodies and assessing the extent of orbital soft tissue and bony injury.

Foreign Bodies

Metal

Metal foreign bodies are best detected by CT. The metal foreign body has a much higher density (Hounsfield unit, HU) than orbital soft tissue or bone and is best identified on wider bone window width of 2000 to 4000 HU. Usually, significant stellate beam hardening artifacts confirm the metallic nature (▶ Fig. 11.37). Localization of the metal foreign body within the anterior, posterior, or central portion of the globe is important for surgical planning (▶ Fig. 11.38). It is also important to localize foreign bodies as posterior to the globe, orbital apex, or transorbital intracranial (▶ Fig. 11.37b; ▶ Fig. 11.39a–f). Thinner slice thickness improves the visibility of streak artifacts in small foreign bodies by eliminating volume averaging of adjacent tissues (▶ Fig. 11.40). MR is generally contraindicated in acute penetrating trauma until any metal foreign bodies are excluded from within or immediately adjacent to the eye and optic nerve.

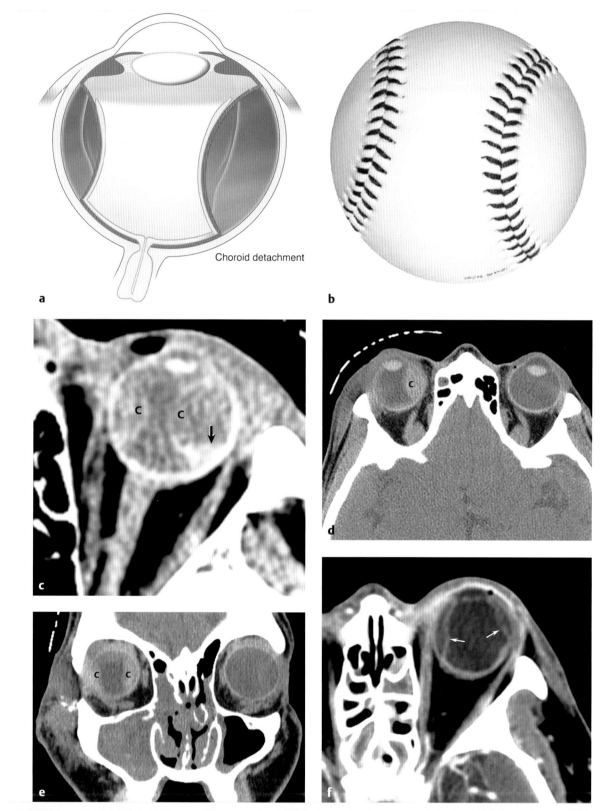

Fig. 11.28 Choroidal detachment. (a) Diagram showing nasal and temporal choroidal detachments, indicating that the posterior margin of the detachment does not extend to the optic nerve head. (b) Baseball stitching mimics the contour of choroidal detachments. (c) Axial computed tomography (CT) of acute post-traumatic choroidal detachments (c) nearly isodense with the central vitreous, with high-density hemorrhage (*arrow*) layering dependently within the choroidal detachment. (d) Axial and (e) coronal CT in another trauma patient showing high-density homogeneous hemorrhage within the nasal and temporal choroidal detachments (c). (f) Chronic choroidal detachments with deflated subchoroidal fluid and wavy choroidal membranes (*arrows*).

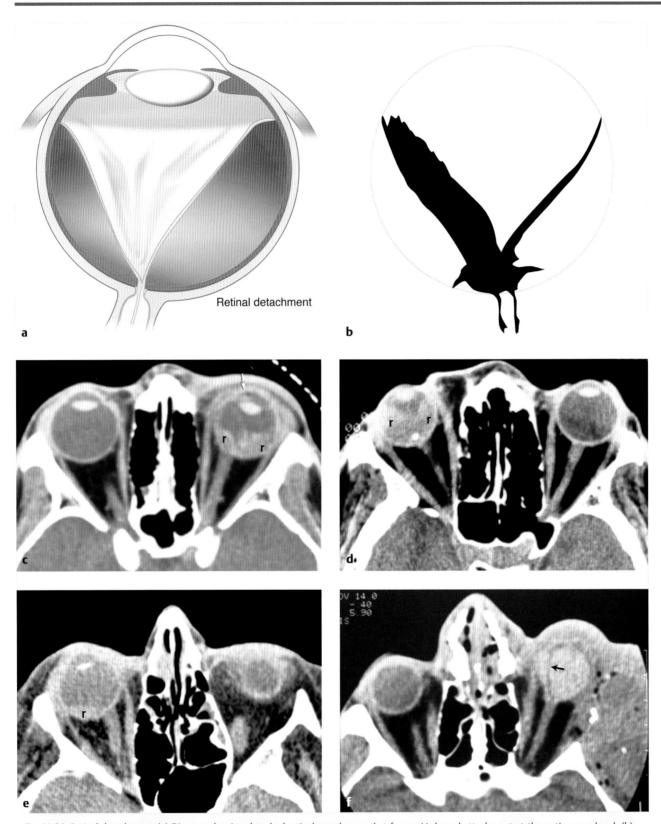

Fig. 11.29 Retinal detachment. (a) Diagram showing detached retinal membranes that form a V-shaped attachment at the optic nerve head. (b) Drawing showing the "gull-wing" appearance of retinal detachment. (c) Axial computed tomography (CT) shows a left retinal detachment (*r*) from a penetrating ocular injury. Note also the hemorrhage (*arrow*) in the anterior chamber. (d) Axial CT demonstrates a large acute retinal detachment with retinal membranes extending posterior to the calcified drusen at the right optic nerve head. (e) Axial CT shows a small subretinal hemorrhage (*r*) extending laterally from the optic nerve head, in a patient with a right plastic lens implant. (f) Axial CT in high-speed accident with ruptured globe and clear visualization of the retinal membrane (*arrow*) extending through the nasal aspect of the eye.

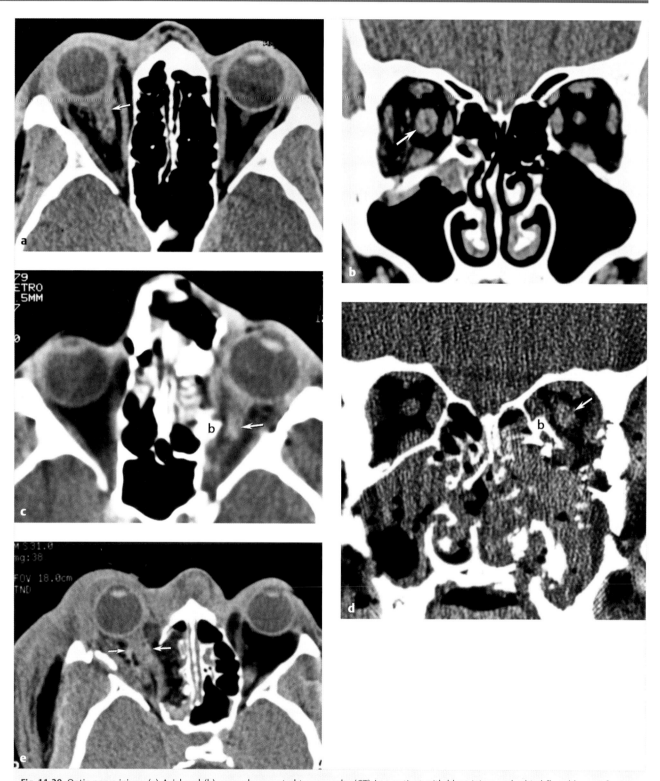

Fig. 11.30 Optic nerve injury. (a) Axial and (b) coronal computed tomography (CT) in a patient with blunt injury and orbital floor blowout fracture shows hemorrhage (*arrow*) in the right dilated optic nerve sheath causing visual loss. (c) Axial and (d) coronal CT demonstrates in a second patient a laterally displaced fragment of bone (*b*) near the optic nerve with high density hemorrhage (*arrow*) within the optic nerve sheath in a patient with a left Le Fort III fracture, associated with complete visual loss in that eye. (e) Axial CT in another patient with a right zygomaticomaxillary complex and large medial orbital wall displaced fracture. Note the focal hemorrhage (*arrows*) within the right optic nerve sheath.

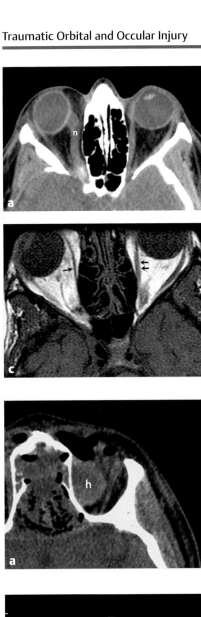

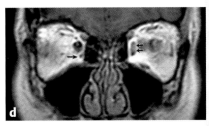

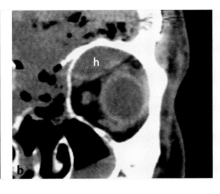

Fig. 11.31 Rectus muscle tear. (a) Axial computed tomography (CT) shows disconjugate gaze with marked lateral rotation of the right globe, medial position of the optic nerve (*n*), and absence of the medial rectus. (b) and (c) Axial T1 W and (d) coronal T1 W MR in the same patient again shows only a thread-like component of the right "lost" medial rectus (*arrow*) muscle. Compare with the normal left medial rectus (*double arrow*).

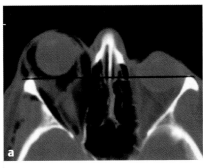

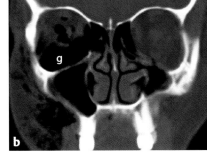

Fig. 11.32 Subperiosteal hematoma. (a) Axial and (b) coronal computed tomographic scans show a subperiosteal hematoma (*h*) in the superior-medial orbit displacing the right superior muscle complex and the superior oblique in a postoperative patient.

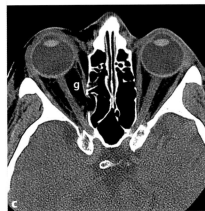

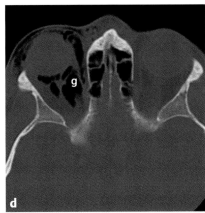

Fig. 11.33 Tension pneumo-orbita. (a) Axial and (b) coronal computed tomography (CT) bone windows demonstrate marked right proptosis (using the interzygomatic reference line) caused by a blowout fracture (not shown) with retro-ocular gas (*g*) filling the orbit and displacing the globe. (c) Soft tissue window axial CT in a different patient shows right proptosis with stretching and thinning of the optic nerve and a small posterior, acute medial orbital blowout fracture. (d) Axial CT bone window clearly reveals the cause of this proptosis is trapping of a large amount of retro-ocular air.

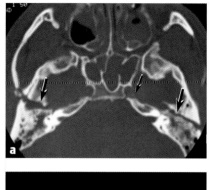
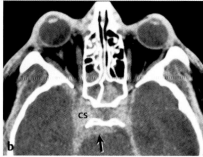
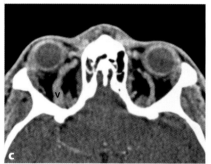
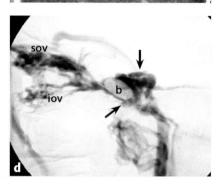
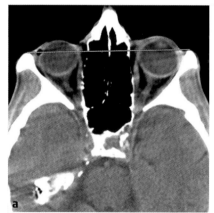
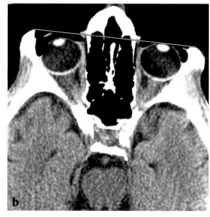
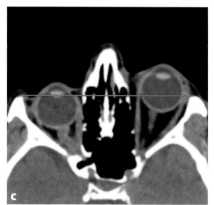
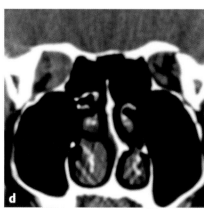

Fig. 11.34 Carotid-cavernous fistula. (a) Axial computed tomography (CT) bone window shows an acute central skull-base fracture traversing through both temporal bones and sphenoid body. (b) Axial CT with contrast shows asymmetric enlargement of the cavernous sinus (cs) on the right, extending into the retroclival venous plexus (arrow). (c) Axial enhanced CT higher in the orbit shows asymmetric enlargement of the right superior ophthalmic vein (v) indicating increased venous pressure and flow on the right. (d) Lateral right internal carotid angiogram demonstrates a partially inflated balloon (b) inserted through the cavernous carotid fistula (arrows) into the cavernous sinus. Note the marked venous flow anteriorly into the superior (sov) and inferior (iov) ophthalmic veins.

Fig. 11.35 Post-traumatic orbital fat atrophy. (a) Axial computed tomography (CT) in a patient with recent facial soft tissue trauma. Note the anterior third of the globes project beyond the interzygomatic line. (b) Axial CT in the same patient 6 months later complains of sunken appearance of eyes. The CT shows the globes are now several millimeters posterior to the interzygomatic line, with an accompanying loss of retro-ocular fat and obscuration of fat planes, bilaterally. (c) Axial CT in a second patient with prior orbital soft tissue trauma, but no fracture, has marked enophthalmos of the right eye, loss of retro-ocular fat, and redundancy of the optic nerve. (d) Coronal CT in the second patient shows normal bony orbital volume, with obscuration of fat planes in the right obital apex.

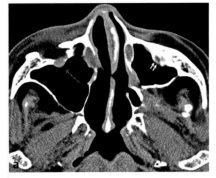
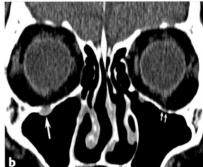
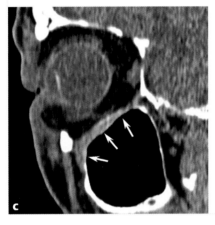

Fig. 11.36 Post-traumantic V2 neuroma. (a) Axial and (b) coronal computed tomographic (CT) scans (CT) show asymmetric enlargement of the right infraorbital branch of the maxillary division of cranial nerve V (V2) in a patient with a prior right zygomaticomaxillary complex and orbital floor fracture. Note the normal left V2 (double arrows). (c) Sagittal CT shows the expansion of V2 (arrows) from the infraorbital foramen to the posterior infraorbital canal.

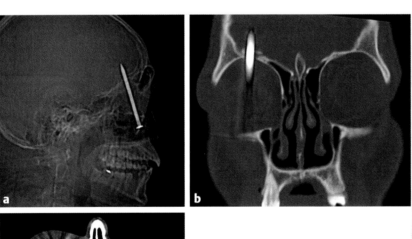

Fig. 11.37 Nail gun injury. (a) Lateral computed tomographic (CT) scout view showing a transorbital nail. The patient was accidentally hit in the eye with a pneumatic nail gun nail. (b) Coronal CT bone window demonstrates the transorbital to intracranial path of the nail foreign body. (c) Axial CT shows the intense streak artifact of the nail within the globe.

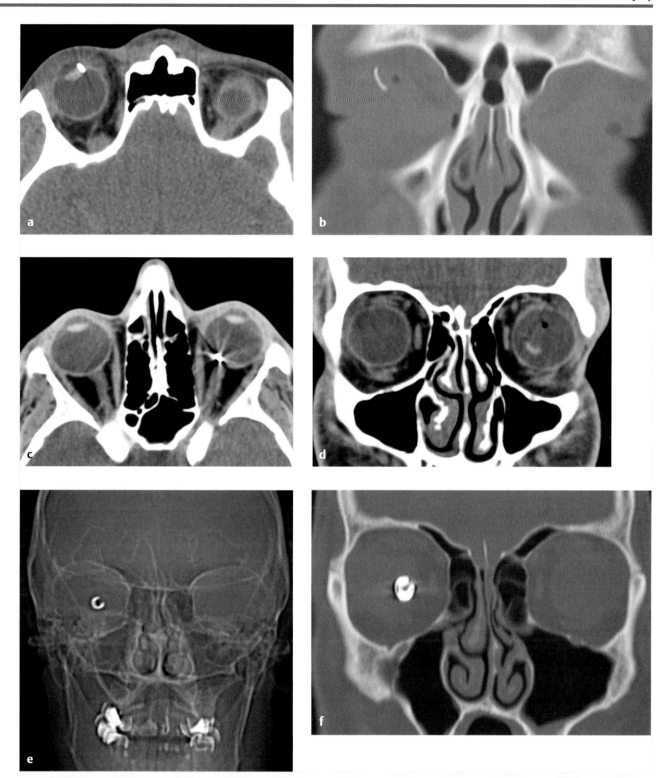

Fig. 11.38 Intraocular metal foreign bodies. (a) Axial and (b) coronal computed tomography (CT) bone window show a curvilinear metal foreign body lodged in the right anterior chamber in a patient who had a guitar string snap. Note the more subtle streak artifact from the small wire on soft tissue windows. (c) Axial CT in another patient demonstrates the metal foreign body lodged in the left retina near the optic nerve head. (d) The coronal CT in this same patient shows the intravitreal gas and bloody tract of the metal projectile. (e) Anteroposterior scout image in a third patient shows a C-shaped metal foreign body from an archer hit in the right eye by his bow-string clip. (f) Coronal CT bone window confirms the bow string clip in the middle of the right globe.

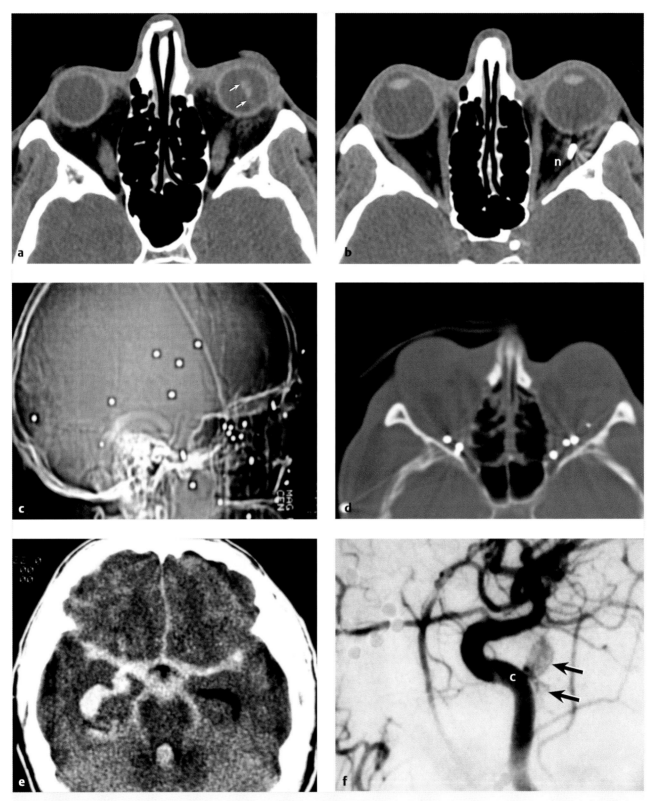

Fig. 11.39 Transorbital metal foreign bodies. (a) Axial computed tomography (CT) shows a linear hemorrhagic penetration tract (*arrows*) through the left globe in a sheet metal grinder. (b) A higher slice reveals the retro-ocular location of the metal fragment adjacent to the optic nerve (*n*). (c) Lateral CT scout view in another patient suffering from a shotgun blast to the face with multiple pellets overlying the orbits and cranium. (d) Axial CT bone window reveals multiple intraorbital pellets in both orbital apices, as well as rupture of the right globe. (e) Axial brain window in same patient shows a large amount of acute subarachnoid hemorrhage. (f) Lateral right internal carotid angiogram shows an abnormal blush (*arrows*) just behind the posterior margin of the precavernous internal carotid (*c*) from a pellet (not shown) passing through the right superior orbital fissure and nicking the vessel, causing the subarachnoid hemorrhage.

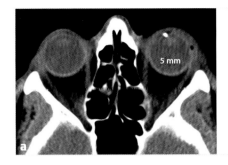
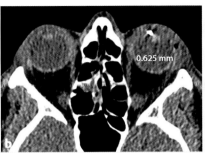

Fig. 11.40 Metal streak artifact on thick and thin-section computed tomography (CT). (a) Axial 5-mm CT slice through a 1-mm-thick metal anterior chamber shunt for glaucoma, showing equivocal metal artifact. (b) Axial retrospective 0.625-mm CT slice eliminates volume averaging to better identify the streak artifact and confirm the foreign body as metal.

Glass/Silicate

Glass foreign bodies often originate from windshields, windows, and glass doors. Rocks and silicates may also be driven into the orbital soft tissues from direct impact against the ground or flying debris from machinery or explosions. Both glass and other silicates are denser (i.e., have higher HUs) than any of the normal orbital soft tissues, but they are less dense than the orbital bones. So CT is excellent in the detection and localization of these foreign bodies (▶ Fig. 11.41).

Wood

Wooden orbital soft tissue foreign bodies may originate in the natural environment from sticks and branches of bushes and trees, or they may originate in a wide variety of wood products for use by humans. These may include pencils, broomsticks, yardsticks, rulers, brush handles, and similar objects (▶ Fig. 11.42). Flying wood debris from explosions can also penetrate the orbit. The interesting CT properties of wood foreign bodies arise from the degree of dryness or hydration of the wood. Dry wood contains gas and appears often as linear or rectangular gas collections on CT (▶ Fig. 11.43a,b). More hydrated wood may be isodense or somewhat hyperdense to orbital soft tissues on CT (▶ Fig. 11.43c,d). The linear or angular margins of the hydrated foreign body should raise suspicion.

Plastic and Miscellaneous

Plastic orbital foreign bodies are uncommon but could result from a stabbing injury with a plastic utensil or pen. However, a common example of plastic intraocular foreign bodies is intraocular lens implants for cataract surgery. Flying debris from an explosion could contain paper, plastic, metal, or chemical foreign material (▶ Fig. 11.44). The CT density (HU) of a plastic may vary from hypodense to isodense to hyperdense relative to orbital soft tissues, but it would always be less dense than bone. Air can rarely be a penetrating force with a pressurize air hose or air gun (▶ Fig. 11.45).

Use of MR for localizing suspected wood or plastic foreign bodies has been used in rare circumstances. In the setting of acute trauma, a CT should always be done first to exclude any metallic foreign body before placing the victim in the high magnetic field of an MR scanner. MR can then be used when the index of suspicion is high for a retained wood or plastic foreign body that is not detected on CT.[11]

Iatrogenic Ocular and Orbital Foreign Bodies

Knowledge of common implants in the orbit and globe is helpful for differentiating a traumatic from an iatrogenic foreign body. Objects implanted by a physician include Silastic or Teflon cosmetic implants in the preseptal soft tissues, gold weight in the upper eyelid of a patient with facial nerve palsy, cataract replacements, scleral bands (buckles) (▶ Fig. 11.46), eye prosthetics, and spacers (▶ Fig. 11.47).

Globe Puncture and Laceration

Rupture of the globe can result from either blunt or penetrating ocular injury. Penetrating injury is sometimes seen in the lens (▶ Fig. 11.25b,c). The usual CT manifestation of globe rupture is a smaller globe size caused by extrusion of the aqueous or vitreous globe fluids and a deformed or deflated appearance ("flat-tire sign"), absence of the lens, or frank disruption of the globe margin. Intraocular hemorrhage will appear more hyperdense than normal vitreous and may outline choroidal or retinal detachments (▶ Fig. 11.48). Gas may also be present in the collapsed globe.

Penetrating Optic Nerve Injury

Optic Nerve Laceration

Traumatic optic nerve laceration is uncommon. It usually occurs with a penetrating injury from a projectile or a sharp, penetrating object such as a knife or glass (▶ Fig. 11.49a). On occasion, a displaced bone fragment from one of the orbital margins can rotate and impact the optic nerve. CT may show perioptic hemorrhage in the nerve or nerve sheath or a complete transection. Once CT has excluded a metal foreign body, then high-resolution MR of the optic nerve with short Tau Inversion Recovery (STIR) or fat saturation T2 imaging in the axial, coronal, or oblique sagittal plane can show a focal injury to the optic nerve (▶ Fig. 11.49b,c,d).

Optic Nerve Compression

Optic nerve compression may be chronic, as seen in thyroid eye disease, or acute in the traumatized patient. The most likely cause of optic nerve compression is either soft tissue injury (such as a subperiosteal hematoma), foreign bodies, or displaced bone fracture fragments that impinge on the optic nerve at the orbital apex or within the optic canal (▶ Fig. 11.43b,d).

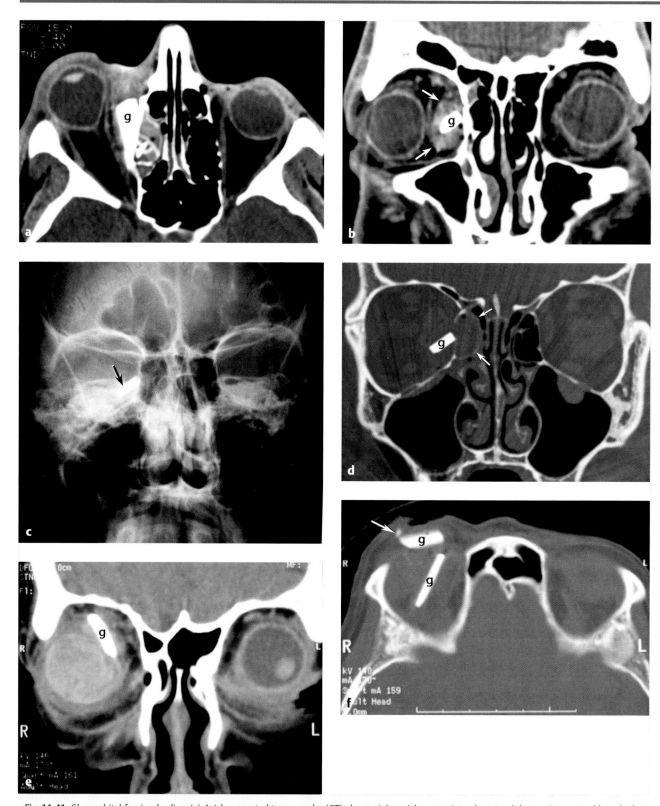

Fig. 11.41 Glass orbital foreign bodies. (a) Axial computed tomography (CT) shows right axial proptosis and acute globe tenting caused by a high density glass (*g*) fragment in the medial orbit, missing the globe, but causing a medial orbital wall fracture. Note the relative lack of streak artifact with glass compared with metal. (b) Coronal CT shows the rectangular cross-section of the glass associated with an extraconal or subperiosteal hematoma (*arrows*) displacing the globe laterally. (c) Anteroposterior CT scout demonstrates the glass fragment (*arrow*) end on. (d) Confirmation of the glass and the medial orbital wall fracture (*arrows*) matching the position of the fragment seen on the scout. (e) Coronal CT soft tissue and (f) axial bone windows showing the glass foreign body lacerating the globe with vitreal hemorrhage caused by a different patient falling on a glass of water. Note even the 2-mm glass fragment (*arrow*) in the preseptal soft tissues is easily seen on CT.

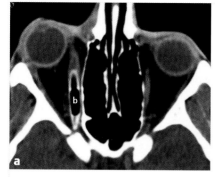
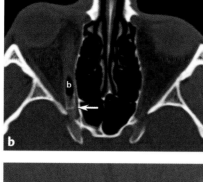
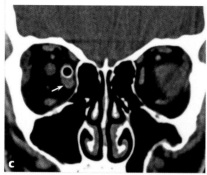
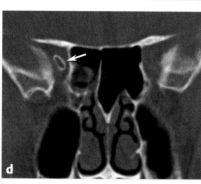

Fig. 11.42 Makeup brush skewering medial rectus. (a) Axial computed tomography (CT) soft tissue and (b) axial bone windows demonstrate the brush end (*arrow*) of a makeup brush (*b*) jammed through the medial rectus into the orbital apex. The girlfriend stabbed her boyfriend during an argument. (c) Coronal CT confirms the right medial rectus (*arrow*) location with muscle swelling and hematoma. Note the extremely dry wood of the makeup brush handle appears as gas density within the metal jacket of the brush holder. (d) Coronal CT bone window localizes the metal bristle containing metal tip (*arrow*) deep in the orbital apex compressing the optic nerve from below.

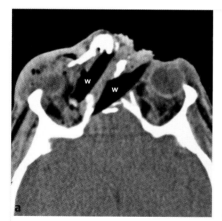
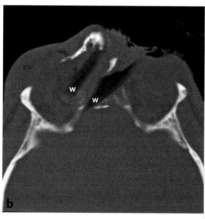
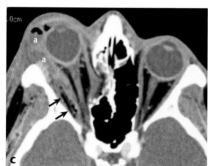
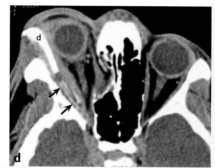

Fig. 11.43 Dry versus hydrated wood foreign bodies. (a) Axial computed tomography (CT) in a patient was hit in the face by a dry log shows frontal bone and orbital injury. Two angular gas density foreign bodies (*w*) are seen traversing the orbits and ethmoid sinuses suggesting dry wood. Gas bubbles should have round contours. (b) Axial CT with bone windowing reveals the subtle striations of the internal wood fibers in this dry wood. (c) Axial CT in a different patient hit in the eye with the end of a broken broomstick 2 days before this CT was performed. Note the periorbital and right lateral subperiosteal abscess (*a*) with some linear gas (*arrows*) near the orbital apex. Right globe tenting is present. (d) Axial CT 3 days after drainage of the subperiosteal abscess; the retained drain (*d*) is seen anteriorly. However, the former gas density area has now become hyperdense with linear margins (*arrows*), confirming a retained subperiosteal wood fragment, which changed from initially dry wood mimicking gas, to denser hydrated wood after 5 days.

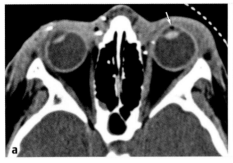

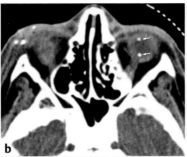

Fig. 11.44 Blasting cap explosive debris in orbit. (a) Axial computed tomography (CT) at lens level shows periorbital soft tissue swelling, with multiple punctate high-density, preseptal foreign bodies that could be metal, plastic, or mineral components of the exploded blasting cap. Note the tiny gas bubble (*arrow*) in the left globe anterior chamber. (b) Axial CT slice seen lower down reveals intraocular penetrating foreign bodies in the left globe.

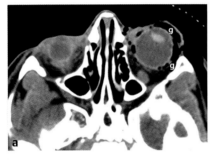

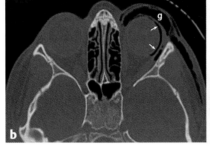

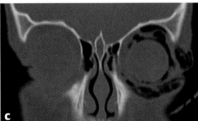

Fig. 11.45 Air-gun orbital injury. (a) Axial computed tomography (CT) soft tissue and (b) bone windows show left preseptal subcutaneous gas (*g*), as well as gas dissecting laterally in the subconjunctival layer (*arrows*) of the left globe, but no intraocular gas or hemorrhage. (c) Coronal CT bone window reveals the extent of the gas blast into the periorbital soft tissues. This was caused by the victim being too close to the muzzle of the air gun when it discharged, with compressed air penetrating the skin and orbital soft tissues.

Extraocular Muscle Laceration

Laceration of one or more of the extraocular muscles is a relatively rare injury. It most often occurs with a penetrating injury. Clinical presentation would include dysfunction of the affected extraocular muscle. CT in the axial or sagittal plane can show a V-shaped partial laceration or a complete tear of the muscle (▶ Fig. 11.50). Eye position during the scan is not usually a diagnostic finding because eye position is extremely variable in normal patients.

Orbital Infection Associated with Penetrating Trauma

Any penetrating orbital injury has the potential for carrying bacteria or fungus into the soft tissues. Wood foreign bodies are most significant, as they frequently result in post-traumatic infection if they are not found and surgically removed. Infections can range from an endophthalmitis of the globe to diffuse orbital cellulitis and/or orbital abscess (▶ Fig. 11.43c,d; ▶ Fig. 11.51).

Postoperative Orbit

Postoperatively, microplates and screws in the orbital rim, as well as Teflon or Porex sheet implants to reinforce the orbital floor or wall, may be seen (▶ Fig. 11.9a,b,c). Postoperative CT can be used to assess the surgical sites for complications. Three-dimensional surface rendering may be helpful in assessing the postoperative bony alignment as well as hardware placement (▶ Fig. 11.52).

11.6 Pearls

- Many types of facial fractures involve the bony orbit. Thus, orbital fractures, hematomas, foreign bodies, and globe injuries should be routinely evaluated.
- Acute orbital mass effect with proptosis, especially with globe tenting, should be considered urgent or emergent, depending on the degree of acute orbital tension. Emergency surgical decompression may be needed.
- If penetrating orbital or ocular injury has occurred or is suspected, CT should be used to identify and localize any retained foreign body. Metal and glass foreign bodies are usually easily seen on CT; however, wood and plastic foreign bodies may be much more challenging to identify.
- Do not perform MR in the setting of trauma if metal foreign bodies are suspected until a CT has been performed. MR can then be done if no metal foreign bodies are seen close to the optic pathway or localized intracranially.

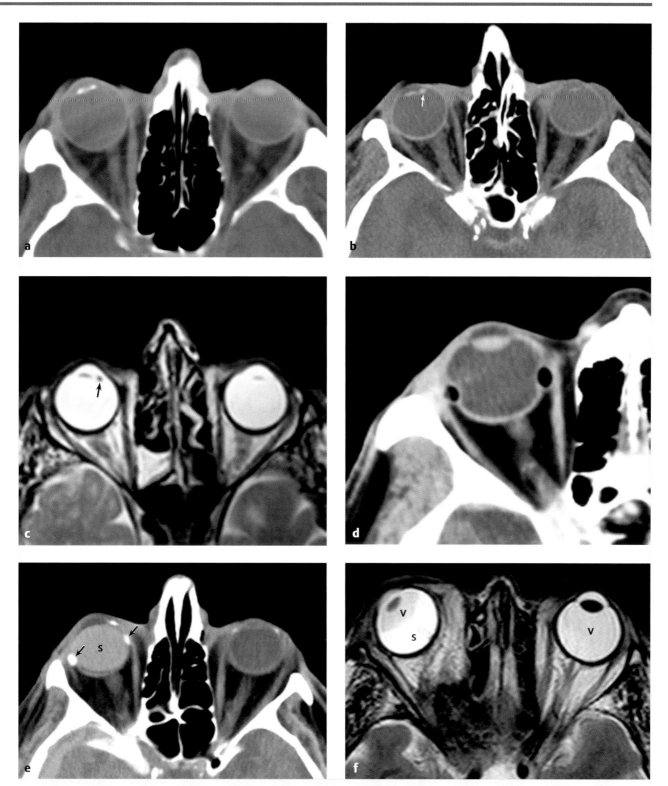

Fig. 11.46 Assorted iatrogenic lens and globe implants and fluids. (a) Axial computed tomography (CT) of unusual right metal lens replacement. (b) Axial CT and (c) axial T2 W magnetic resonance (MR) of bilateral plastic intraocular lenses, with a small right adjacent ganciclovir implant (*arrow*) on the nasal side of the right lens implant for intraocular cytomegalovirus infection. Note the plastic lenses are easily identified on both CT and MR. (d) Axial CT of gas-filled scleral band. (e) Axial CT shows a right Silastic scleral band (*arrows*) with high-density intraocular silicone oil (*s*) after vitrectomy. (f) Axial T2 W MR reveals a right mixture of moderately high signal native vitreous (*v*) and very high T2 signal silicone oil (*s*) after partial vitrectomy.

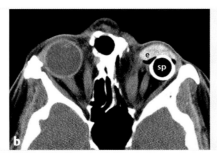

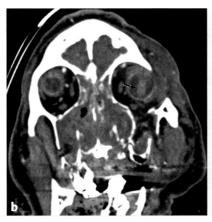

Fig. 11.47 Globe prostheses. (a) Axial computed tomography (CT) demonstrates a high-density porcelain sphere spacer (*sp*) implant supporting the external glass eye (*e*) prosthesis. (b) Axial CT shows a left hollow porcelain sphere containing gas, supporting the external glass eye prosthesis.

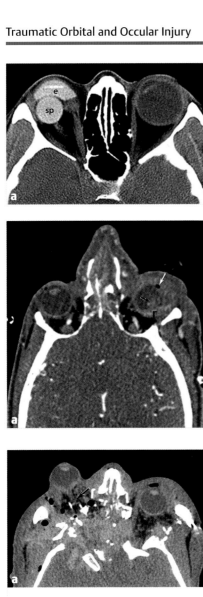

Fig. 11.48 Punctured globe. (a) Axial and (b) coronal computed tomography (CT) in a victim mauled by a grizzly bear biting his face and left orbit, resulting in a left Le Fort III fracture. Note the left vitreal hemorrhage (*black arrow*), subretinal bleed (*r*), absence of the lens, and the slightly deflated globe and gas (*white arrow*) adjacent to the cornea.

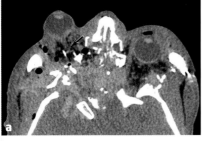

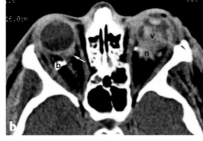

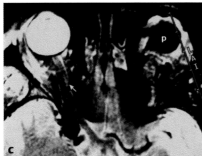

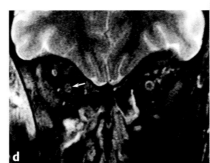

Fig. 11.49 Gunshot injuries to optic nerve. (a) Axial computed tomography (CT) shows the destructive path of the gunshot wound (GSW) traversing the orbital apices bilaterally. Note the complete transection of the right optic nerve (*arrow*) with the right globe dangling anterior to the eyelids, with subretinal and anterior chamber hemorrhage. (b) Axial CT in another patient the bullet traversed the midright orbit and struck the posterior left globe. A bone (*b*) fragment abuts the midright optic nerve with some retro-ocular hemorrhage (*arrow*). The left globe is ruptured posteriorly with vitreal (*v*) and optic nerve (*n*) head hemorrhage. (c) Axial and (d) coronal fat saturated T2 W images after left globe enucleation with prosthesis (*p*). Note the focal high T2 signal within the midright optic nerve (*arrow*) on the axial slice, which is confirmed as a horizontal optic nerve tear on the coronal slice.

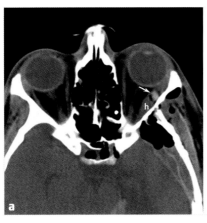

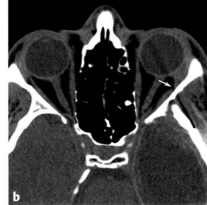

Fig. 11.50 Acute and chronic rectus muscle laceration. (a) Axial computed tomography (CT) immediately postoperatively after surgical misadventure shows left extraconal hemorrhage (*h*) obscuring the left lateral rectus muscle, with a focal higher density clot (*arrow*) and laceration at the junction of the anterior third of the lateral rectus. (b) Axial CT 1 month later demonstrates a focal interruption (*arrow*) of the left lateral rectus muscle with unopposed medial rotation of the left globe.

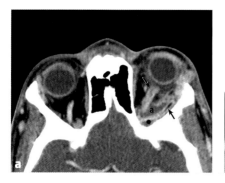
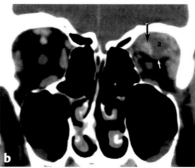

Fig. 11.51 Subperiosteal abscess from penetrating wood stick. (a) Axial contrast enhanced computed tomography (CT) shows a left subperiosteal abscess (a) in the superior orbit surrounding hydrated wood stick fragments (*arrows*) with parallel straight high-density margins, which are nonanatomic. The left globe is proptotic on the axial. (b) Coronal CT shows the mass effect of the abscess (a) surrounding the hydrated stick (*black arrow*) displacing the superior muscle complex (*white arrow*) inferiorly.

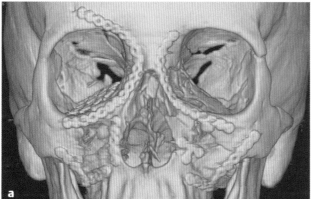

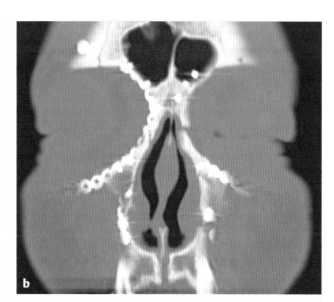

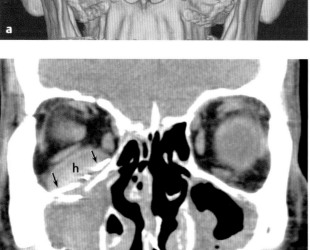

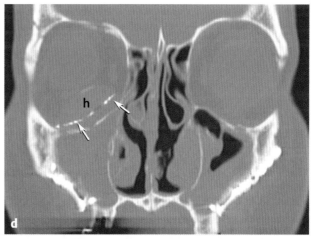

Fig. 11.52 Post open reduction internal fixation of facial fractures. (a) Three-dimensional computed tomography (CT) bone surface reconstruction in a patient with right Le Fort I/II and left Le Fort I-III fractures and right orbital implant placement to repair an orbital floor depressed fracture. The patient went to the emergency department 1 day postoperatively with new right-eye proptosis. Note the microplates and screws across the various fracture lines. (b) Coronal CT shows the microplates and screws along the medial buttresses. (c) Coronal soft tissue and (d) bone windows show a large right inferior postoperative subperiosteal hematoma (*h*) elevating the inferior rectus. The right orbital floor implant (*arrows*) repairing the depressed floor fracture is within the hematoma.

Table 12.1 Summary of potential changes in diffusion tensor imaging metrics in the setting of acute and chronic mild traumatic brain injury (mTBI)

	Acute mTBI	Chronic mTBI
Fractional anisotropy	↑	↓
Radial diffusivity	↓	↔ or ↑
Axial diffusivity	↔ or ↓	↔ or ↑

DTI pulse sequence is used to elucidate the orientation and integrity of white matter tracts by mathematically modeling the diffusion profile on a per voxel basis. A minimum of six noncollinear measurements (or directions) is required to generate a tensor model for a given voxel, which is then used to generate several descriptive scalar metrics. The most common of these include apparent diffusion coefficient (ADC); the mean diffusivity (MD) averaged over all interrogated directions; and fractional anisotropy (FA), a normalized measure that describes the degree of directionality of diffusion, assuming a Gaussian distribution. Axial diffusivity (AD), a measure of the magnitude of diffusion in the direction of the fiver orientation, and radial diffusivity (RD), a measure of the average sum of diffusivity orthogonal to the fiber orientation, are additional commonly obtained metrics. By using these parameters, healthy brain tissue is normally associated with lower ADC values and higher FA values (the latter potentially approaching unity, indicative of increased directionality and nonuniformity). In the setting of traumatic injury, expected changes include a rise in ADC values and a decrease in FA (the latter might approach zero, indicative of uniform diffusion in all directions, and loss of directionality). A summary of expected changes in DTI metrics at acute and chronic time points is presented in ▶ Table 12.1.

A general review of the literature unveils four common forms of DTI analysis that are routinely used to evaluate patients with suspected acute versus chronic mTBI. These include (1) whole-brain histogram, (2) region of interest (ROI), (3) voxel-based morphometry (VBM); and (4) quantitative tractography analyses.[15] Some have performed an atlas-based approach, illustrated in ▶ Fig. 12.4.

Of note, somewhat conflicting reports have been published describing use of the whole-brain histogram analysis, which cannot provide regionally specific information, and represents a limitation in the application of this analytical approach for prognostic utility. ROI analysis is the most commonly reported method of data analysis and is relatively easy to perform, but it is time-consuming, limited in application for individual cases, and has been criticized for possible introduction of sampling error. VBM, on the other hand, is an automated data-driven analytical method that is reproducible and able to interrogate the entire brain. The shortcomings of this technique include variable spatial smoothing and requisite (and potentially error-prone) spatial normalization and statistical correction. This technique is well-suited for group analysis, but intersubject differences are often lost in the analysis, thus reducing the apparent sensitivity for detecting differences in findings related to mTBI. Quantitative tractography is able to identify fiber tract discontinuity, which has been identified in the setting of TBI,[45,46] and may hold promise as a technique to better assess loss of fiber tract coherence but remains underinvestigated in mTBI.

Older DTI pulse sequences were more prone to geometric distortion related to the slow phase-encoding bandwidth of traditional EPI sequences. Recent advances in imaging with DTI, however, has allowed for improved characterization of brain injuries in mTBI, including the ability to detect subtle changes in white matter fiber tracts and microstructural axonal injury.[47,48] The use of parallel imaging, increased matrix size, motion correction, and alternate readout schemes have allowed for reduction in geometric distortion and increased fidelity of the DTI data set. However, performing DTI near the skull base, for example, is still challenged by relatively low signal-to-noise ratio (SNR) and residual geometric distortion, which reduces the reliability of tractography results because eigenvector orientation fluctuations are exacerbated considerably by low SNR. Therefore, it is imperative to monitor SNR levels and evaluate the raw DWIs or FA and color-FA maps for the presence of corruption by noise. A healthy skepticism should be maintained regarding tractography results. Furthermore, the lack of normative data and inconsistent methods of DTI acquisition (including number of directions, b-value, and voxel size) and analysis used in many studies prevent direct comparison of the respective results.[49]

Standard DTI analysis methods are compromised by the inability to accurately distinguish crossing fibers[50] and the observation that derived values for FA erroneously assume that water diffusion has a Gaussian profile. These observations have led to the use of more complex tensor models, as suggested by Shenton et al (▶ Fig. 12.5),[47] including Q-ball and other high-angular-resolution diffusion imaging (HARDI) techniques,[51,52] which can provide diffusion measurements that can be used to infer the underlying tissue microstructure, such as orientation of crossing fibers. Thus, in evaluating DTI applications of mTBI, it is imperative to consider the metrics being investigated. FA, for example, is a measure derived from the diffusion tensor model, whereas f1 and f2 are derived from the partial volume model and have significant implications with respect to observed results (▶ Fig. 12.6).[53,54]

In a seminal study by Morey et al evaluating DTI metrics of chronic mTBI in military veterans who participated in the Iraq and Afghanistan wars (including veterans suffering from blast-related TBI), 30 subjects were compared with 42 primary and 28 confirmatory controls.[55] These researchers used a HARDI diffusion model and obtained partial volume fractions for primary (f1) and secondary/crossing (f2) fibers modeled with second-order tensor modeling, followed by whole-brain voxel-wise analysis of crossing fibers as a metric of primary and secondary (crossing) fiber integrity. Their findings demonstrated that chronic mTBI was associated with loss of white matter integrity in primary fibers of major fiber bundles and smaller peripheral tracts, including the CC (genu, body, and splenium), forceps major and minor, superior and inferior corona radiata, internal capsule, superior longitudinal fasciculus, and others (▶ Fig. 12.7).

Notably, conventional three-dimensional (3D)-FSPGR (Fast Spoiled Gradient Echo) T1-weighted images failed to reveal any abnormalities.[55] They reported that the distributed loss of white matter integrity correlated with subjects' "feeling dazed or confused" and, to a slightly lesser extent, with duration of LOC, but not with the diagnosis of PTSD or depressive

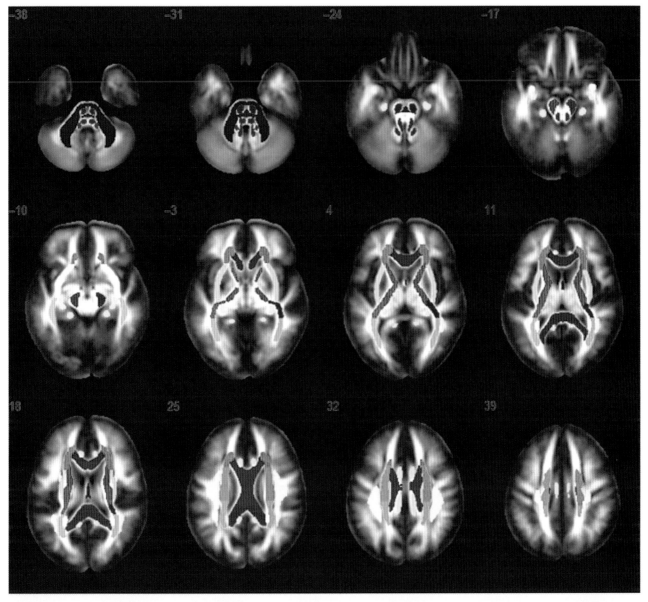

Fig. 12.4 Atlas-based regional approach: atlas with regions denoted by color to show major white matter tracts as regions of interest. (Used with permission from Kou Z, Wu Z, Tong KA, et al. The role of advanced MR imaging findings as biomarkers of traumatic brain injury. J Head Trauma Rehabil. 2010;25:267-282.)

symptoms.[55] In conclusion, compared with DTI, the measured variable, f1, was more specific to mTBI than DTI-derived FA.

Serial short-term DTI assessment of brain structural changes were performed by Wilde, McCauley, and colleagues in evaluating eight subjects with uncomplicated mTBI over the first 8 days after injury.[56] Imaging metrics, including DTI-derived FA, ADC, AD, and RD (of the left cingulum), at four time points were compared with neuropsychological testing and memory performance (via Hopkins Verbal Learning Test—Revised). The DTI sequence acquired 70 slices, obtained with 30 diffusion-encoding directions, a sensitivity encoding reduction factor of 2, and averaged two combined acquisitions to improve the SNR. The results of this study demonstrated that memory performance was transiently affected throughout the week, was most affected at the second assessment (between days 3 and 4 or 97 to 144 hours after injury), and returned to baseline by 8 days after injury. FA transiently increased in some participants, but the pattern and degree of symmetry between FA and memory performance were complex and did not always correlate.[56] Although the authors cite the small sample and short imaging interval as limitations to the study, the results highlight the degree of complex variability within and between subjects, depending on time of imaging post injury, as demonstrated in ▶ Fig. 12.8. Although several confounding variables are acknowledged, these results support the overall assumption that most patients with sports-related mTBI may exhibit transient symptoms that appear to spontaneously and completely resolve within 2 to 14 days after their injury[57-60] and up to 3 months after alternate mechanisms of injury.[61] A subset of subjects may demonstrate PPCS beyond 3 months, as previously described.

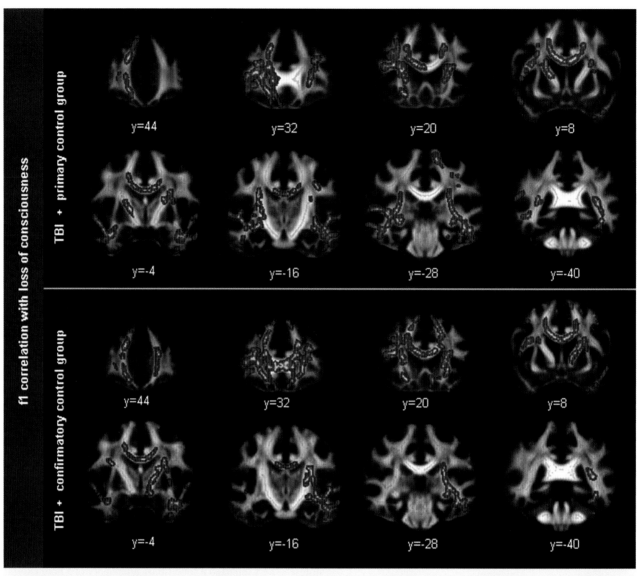

Fig. 12.7 Regarding f1 correlation with loss of consciousness, a significant correlation showed lower partial volume fraction (P < 0.05; corrected TFCE) in the primary fibers (f1) and duration of loss of consciousness in a widespread distribution of voxels in the analysis using the primary control group (top) and the confirmatory control group (bottom). Skeleton voxels are highlighted in green and correlated voxels are in blue. (Used with permission from Mosey et al. Morey RA, Haswell CC, Selgrade ES, et al. Effects of chronic mild traumatic brain injury on white matter integrity in Iraq and Afghanistan war veterans. Human brain mapping, 2012.)

demonstrated,[71] reported qualitatively,[74] or not reported. Studies performed to evaluate chronic mTBI (6 months or more post injury) usually focused on symptomatic subjects and have also demonstrated hypoperfusion on SPECT imaging (generally involving the frontal and temporal lobes), but the relationship between findings identified on SPECT imaging and neuropsychological testing as well as reported symptoms and the clinical picture remain inconsistent.[76–80] Future studies are required to better answer these questions.

12.3.3 Positron Emission Tomography

PET imaging uses positron emitting tracers (most commonly 2-deoxy-2-(^{18}F)-fluoro-D-glucose [FDG]) that annihilate with electrons within millimeters from their site of emission. This annihilation results in two gamma photons being emitted at 180 degrees relative to one another, which are subsequently temporally detected in "coincident" fashion via rings of radiation detectors in the gantry of the PET scanner. The coincident detection provides higher spatial resolution than SPECT images (usually on the order of 1 cm). FDG PET assesses regional brain glucose metabolism since the FDG ligand behaves much like glucose in the body, which crosses the blood-brain barrier and is taken up and trapped by the brain cells. In this capacity, the trapped FDG (a nonmetabolized molecule) can be used for glucose metabolic imaging to evaluate local brain damage, providing information that is not significantly dissimilar from that obtained with ^{99m}Tc HMPAO SPECT. However, the PET isotopes have a shorter half-life than those used in SPECT imaging and require that the radiopharmaceutical be more readily available, increasing the cost of the examination.

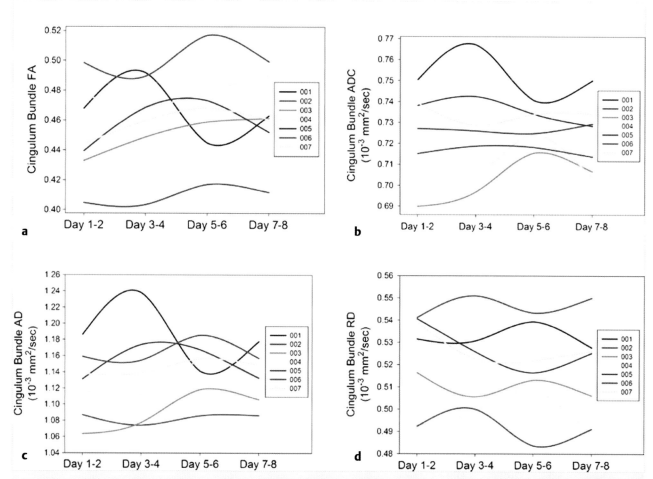

Fig. 12.8 Line graphs illustrating measurement of (a) fractional anisotropy (*FA*), (b) apparent diffusion coefficient (*ADC*), (c) axial diffusivity (*AD*), and (d) radial diffusivity (*RD*) in the left cingulum bundle over the four assessment occasions in each participant. Comparison of the trajectories of apparent diffusion coefficient (b), axial diffusivity (c), and radial diffusivity (d) for each participant highlights the complex and variable nature of change as measured by diffusion tensor imaging. Considerable qualitative differences in the pattern of change are noted between metrics and between subjects, in which some metrics indicate a more prominent change within each individual, varying by the metric used. (Modified from Wilde EA, McCauley SR, Barnes A, et al. Serial measurement of memory and diffusion tensor imaging changes within the first week following uncomplicated mild traumatic brain injury. Brain Imaging Behav. 2012;6:319-328.)

For these reasons, few studies have been performed with FDG PET in mTBI. In fact, no acute mTBI cohort FDG PET studies have been published to date. Of the chronic mTBI studies performed with FDG PET, all evaluated mTBI months to years after the initial injury. Early studies provided quantitative corroboration of neuropsychological testing in attention and memory such that mTBI subjects demonstrated significantly worse performance, but these studies were faulted for lack of direct correlation between PET measures with testing results.[81,82] In a separate study evaluating 20 chronic mTBI patients, a total of 82 ROIs were compared, revealing foci of hypometabolism within the midtemporal lobe in three patients and foci of hypermetabolism within the midtemporal lobe in another 12 patients.[83] Similar contradictory findings were identified in other brain regions, although all 20 subjects demonstrated some notable FDG PET abnormalities. Surprisingly, the combination of these presumably discordant findings correlated with neuropsychological testing.[83] Combined PET-SPECT studies have revealed similar contradictory

findings such that one study identified changes in the bilateral temporal lobes,[80] whereas a similar study found no such changes.[84]

Most recently, Peskind et al studied repeated episodes of explosive blast-related chronic mTBI in Iraq combat Veterans evaluated with whole-brain FDG-PET, correlated with neuropsychological assessments and completed PCS and psychiatric symptom rating scales.[85] These researchers observed that veterans with or without PTSD demonstrated decreased cerebral metabolic rate of glucose in the cerebellar vermis, pons, and medial temporal lobe (▶ Fig. 12.11) and exhibited subtle impairments in verbal fluency, cognitive processing speed, attention, and working memory, similar to those reported in the literature for patients with cerebellar lesions. These recent results, correlating FDG-PET imaging findings with neuropsychological assessment, provide new insights into blast-related mTBI and underscore the need for further investigation in this area while increasing interest in FDG-PET as a potentially useful biomarker for evaluating this population.

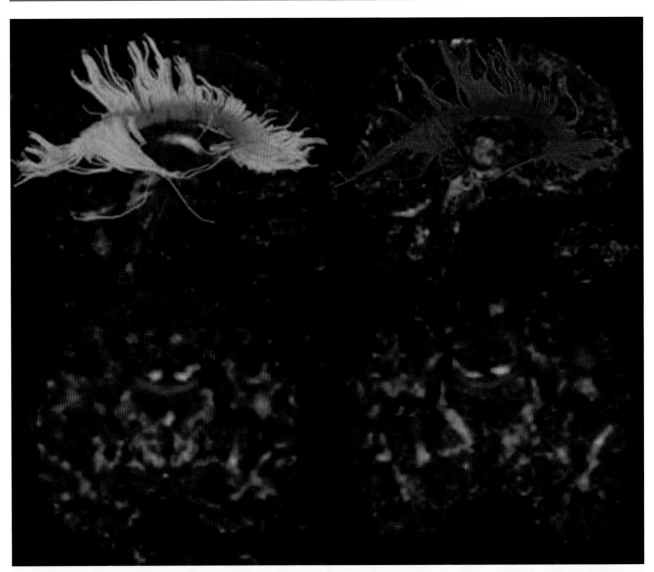

Fig. 12.9 Diffusion tensor images captured on a 3 T magnet analyzed with streamline tractography using Slicer 3. Control brain on the left and the brain of a former professional boxer in his 40 s on the right. The top two images are sagittal views with the callosal fiber tracts delineated; it is notable that the boxer's fiber tracts are markedly shorter than the control. The bottom two images are a coronal view of the same two individuals, and it can be seen that the athlete's corpus callosum (red structure in the middle of the brain) is noticeably thinner than the control. (Used with permission from Baugh. Brain Imaging and Behavior (2012) 6:244–254.)

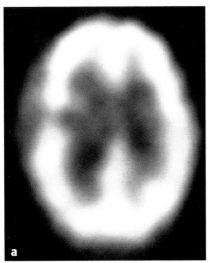

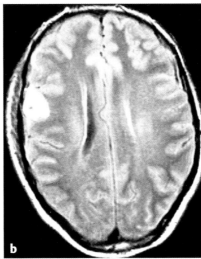

Fig. 12.10 Images obtained from a 37-year-old bicyclist. (a) Single-photon emission computed tomography image shows a right frontal perfusion deficit. (b) Corresponding fluid-attenuated inversion recovery (FLAIR) image shows a hemorrhagic contusion. (Used with permission from Hofman PA et al. Am J Neuroradiol 2001;22:441-449.)

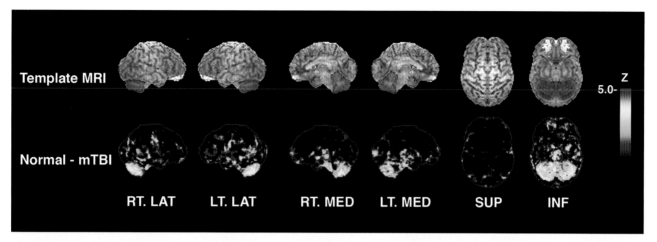

Fig. 12.11 Magnetic resonance imaging (MRI) brain template (top row) and three-dimensional SSP Z-score map of cerebral glucose metabolism difference between mild traumatic brain injury (mTBI) veterans group (n = 12) and community volunteer control group (n = 12) (bottom row) showing patterns of hypometabolism in the mTBI veterans group relative to the latter. Views are right lateral (*RT LAT*), left lateral (*LT LAT*), right medial (*RT MED*), left medial (*LT MED*), superior (*SUP*), and inferior (*INF*). Vertical bar shows image color vs. Z-score scale. (Modified with permission from Peskind ER, Petrie EC, Cross DJ, et al. Cerebrocerebellar hypometabolism associated with repetitive blast exposure mild traumatic brain injury in 12 Iraq war Veterans with persistent post-concussive symptoms. Neuroimage 2011;54 Suppl 1:S76-82.)

Current specific PET ligands are available and useful in assessing general brain function and in assessing for Alzheimer disease, but no specific ligands have yet been developed for chronic traumatic encephalopathy (often considered the sequelae of mTBI). Although the results of FDG PET studies in mTBI have been historically inconsistent, the strong correlation with neuropsychological performance does provide incentive for further investigation, especially with the advent of specialized ligands that may be highly sensitive and specific for mTBI. Until recently, FDG PET did not appear to be diagnostic for mTBI, but perhaps this will change in the near future.

12.3.4 Arterial Spin Labeling

Arterial spin labeling (ASL) is often described as a relatively new MRI technique, but it has been used experimentally for more than 20 years. ASL employs radiofrequency (RF) pulses to electromagnetically label water molecules contained within arterial blood in the neck (the usual placement of the labeling slab) en route to the brain. The labeled water molecules in the blood, unrestricted by the presence of the blood-brain barrier, act as a diffusible tracer to assess CBF. Labeled images are then compared with control (nonlabeled) images otherwise acquired in the same fashion. Because ASL relies on RF pulses to label water, it is an attractive alternative to other perfusion techniques such as gadolinium-based perfusion-weighted imaging (T2-based dynamic susceptibility contrast or T1-based dynamic contrast enhancement) techniques or nuclear medicine studies (PET and SPECT), which are dependent on the requisite intravenous injection of an exogenous substance to act as the detectable perfusion agent. With ASL, knowable variables such as the decay rate of the label and the T1 of blood relative to magnetic field strength are abstracted from the literature.[86] Multiple iterations of the ASL sequence are available, but all are based on three general techniques: pulsed ASL (PASL), continuous ASL (CASL), and pseudocontinuous ASL (pCASL). A newer velocity-selective labeling technique has been more recently introduced (velocity-selective ASL), but PASL remains the most commonly used clinical technique.

Although ASL has been used in the study of animal models[87, 88] of TBI and in human studies,[89] little research has specifically looked at ASL in the context of mTBI. The Rafols laboratory demonstrated that endothelin-1 (a powerful vasoconstrictor) and its associated receptors (endothelin receptors A and B, respectively) are upregulated after brain trauma, identifying a direct association with chronic hypoperfusion up to 48 hours after TBI.[90] Given these findings, they used a closed head acceleration impact model of TBI in rats to evaluate TBI-induced hypoperfusion and cell injury in the sensory motor cortex and hippocampus using ASL measures of CBF.[87] By selectively blocking endothelin-1 receptor A or B individually, 24 hours before TBI, they demonstrated that only blockage of endothelin-1 receptor A prevented the (> 35%) reduction in CBF identified in nontreated injured rats, thereby also highlighting the use of ASL in detecting TBI-related changes in CBF.[87]

A more recent study conducted in humans using ASL at 3 teslas (T) to assess the relative differences in regional CBF in the setting of chronic mTBI demonstrated significant reduction in bilateral mean thalamic CBF (▸ Fig. 12.12).[91]

Compared with 18 age-matched healthy controls, the evaluated 21 subjects (with median time from prior mTBI of 24.6 months) also demonstrated relative decreased CBF involving the caudate heads and bilateral frontal-lobe gray matter, although these findings did not reach statistical significance when Bonferroni correction was applied. However, the observed relative decrease in bilateral thalamic CBF was significantly correlated with neuropsychological testing results, including measures of processing and response speed, memory and learning, verbal fluency, and executive function.[91] These results suggest that regional chronic hypoperfusion is a possible sequela of mTBI, may be associated with measurable clinical impairment and neurocognitive dysfunction, and may be radiographically detected with perfusion metrics such as ASL. It is worth noting that relative hypoperfusion affecting the thalami

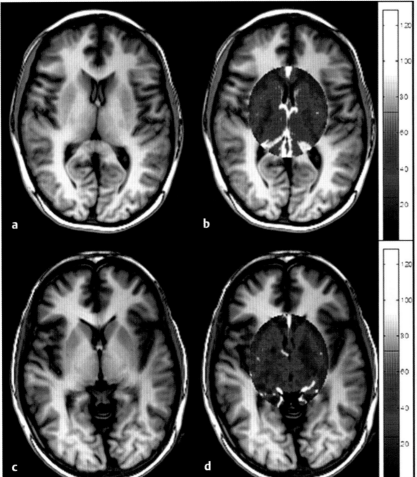

Fig. 12.12 True FISP ASL perfusion images and regional cerebral blood flow (CBF) maps in an age-matched normal control (a, b) and in a patient (c, d) with mild traumatic brain injury. Note the decreased level of CBF within the thalamic region in the patient (d) compared with the normal control (b). (Used with permission from Ge Y, Patel MB, Chen Q, et al. Assessment of thalamic perfusion in patients with mild traumatic brain injury by true FISP arterial spin labelling MR imaging at 3T. Brain Inj. 2009;23:666-674.)

(and posterior cingulate and bilateral frontal cortices) was also identified in a separate study evaluating a cohort of moderate and severe chronic TBI patients using ASL.[89]

Thus, ASL appears to be a promising technique for use in mTBI research based on the ability to characterize regional brain perfusion, the potential to conduct serial measurements of CBF in the same imaging session, the relative reproducibility of the technique, and the use of ASL as a biomarker for pharmaceutical trials. Given the relatively elevated baseline perfusion of gray matter relative to white matter, ASL might be better suited to specifically assess alterations in gray matter CBF and suspected regional hypoperfusion after mTBI. Furthermore, the ability to correlate changes in regional blood flow with cognitive deficits is an attractive feature of this technique. In addition to quantitative CBF maps, ASL can provide oxygen extraction fraction measurements and may be used to assess cerebral blood volume in the foreseeable future. Thus, ASL is a promising technique for evaluating acute, subacute, and chronic mTBI and may play a more significant role in assessing mTBI in the near future.

12.3.5 Susceptibility-Weighted Imaging

Susceptibility-weighted imaging (SWI) has been shown to be sensitive to microhemorrhages that can occur in mTBI, as demonstrated in ▶ Fig. 12.1.[92-94] The SWI technique is traditionally performed after the acquisition of a high-resolution 3D gradient recalled echo data set, for which additional phase and magnitude postprocessing is performed to accentuate the paramagnetic properties of mineralization and hemorrhagic products, thereby providing an alternate type of MR contrast.[95,96]

In the context of mTBI, the method is potentially useful in detecting tiny hemorrhagic foci (microhemorrhages) within white matter structures, which are thought to be a marker for TAI, often not detectable on conventional imaging.[3] Whereas SWI affords increased sensitivity in detecting hemorrhagic TAI relative to more conventional MRI techniques, the potential prognostic value of this sequence (in the context of mTBI) remains unclear because the technique is relatively insensitive for the detection of nonhemorrhagic TAI.[97] This insensitivity is complicated by the observation that TAI is not definitively associated with microhemorrhage,[98] an observation supported by other mTBI studies that have reported no detectable postinjury microhemorrhages or significant brain parenchymal changes when assessed with SWI.[99] Thus, SWI appears to increase the sensitivity for detecting hemorrhagic TAI, likely of added value in moderate and severe TBI (▶ Fig. 12.13), but future studies will be required to further delineate the potential prognostic value of this technique as applied to mTBI.

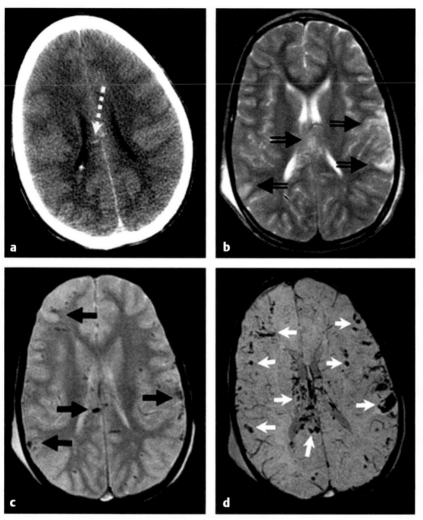

Fig. 12.13 Computed tomography (a) shows only a few small hyperdense hemorrhages in the corpus callosum (*dashed white arrow*) of a child with traumatic brain injury. Axial T2-weighted image (b) is not sensitive to hemorrhage, although ill-defined T2 hyperintense areas of edema are detected in the corpus callosum and the periphery of the hemispheres (*double-line black arrows*). Conventional gradient recalled echo (GRE) image (c) is routinely used to detect hemorrhage, which demonstrates small hypointense hemorrhagic contusions along the brain surface as well as hemorrhagic shearing injury in the corpus callosum (*solid black arrows*). However, susceptibility-weighted imaging (d) is significantly more sensitive to hemorrhage, and shows many more hemorrhages (*white arrows*) than any of the other images. (Adapted from Hunter JV, Wilde EA, Tong KA, et al. Emerging imaging tools for use with traumatic brain injury research. J Neurotrauma. 2012;29:654–671.)

12.3.6 Functional Magnetic Resonance Imaging

Functional magnetic resonance imaging (fMRI) is based on blood oxygen level–dependent (BOLD) signal alterations that result from activated neurons with increased metabolic demands, which divert a surfeit delivery of oxygenated arterial blood to their immediate surroundings, resulting in a detectable overabundance of oxygenated venous blood in the effluent leaving these regions. The resulting conversion of oxyhemoglobin to deoxyhemoglobin in the immediate surroundings alters the paramagnetic and diamagnetic properties of the tissue, resulting in decreased signal, which can be detected using a T2*-based acquisition.[100] Thus, the higher concentration of oxyhemoglobin resulting from increased neuronal activity results in higher signal intensities that result from a reduction in local field inhomogeneities and signal dephasing caused by deoxyhemoglobin. In this way, it is postulated that fMRI detects the secondary effects of neuronal firing, allowing an indirect assessment of responses to paradigms (specific cognitive or sensory patient tasks).[101] These paradigms are then applied to generate repeatable stimuli, allowing for alternating periods of rest and stimulation, which are summed to generate statistical parametric maps. The T2*-based parametric maps are generally reapplied as an overlay to high spatial resolution T1-weighted anatomic images.

In the context of mTBI, fMRI has shown promise in the ability to detect subtle, early, and chronic alterations in BOLD signal, which has been previously used to successfully differentiate among various forms of neurodegenerative diseases, including Lewy body, Alzheimer disease, and frontotemporal dementia.[102] Alterations in functional connectivity have been demonstrated with fMRI in mTBI,[103] as well as disruption of thalamic resting state.[104] In the context of sports-related mTBI, a recent study evaluated repetitive subconcussive trauma (determined by helmet accelerometer data) in high school football players and demonstrated significant changes in preseason fMRI results compared with postseason results in the same athletes, including four of eight athletes who showed no clinically observable cognitive impairment (▶ Fig. 12.14).[105]

Functional MRI has also been used to examine resting state functional connectivity (also known as resting state or rs-fMRI), which examines the interconnectedness and function of sets of neural networks, including the "default-mode network" (DMN) while subjects lie passively in the MR scanner.[106] These networks appear to represent an orderly set or cluster of regions that have a particularly high local connectedness, with a limited number of relay stations or hubs. The DMN is thought

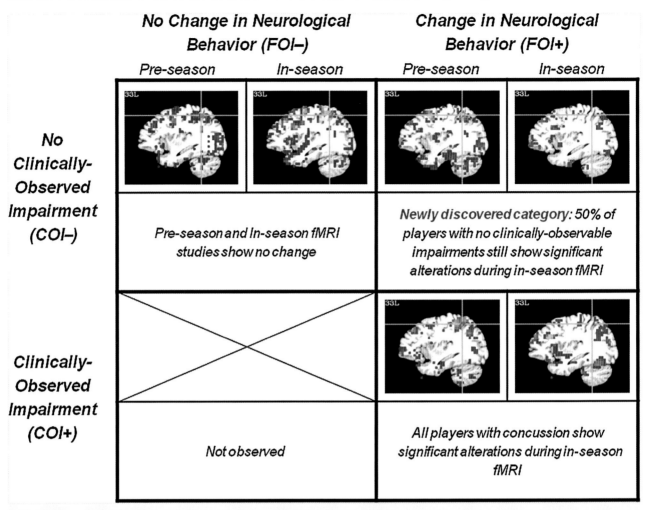

Fig. 12.14 Summary of observed football player categories, with representative function magnetic resonance imaging (fMRI) observations. Categories are based on both clinical observations by the team physician of impairment associated with concussion (clinically observed impairment; COI+ or COI-) and the presence or absence of significant neurocognitive impairment via ImPACT (functionally observed impairment; FOI+ or FOI-). fMRI activations are depicted for all players using a sagittal slice through the left inferior parietal lobule (L IPL) to illustrate the presence of many changes, relative to preseason assessment, for FOI+ players. Bottom right: As expected, all (three of three) players who were diagnosed by the team physician as having experienced a concussion (COI+) were also found to exhibit significantly reduced ImPACT scores (FOI+) and are categorized as COI+/FOI+. Top left: Half (four of eight) of the players brought in for assessment, ostensibly for control purposes (i.e., presenting with no clinically observable impairments, COI-) were found to be neurocognitively consistent with preseason assessment (FOI-) and are categorized as COI-/FOI-. Top right: The other half (four of eight) of the intended control group, studied in the absence of diagnosed concussion (COI-), were found to exhibit significantly impaired ImPACT performance (FOI +) and are categorized as COI-/FOI+. This group represents a newly observed category of possible neurological injury. Bottom left: No players who were diagnosed with a concussion (COI+) were found to exhibit ImPACT scores consistent with preseason assessments (FOI-). (Modified from Talavage TM, Nauman E, Breedlove EL, et al. Functionally-Detected Cognitive Impairment in High School Football Players Without Clinically-Diagnosed Concussion. J Neurotrauma, 2014;31(4):327-338.)

to represent one of the resting state networks of the brain, and it includes structures such as the precuneous or posterior cingulate cortex), the medial prefrontal cortex, and medial, lateral, and inferior parietal cortex. The DMN is active during rest but deactivated during specific tasks and has been related to introspection, self-referential thought, and mind wandering.

Mayer et al recently evaluated functional connectivity in 27 subacute noncomplicated mTBI patients using rs-fMRI correlated to self-reported subjective emotional, cognitive, and somatic complaints.[103] They evaluated subjects less than 3 weeks after injury and at 3 to 5 months after injury and compared results with age-matched controls. Although only 15 subjects returned for follow-up imaging, these authors identified

decreased functional connectivity within the DMN and increased connectivity between the DMN and lateral prefrontal cortex in mTBI patients.[103] Although the study identified associations between functional connectivity and predicted cognitive complaints at less than 3 weeks after injury, no changes in functional connectivity were identified at a 4-month recovery period. Interestingly, these authors report that functional connectivity measurements were able to correctly classify mTBI patients and healthy, age-matched controls in 84.3% of the time and were predictive of cognitive complaints.[103]

In a follow-up study, these same investigators used fMRI to evaluate potential differences in hemodynamic activation in mTBI patients and matched healthy controls during a multimodal selective attention task,[107] based on the observation that impaired selective attention is one of the more enduring behavioral sequelae after mTBI.[108] These investigators observed abnormalities in DMN regulation and in the top-down allocation of visual attention during the semiacute stage of mTBI despite near-normal behavioral performance in these patients.[107] More specifically, the mTBI patients failed to exhibit task-induced deactivation of the DMN during higher attention load and failed to demonstrate attention-related modulations during top-down visual attention.

In a seminal study, Stevens et al sought to evaluate the extensiveness of functional connectivity abnormalities in uncomplicated mild TBI using independent component analysis based on the observation that moderate to severe TBI results in abnormalities in coordinated activation among brain regions.[109] They evaluated 12 independent networks from fMRI data obtained with patients in a task-unconstrained resting state (30 mTBI patients and 30 demographically matched healthy control subjects; see ▶ Fig. 12.15). Abnormal functional connectivity was identified in every evaluated brain network in these mTBI patients and included networks related to visual processing, motor and limbic systems, and other circuits considered relative to executive function. Enhancements in several of these networks were also identified, suggesting possible compensatory neural processes. For nearly all interrogated brain networks, aberrant regional connectivity correlated with PCS severity.[109]

The role of fMRI in evaluating and better-defining suspected mTBI appears to be increasing, based on the added sensitivity of this technique in detecting aberrant BOLD signal, considered an indirect marker for altered neuronal activity. Continued work in rs-fMRI is anticipated to be of added future clinical utility.

12.3.7 Magnetoencephalography

Magnetoencephalography (MEG) allows the detection of magnetic flux about the surface of the head, associated with intracranial electrical currents produced between synapses or within the axons or dendrites. As with electroencephalography and evoked potential recordings, MEG can detect abnormalities in spontaneous brain activity. In addition, MEG can be used for localization, magnitude, and temporalizing the signals, allowing the generation of brain activity maps often referred to as magnetic source imaging.

Few imaging studies have been performed that evaluated mTBI with MEG.[37,110] However, one study found MEG to be superior to conventional MRI and marginally better than SPECT imaging in identifying abnormalities related to mTBI.[111] Furthermore, MEG abnormalities identified in the frontal, temporal, and parietal lobes were associated with cognitive impairment.[111] In a separate study, MEG was able to detect abnormalities in select mTBI subjects that were not detectable by DTI, suggesting that MEG may be sensitive in assessing for mTBI.[37] However, MEG is reportedly suboptimal at evaluating subcortical structures such as the deep gray nuclei, compromising its utility.[111] The limited availability of the technique, confined to major research institutions, also decreases its clinical applicability.

12.3.8 Magnetic Resonance Spectroscopy

Magnetic resonance spectroscopy (MRS) is a powerful, noninvasive technique for examining brain metabolism using clinically available MR scanners. It has shown increased sensitivity in the evaluation of mTBI by detection of brain chemistry in the setting of neuronal injury, especially related to DAI.[112–115] Unlike more traditional neuroimaging techniques, which often provide only structural detail, MRS can allow for in vivo assessment of neurochemistry by detecting individual solute-derived signals in neuronal tissue, and it can thus be used to assess for the presence of metabolic abnormalities after mTBI. Signal is most commonly derived (in experiments evaluating mTBI) from measuring hydrogen nuclei (1H) or after radiofrequency excitation and allows for repeated measurements and therapeutic monitoring. Commonly measured metabolites in 1 H MRS include the following:

- *N*-acetylaspartate (NAA): A quantitative marker of general neuronal, axonal, and dendritic viability, commonly decreased in primary brain tumors, areas of demyelination in the setting of multiple sclerosis, and brain injury.[116,117]
- Choline (Cho): A general marker for membrane disruption, synthesis, or repair and a marker of inflammation. Cho is increased in cell proliferation and membrane turnover and often is described as a marker of DAI in the context of brain injury.[118,119]
- Myo-inositol (mI): A glial cell marker involved in metabolism, expected to increase after TBI resulting from membrane damage.[120]
- Creatine (Cr) and phosphocreatine: Markers of, and proportional to, energy metabolism. Creatine is routinely used as an internal reference for the measurement of other MRS peaks.[121]
- Lactate: An indirect marker of ischemia and hypoxia, generally signaling a shift to anaerobic cellular metabolism. Its presence in the spectra is reportedly indicative of a poor outcome (in brain injury).[122]
- Glutamate/glutamine (Glx): Coupled metabolites found in astrocytes. Elevation of the Glx peak is reportedly predictive of poor outcome in severe TBI.[123]

In MRS, the preceding metabolites are usually reported as ratios, such as NAA:Cho and NAA:Cr ratios, to allow for concentration differences related to cell density rather than metabolic abnormalities.

Several techniques are used to interrogate MRS data in clinical practice; the most commonly used method is single-voxel spectroscopy (SVS), demonstrated in ▶ Fig. 12.16. This technique defines a single three-dimensional cubic ROI, usually 8 cc or larger, from which to inte a single MR spectrum. Of the various MRS techniques, SVS offers an optimal SNR and is relatively easy to perform. However, it has been criticized for being time consuming compared with other techniques because comparison with other regions of the brain requires the placement of additional voxels, each with a requisite 2 to 5 minutes of imaging time, depending on scanner parameters. Chemical shift imaging (CSI), on the other hand, allows for a larger ROI to be

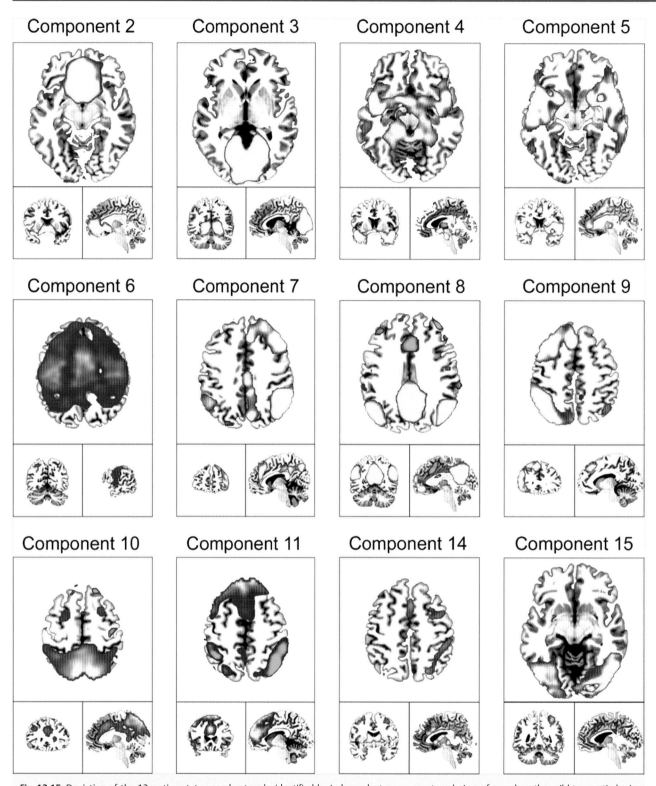

Fig. 12.15 Depiction of the 12 resting-state neural networks identified by independent component analysis performed on the mild traumatic brain injury and healthy control participants. All images are thresholded at p < 0.05 (FWE). (Used with permission from Stevens MC, Lovejoy D, Kim J, et al. Multiple resting state network functional connectivity abnormalities in mild traumatic brain injury. Brain Imaging Behav. 2012;6:293-318.)

defined by use of an additional phase encoding step and offers the advantage of allowing smaller "sub-ROIs" to be defined following the MR examination such that "retrospective" analysis can be performed. Furthermore, use of this technique allows evaluation of a more regional distribution of metabolic alterations rather than that of a single voxel (ROI). The shortcomings of this technique include decreased per-voxel SNR, such that variability of metabolite measurements is greater than with the

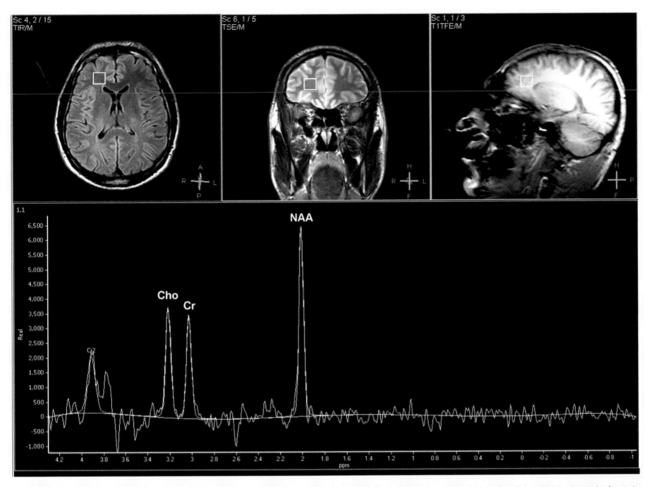

Fig. 12.16 Axial magnetic resonance imaging of a normal volunteer showing the single volume of interest (single voxel) located in the right frontal lobe, along with the corresponding proton spectrum. The tallest peak on the right represents N-acetylaspartate (*NAA*), the middle peak creatine-containing compounds (*Cr*), and left-most choline-containing compounds (*Cho*).

SVS technique, and the limitations of the two-dimensional (2D) acquisition (metabolite analysis is limited to one slice only). 3D CSI methods are becoming more readily available but lack the rigorous testing and familiarity of the former-mentioned techniques. Both the 2D- and 3D CSI techniques suffer from the contribution of metabolite signals arising from both gray matter and white matter within the same voxel and possible unwanted CSF sampling.

In the setting of moderate and severe TBI, significantly decreased NAA with associated increased Cho have been reported in both gray and white matter after injury (▶ Fig. 12.17).[124–128] It is thought that reduction of NAA in regions of visibly injured brain are likely the result of the primary impact, whereas decreased NAA in regions of normal appearing tissue may result from Wallerian degeneration versus DAI.[128] The increased Cho within white matter is thought to represent a metabolic by-product of myelin shear injury.[129]

In evaluating mTBI, several longitudinal studies have been performed that have demonstrated a relative decrease in NAA with an increase in white matter Cr in the acute stages of mTBI, both of which reportedly return to normal levels by the conclusion of the respective longitudinal study.[115,130–133] In one such study, for example, Vagnozzi et al used single-voxel MRS

performed at 1.5 T and 3 T and multivoxel MRS performed at 3 T to prospectively evaluate 40 concussed athletes (and 30 control subjects) 3, 15, 22, and 30 days after injury.[115] Athletes and control subjects were imaged at three different institutions with differing field-strength MRI systems for which the MR spectra (focused on NAA-, Cr-, and Cho-containing compounds) were compared. These authors reported that spectroscopic data obtained from controls using differing field strengths or modes of acquisition did not reveal any differences in brain metabolite ratios. Compared with normal controls, the most significant alteration in metabolite ratios in concussed athletes was noted at postinjury day 3 (NAA: Cr = 17.6%, NAA:Cho = 21.4%). The authors reported that metabolic disturbances gradually recovered in these athletes, initially slowly until day 15, then more rapidly, such that all athletes demonstrated normal metabolic ratios at day 30, comparable with values detected in normal controls.[115]

Interestingly, if a second traumatic insult is obtained during the initial recovery period in adults with acute mTBI, there is evidence to suggest prolongation of decreased NAA values after the initial traumatic insult, which may take up to 45 days to approach, but not necessarily reach, baseline levels.[130] This evidence has important implications for a hypothesized

¹H-MRS Spectra

NV

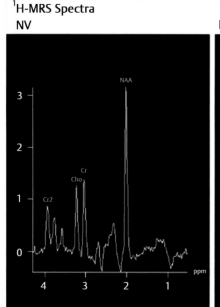

MTBI

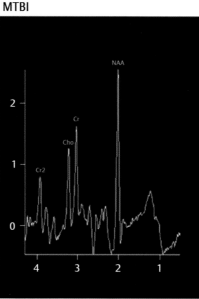

Fig. 12.17 Examples of 1H-MRS spectra acquired from one voxel for mTBI (*MTBI*) and normal volunteer (*NV*) group. Notice the increased Cho and decreased NAA peaks in the MTBI subjects compared to NV. (Modified from Brian Johnson, Kai Zhang, Michael Gay, et al. Metabolic alterations in corpus callosum may compromise brain functional connectivity in MTBI patients: An 1H-MRS study, Neuroscience Letters. 2012; 509 (1):5-8.)

cumulative effect in mTBI. At the same time, Maugans et al used a similar longitudinal study design in a pediatric population and identified no significant change in NAA concentrations after acute mTBI, suggesting some possible age-related neuroprotection.[133] This observation, although promising, warrants further investigation to substantiate these claims.

With respect to chronic mTBI, several studies have suggested that NAA is generally decreased in white matter structures, including the splenium, centrum semiovale, and frontal white matter,[125,130,134] This observation has also been confirmed in CSI studies of mTBI[135,136] and is supported by evaluations of whole-brain NAA using volumetric spectroscopy.[137] DTI studies evaluating mTBI corroborate these observations, demonstrating a similar distribution of injury and loss of neurons within the gray and white matter.[138]

The often reported general increase in Cho levels in the setting of chronic TBI is thought to reflect diffuse glial proliferation, supported by concomitantly increased mI, which persists months after the initial injury.[139,140] However, further studies are needed to substantiate these observations. In a select few studies performed in the evaluation of mTBI using MRS have demonstrated somewhat conflicting results. For example, one study by Son et al determined that lactate levels are elevated acutely in mTBI,[141] whereas a similar study by Garnett et al revealed no such lactate elevation.[142]

Use of MRS in mTBI is advantageous because it can be easily performed, is safely repeatable because it does not require the use of ionizing radiation, and can be used in longitudinal studies. Further investigation is needed to evaluate the sensitivity and specificity of MRS in the context of mTBI and establish its prognostic value. Although it is a relatively nonspecific tool, NAA evaluation by MRS represents a noninvasive manner with which to measure transient changes in energy metabolism in the setting of mTBI. Further studies are needed to verify the effects of a second traumatic insult within the recovery period

and to define more clearly the observed differences in MR spectra in adults versus children.

12.4 Conclusion

Advanced MRI techniques have significantly contributed to recent research in mTBI and have at times suggested mechanistic, as well as structural, correlates to clinical observations and neuropsychological testing results. DTI, MRS, and fMRI appear optimal at evaluating for mTBI, based on their individual sensitivities and specificities in detecting mTBI, as well as the potential prognostic value and strong correlation with patient symptoms. Research in these techniques has revealed that what was once considered *mild* traumatic brain injury (implicit in the name: mTBI) may have more significant long-term consequences and that even subconcussive blows may contribute to declines in various performance and cognitive metrics. The detection of abnormalities using these advanced imaging techniques, in the setting of normal-appearing morphologic MRI, suggests a new baseline on which to assess changes related to mTBI. The increasing use of these advanced imaging techniques provides new insights into better identifying abnormalities related to suspected parenchymal injury, possibly allowing for more appropriate triage and earlier treatment of patients suffering from suspected TBI-related symptoms. Furthermore, specific research in sports-related concussion has unveiled substantive, specific concerns regarding the role of cumulative blows and multiple concussions that may increase the risk for developing chronic traumatic encephalopathy, psychiatric illnesses such as depression, and the possibility of long-term mild cognitive impairment. Although many unanswered questions remain, it is likely that advanced MRI techniques will continue to contribute to the current understanding and pathophysiology of mTBI and will become more commonplace in the clinical workflow.

References

[1] Bazarian JJ, Zhong J, Blyth B, Zhu T, Kavcic V, Peterson D. Diffusion tensor imaging detects clinically important axonal damage after mild traumatic brain injury: a pilot study. J Neurotrauma 2007; 24: 1447–1459

[2] Inglese M, Makani S, Johnson G et al. Diffuse axonal injury in mild traumatic brain injury: a diffusion tensor imaging study. J Neurosurg 2005; 103: 298–303

[3] Scheid R, Preul C, Gruber O, Wiggins C, von Cramon DY. Diffuse axonal injury associated with chronic traumatic brain injury: evidence from T2*-weighted gradient-echo imaging at 3 T. AJNR Am J Neuroradiol 2003; 24: 1049–1056

[4] Faul MXL, Wald MM, Coronado VG. Traumatic Brain Injury in the United States: Emergency Department Visits, Hospitalizations and Deaths 2002–2006. Atlanta, GA: Centers for Disease Control and Prevention, National Center for Injury Prevention and Control; 2010.

[5] Thurman DJ, Alverson C, Dunn KA, Guerrero J, Sniezek JE. Traumatic brain injury in the United States: A public health perspective. J Head Trauma Rehabil 1999; 14: 602–615

[6] Bazarian JJ, Blyth B, Cimpello L. Bench to bedside: evidence for brain injury after concussion—looking beyond the computed tomography scan. Acad Emerg Med. 2006; 13: 199–214

[7] Sosin DM, Sniezek JE, Thurman DJ. Incidence of mild and moderate brain injury in the United States, 1991. Brain Inj. 1996; 10: 47–54

[8] Ruff RM, Camenzuli L, Mueller J. Miserable minority: emotional risk factors that influence the outcome of a mild traumatic brain injury. Brain Inj. 1996; 10: 551–565

[9] Bazarian JJ, Wong T, Harris M, Leahey N, Mookerjee S, Dombovy M. Epidemiology and predictors of post-concussive syndrome after minor head injury in an emergency population. Brain Inj. 1999; 13: 173–189

[10] Vanderploeg RD, Curtiss G, Luis CA, Salazar AM. Long-term morbidities following self-reported mild traumatic brain injury. J Clin Exp Neuropsychol 2007; 29: 585–598

[11] Belanger HG, Kretzmer T, Vanderploeg RD, French LM. Symptom complaints following combat-related traumatic brain injury: relationship to traumatic brain injury severity and posttraumatic stress disorder. J Int Neuropsychol Soc 2010; 16: 194–199

[12] Hoge CW, McGurk D, Thomas JL, Cox AL, Engel CC, Castro CA. Mild traumatic brain injury in U.S. Soldiers returning from Iraq. N Engl J Med 2008; 358: 453–463

[13] Hoge CW, Goldberg HM, Castro CA. Care of war veterans with mild traumatic brain injury—flawed perspectives. N Engl J Med. 2009; 360: 1588–1591

[14] FitzGerald DB, Crosson BA. Diffusion weighted imaging and neuropsychological correlates in adults with mild traumatic brain injury. Int J Psychophysiol 2011; 82: 79–85

[15] Niogi SN, Mukherjee P. Diffusion tensor imaging of mild traumatic brain injury. J Head Trauma Rehabil. 2010; 25: 241–255

[16] Green R, Koshimori Y, Turner G. Research digest: understanding the organic basis of persistent complaints in mTBI: findings from functional and structural neuroimaging. Neuropsychol Rehabil. 2010; 20: 471–478

[17] Mittl RL, Grossman RI, Hiehle JF et al. Prevalence of MR evidence of diffuse axonal injury in patients with mild head injury and normal head CT findings. AJNR Am J Neuroradiol 1994; 15: 1583–1589

[18] Gentry LR, Godersky JC, Thompson B, Dunn VD. Prospective comparative study of intermediate-field MR and CT in the evaluation of closed head trauma. AJR Am J Roentgenol 1988; 150: 673–682

[19] Benson RR, Meda SA, Vasudevan S et al. Global white matter analysis of diffusion tensor images is predictive of injury severity in traumatic brain injury. J Neurotrauma. 2007; 24: 446–459

[20] Hammoud DA, Wasserman BA. Diffuse axonal injuries: pathophysiology and imaging. Neuroimaging Clin N Am. 2002; 12: 205–216

[21] Vos PE, Battistin L, Birbamer G et al. European Federation of Neurological Societies. EFNS guideline on mild traumatic brain injury: report of an EFNS task force. Eur J Neurol. 2002; 9: 207–219

[22] Belanger HG, Vanderploeg RD, Curtiss G, Warden DL. Recent neuroimaging techniques in mild traumatic brain injury. J Neuropsychiatry Clin Neurosci. 2007; 19: 5–20

[23] Bigler ED. Neuropsychology and clinical neuroscience of persistent post-concussive syndrome. J Int Neuropsychol Soc. 2008; 14: 1–22

[24] Blumbergs PC, Scott G, Manavis J, Wainwright H, Simpson DA, McLean AJ. Topography of axonal injury as defined by amyloid precursor protein and the sector scoring method in mild and severe closed head injury. J Neurotrauma 1995; 12: 565–572

[25] Adams JH, Doyle D, Ford I, Gennarelli TA, Graham DI, McLellan DR. Diffuse axonal injury in head injury: definition, diagnosis and grading. Histopathology. 1989; 15: 49–59

[26] Sheedy J, Geffen G, Donnelly J, Faux S. Emergency department assessment of mild traumatic brain injury and prediction of post-concussion symptoms at one month post injury. J Clin Exp Neuropsychol 2006; 28: 755–772

[27] Lundin A, de Boussard C, Edman G, Borg J. Symptoms and disability until 3 months after mild TBI. Brain Inj 2006; 20: 799–806

[28] Iverson GL. Misdiagnosis of the persistent postconcussion syndrome in patients with depression. Arch Clin Neuropsychol 2006; 21: 303–310

[29] Begaz T, Kyriacou DN, Segal J, Bazarian JJ. Serum biochemical markers for post-concussion syndrome in patients with mild traumatic brain injury. J Neurotrauma. 2006; 23: 1201–1210

[30] McCauley SR, Boake C, Pedroza C et al. Correlates of persistent postconcussional disorder: DSM-IV criteria versus ICD-10. J Clin Exp Neuropsychol 2008; 30: 360–379

[31] Lannsjö M, af Geijerstam JL, Johansson U, Bring J, Borg J. Prevalence and structure of symptoms at 3 months after mild traumatic brain injury in a national cohort. Brain Inj. 2009; 23: 213–219

[32] King NS, Kirwilliam S. Permanent post-concussion symptoms after mild head injury. Brain Inj. 2011; 25: 462–470

[33] Ponsford J, Willmott C, Rothwell A et al. Factors influencing outcome following mild traumatic brain injury in adults. J Int Neuropsychol Soc 2000; 6: 568–579

[34] Kou Z, Wu Z, Tong KA et al. The role of advanced MR imaging findings as biomarkers of traumatic brain injury. J Head Trauma Rehabil 2010; 25: 267–282

[35] Arfanakis K, Haughton VM, Carew JD, Rogers BP, Dempsey RJ, Meyerand ME. Diffusion tensor MR imaging in diffuse axonal injury. AJNR Am J Neuroradiol 2002; 23: 794–802

[36] Lipton ML, Gellella E, Lo C et al. Multifocal white matter ultrastructural abnormalities in mild traumatic brain injury with cognitive disability: a voxel-wise analysis of diffusion tensor imaging. J Neurotrauma 2008; 25: 1335–1342

[37] Huang MX, Theilmann RJ, Robb A et al. Integrated imaging approach with MEG and DTI to detect mild traumatic brain injury in military and civilian patients. J Neurotrauma 2009; 26: 1213–1226

[38] Niogi SN, Mukherjee P, Ghajar J et al. Extent of microstructural white matter injury in postconcussive syndrome correlates with impaired cognitive reaction time: a 3 T diffusion tensor imaging study of mild traumatic brain injury. AJNR Am J Neuroradiol. 2008; 29: 967–973

[39] Moseley ME, Wendland MF, Kucharczyk J. Magnetic resonance imaging of diffusion and perfusion. Top Magn Reson Imaging 1991; 3: 50–67

[40] Lutsep HL, Albers GW, DeCrespigny A, Kamat GN, Marks MP, Moseley ME. Clinical utility of diffusion-weighted magnetic resonance imaging in the assessment of ischemic stroke. Ann Neurol 1997; 41: 574–580

[41] van Doorn ABP, Bovendeerd PH, Nicolay K, Drost MR, Janssen JD. Determination of muscle fibre orientation using diffusion-weighted MRI. Eur J Morphol 1996; 34: 5–10

[42] Le Bihan D. Molecular diffusion nuclear magnetic resonance imaging. Magn Reson Q 1991; 7: 1–30

[43] Bammer R. Basic principles of diffusion-weighted imaging. Eur J Radiol. 2003; 45: 169–184

[44] Povlishock JT, Katz DI. Update of neuropathology and neurological recovery after traumatic brain injury. J Head Trauma Rehabil 2005; 20: 76–94

[45] Rutgers DR, Fillard P, Paradot G, Tadié M, Lasjaunias P, Ducreux D. Diffusion tensor imaging characteristics of the corpus callosum in mild, moderate, and severe traumatic brain injury. AJNR Am J Neuroradiol 2008; 29: 1730–1735

[46] Rutgers DR, Toulgoat F, Cazejust J, Fillard P, Lasjaunias P, Ducreux D. White matter abnormalities in mild traumatic brain injury: a diffusion tensor imaging study. AJNR Am J Neuroradiol 2008; 29: 514–519

[47] Shenton ME, Hamoda HM, Schneiderman JS et al. A review of magnetic resonance imaging and diffusion tensor imaging findings in mild traumatic brain injury. Brain Imaging Behav 2012; 6: 137–192

[48] Pierpaoli C, Basser PJ. Toward a quantitative assessment of diffusion anisotropy. Magn Reson Med 1996; 36: 893–906

[49] Hunter JV, Wilde EA, Tong KA, Holshouser BA. Emerging imaging tools for use with traumatic brain injury research. J Neurotrauma 2012; 29: 654–671

[50] Watts R, Liston C, Niogi S, Uluğ AM. Fiber tracking using magnetic resonance diffusion tensor imaging and its applications to human brain development. Ment Retard Dev Disabil Res Rev 2003; 9: 168–177

[51] Tuch DS. Q-ball imaging. Magn Reson Med. 2004; 52: 1358–1372

[52] Frank LR. Characterization of anisotropy in high angular resolution diffusion-weighted MRI. Magn Reson Med 2002; 47: 1083–1099

[53] Behrens TE, Woolrich MW, Jenkinson M et al. Characterization and propagation of uncertainty in diffusion-weighted MR imaging. Magn Reson Med 2003; 50: 1077–1088

[54] Behrens TE, Johansen-Berg H, Woolrich MW et al. Non-invasive mapping of connections between human thalamus and cortex using diffusion imaging. Nat Neurosci. 2003; 6: 750–757

[55] Morey RA, Haswell CC, Selgrade ES et al. Effects of chronic mild traumatic brain injury on white matter integrity in Iraq and Afghanistan war veterans. Hum Brain Mapp. 2013;34(11):2986–2999

[56] Wilde EA, McCauley SR, Barnes A et al. Serial measurement of memory and diffusion tensor imaging changes within the first week following uncomplicated mild traumatic brain injury. Brain Imaging Behav 2012; 6: 319–328

[57] Covassin T, Elbin RJ, Nakayama Y. Tracking neurocognitive performance following concussion in high school athletes. Phys Sportsmed 2010; 38: 87–93

[58] Iverson GL. Complicated vs uncomplicated mild traumatic brain injury: acute neuropsychological outcome. Brain Inj. 2006; 20: 1335–1344

[59] Sim A, Terryberry-Spohr L, Wilson KR. Prolonged recovery of memory functioning after mild traumatic brain injury in adolescent athletes. J Neurosurg. 2008; 108: 511–516

[60] Thomas D. A structured approach to brain injury rehabilitation. J Neurosci Rural Pract 2011; 2: 112–114

[61] Kwok FY, Lee TM, Leung CH, Poon WS. Changes of cognitive functioning following mild traumatic brain injury over a 3-month period. Brain Inj 2008; 22: 740–751

[62] Betz J, Zhuo J, Roy A, Shanmuganathan K, Gullapalli RP. Prognostic value of diffusion tensor imaging parameters in severe traumatic brain injury. J Neurotrauma 2012; 29: 1292–1305

[63] Aoki Y, Inokuchi R, Gunshin M, Yahagi N, Suwa H. Diffusion tensor imaging studies of mild traumatic brain injury: a meta-analysis. J Neurol Neurosurg Psychiatry. 2012; 83: 870–876

[64] Salmond CH, Menon DK, Chatfield DA et al. Diffusion tensor imaging in chronic head injury survivors: correlations with learning and memory indices. Neuroimage. 2006; 29: 117–124

[65] Caeyenberghs K, Leemans A, Geurts M et al. Brain-behavior relationships in young traumatic brain injury patients: fractional anisotropy measures are highly correlated with dynamic visuomotor tracking performance. Neuropsychologia. 2010; 48: 1472–1482

[66] Caeyenberghs K, Leemans A, Geurts M et al. Brain-behavior relationships in young traumatic brain injury patients: DTI metrics are highly correlated with postural control. Hum Brain Mapp 2010; 31: 992–1002

[67] Wozniak JR, Krach L, Ward E et al. Neurocognitive and neuroimaging correlates of pediatric traumatic brain injury: a diffusion tensor imaging (DTI) study. Arch Clin Neuropsychol 2007; 22: 555–568

[68] Bergsneider M, Hovda DA, McArthur DL et al. Metabolic recovery following human traumatic brain injury based on FDG-PET: time course and relationship to neurological disability. J Head Trauma Rehabil 2001; 16: 135–148

[69] Masterman DL, Mendez MF, Fairbanks LA, Cummings JL. Sensitivity, specificity, and positive predictive value of technetium 99-HMPAO SPECT in discriminating Alzheimer's disease from other dementias. J Geriatr Psychiatry Neurol 1997; 10: 15–21

[70] Amen DG, Newberg A, Thatcher R et al. Impact of playing American professional football on long-term brain function. J Neuropsychiatry Clin Neurosci 2011; 23: 98–106

[71] Hofman PA, Stapert SZ, van Kroonenburgh MJ, Jolles J, de Kruijk J, Wilmink JT. MR imaging, single-photon emission CT, and neurocognitive performance after mild traumatic brain injury. AJNR Am J Neuroradiol 2001; 22: 441–449

[72] Jacobs A, Put E, Ingels M, Put T, Bossuyt A. One-year follow-up of technetium-99m-HMPAO SPECT in mild head injury. J Nucl Med 1996; 37: 1605–1609

[73] Report of the Therapeutics and Technology Assessment Subcommittee of the American Academy of Neurology. Assessment of brain SPECT. Neurology. 1996; 46: 278–285

[74] Audenaert K, Jansen HM, Otte A et al. Imaging of mild traumatic brain injury using 57Co and 99mTc HMPAO SPECT as compared to other diagnostic procedures. Med Sci Monit. 2003; 9: MT112–MT117

[75] Nedd K, Sfakianakis G, Ganz W et al. 99mTc-HMPAO SPECT of the brain in mild to moderate traumatic brain injury patients: compared with CT—a prospective study. Brain Inj. 1993; 7: 469–479

[76] Umile EM, Plotkin RC, Sandel ME. Functional assessment of mild traumatic brain injury using SPECT and neuropsychological testing. Brain Inj. 1998; 12: 577–594

[77] Bonne O, Gilboa A, Louzoun Y et al. Cerebral blood flow in chronic symptomatic mild traumatic brain injury. Psychiatry Res. 2003; 124: 141–152

[78] Ichise M, Chung DG, Wang P, Wortzman G, Gray BG, Franks W. Technetium-99m-HMPAO SPECT, CT and MRI in the evaluation of patients with chronic traumatic brain injury: a correlation with neuropsychological performance. J Nucl Med 1994; 35: 217–226

[79] Kant R, Smith-Seemiller L, Isaac G, Duffy J. Tc-HMPAO SPECT in persistent post-concussion syndrome after mild head injury: comparison with MRI/CT. Brain Inj. 1997; 11: 115–124

[80] Umile EM, Sandel ME, Alavi A, Terry CM, Plotkin RC. Dynamic imaging in mild traumatic brain injury: support for the theory of medial temporal vulnerability. Arch Phys Med Rehabil 2002; 83: 1506–1513

[81] Ruff RM, Crouch JA, Tröster AI et al. Selected cases of poor outcome following a minor brain trauma: comparing neuropsychological and positron emission tomography assessment. Brain Inj. 1994; 8: 297–308

[82] Roberts MA, Manshadi FF, Bushnell DL, Hines ME. Neurobehavioural dysfunction following mild traumatic brain injury in childhood: a case report with positive findings on positron emission tomography (PET). Brain Inj. 1995; 9: 427–436

[83] Gross H, Kling A, Henry G, Herndon C, Lavretsky H. Local cerebral glucose metabolism in patients with long-term behavioral and cognitive deficits following mild traumatic brain injury. J Neuropsychiatry Clin Neurosci. 1996; 8: 324–334

[84] Chen SH, Kareken DA, Fastenau PS, Trexler LE, Hutchins GD. A study of persistent post-concussion symptoms in mild head trauma using positron emission tomography. J Neurol Neurosurg Psychiatry 2003; 74: 326–332

[85] Peskind ER, Petrie EC, Cross DJ et al. Cerebrocerebellar hypometabolism associated with repetitive blast exposure mild traumatic brain injury in 12 Iraq war Veterans with persistent post-concussive symptoms. Neuroimage. 2011; 54 Suppl 1: S76–S82

[86] Buxton RB. Quantifying CBF with arterial spin labeling. J Magn Reson Imaging. 2005; 22: 723–726

[87] Kreipke CW, Schafer PC, Rossi NF, Rafols JA. Differential effects of endothelin receptor A and B antagonism on cerebral hypoperfusion following traumatic brain injury. Neurol Res 2010; 32: 209–214

[88] Kochanek PM, Hendrich KS, Dixon CE, Schiding JK, Williams DS, Ho C. Cerebral blood flow at one year after controlled cortical impact in rats: assessment by magnetic resonance imaging. J Neurotrauma 2002; 19: 1029–1037

[89] Kim J, Whyte J, Patel S et al. Resting cerebral blood flow alterations in chronic traumatic brain injury: an arterial spin labeling perfusion FMRI study. J Neurotrauma. 2010; 27: 1399–1411

[90] Rafols JA. Editorial: microvascular and neuronal responses in a model of diffuse brain injury: therapeutic implications. Neurol Res 2007; 29: 337–338

[91] Ge Y, Patel MB, Chen Q et al. Assessment of thalamic perfusion in patients with mild traumatic brain injury by true FISP arterial spin labelling MR imaging at 3 T. Brain Inj. 2009; 23: 666–674

[92] Babikian T, Freier MC, Tong KA et al. Susceptibility weighted imaging: neuropsychologic outcome and pediatric head injury. Pediatr Neurol 2005; 33: 184–194

[93] Scheid R, Ott DV, Roth H, Schroeter ML, von Cramon DY. Comparative magnetic resonance imaging at 1.5 and 3 Tesla for the evaluation of traumatic microbleeds. J Neurotrauma. 2007; 24: 1811–1816

[94] Park JH, Park SW, Kang SH, Nam TK, Min BK, Hwang SN. Detection of traumatic cerebral microbleeds by susceptibility-weighted image of MRI. J Korean Neurosurg Soc. 2009; 46: 365–369

[95] Haacke EM, Xu Y, Cheng YC, Reichenbach JR. Susceptibility weighted imaging (SWI). Magn Reson Med. 2004; 52: 612–618

[96] Haacke EM, Mittal S, Wu Z, Neelavalli J, Cheng YC. Susceptibility-weighted imaging: technical aspects and clinical applications, part 1. AJNR Am J Neuroradiol. 2009; 30: 19–30

[97] Chastain CA, Oyoyo UE, Zipperman M et al. Predicting outcomes of traumatic brain injury by imaging modality and injury distribution. J Neurotrauma. 2009; 26: 1183–1196

[98] Kinnunen KM, Greenwood R, Powell JH et al. White matter damage and cognitive impairment after traumatic brain injury. Brain. 2011; 134: 449–463

[99] Toth A, Kovacs N, Perlaki G et al. Multi-modal magnetic resonance imaging in the acute and sub-acute phase of mild traumatic brain injury: Can we see the difference? J Neurotrauma. 2013;

[100] Ogawa S, Menon RS, Tank DW et al. Functional brain mapping by blood oxygenation level-dependent contrast magnetic resonance imaging: a comparison of signal characteristics with a biophysical model. Biophys J. 1993; 64: 803–812

[101] Jueptner M, Weiller C. Review: does measurement of regional cerebral blood flow reflect synaptic activity? Implications for PET and fMRI. Neuroimage. 1995; 2: 148–156

[102] Galvin JE, Price JL, Yan Z, Morris JC, Sheline YI. Resting bold fMRI differentiates dementia with Lewy bodies vs Alzheimer disease. Neurology 2011; 76: 1797–1803

[103] Mayer AR, Mannell MV, Ling J, Gasparovic C, Yeo RA. Functional connectivity in mild traumatic brain injury. Hum Brain Mapp. 2011; 32: 1825–1835

[104] Tang L, Ge Y, Sodickson DK et al. Thalamic resting-state functional networks: disruption in patients with mild traumatic brain injury. Radiology. 2011; 260: 831–840

[105] Talavage TM, Nauman E, Breedlove EL et al. Functionally-detected cognitive impairment in high school football players without clinically-diagnosed concussion (abstract). J Neurotrauma. 2013;E-pub ahead of print.

[106] Greicius MD, Krasnow B, Reiss AL, Menon V. Functional connectivity in the resting brain: a network analysis of the default mode hypothesis. Proc Natl Acad Sci U S A. 2003; 100: 253–258

[107] Mayer AR, Yang Z, Yeo RA et al. A functional MRI study of multimodal selective attention following mild traumatic brain injury. Brain Imaging Behav 2012; 6: 343–354

[108] Halterman CI, Langan J, Drew A et al. Tracking the recovery of visuospatial attention deficits in mild traumatic brain injury. Brain. 2006; 129: 747–753

[109] Stevens MC, Lovejoy D, Kim J, Oakes H, Kureshi I, Witt ST. Multiple resting state network functional connectivity abnormalities in mild traumatic brain injury. Brain Imaging Behav. 2012; 6: 293–318

[110] Huang MX, Nichols S, Robb A et al. An automatic MEG low-frequency source imaging approach for detecting injuries in mild and moderate TBI patients with blast and non-blast causes. Neuroimage. 2012; 61: 1067–1082

[111] Lewine JD, Davis JT, Bigler ED et al. Objective documentation of traumatic brain injury subsequent to mild head trauma: multimodal brain imaging with MEG, SPECT, and MRI. J Head Trauma Rehabil 2007; 22: 141–155

[112] Babikian T, Freier MC, Ashwal S, Riggs ML, Burley T, Holshouser BA. MR spectroscopy: predicting long-term neuropsychological outcome following pediatric TBI. J Magn Reson Imaging. 2006; 24: 801–811

[113] Ross BD, Bluml S, Cowan R, Danielsen E, Farrow N, Tan J. In vivo MR spectroscopy of human dementia. Neuroimaging Clin N Am 1998; 8: 809–822

[114] Lin A, Ross BD, Harris K, Wong W. Efficacy of proton magnetic resonance spectroscopy in neurological diagnosis and neurotherapeutic decision making. NeuroRx. 2005; 2: 197–214

[115] Vagnozzi R, Signoretti S, Cristofori L et al. Assessment of metabolic brain damage and recovery following mild traumatic brain injury: a multicentre, proton magnetic resonance spectroscopic study in concussed patients. Brain 2010; 133: 3232–3242

[116] Barker PB, Gillard JH, van Zijl PC et al. Acute stroke: evaluation with serial proton MR spectroscopic imaging. Radiology. 1994; 192: 723–732

[117] Signoretti S, Marmarou A, Tavazzi B, Lazzarino G, Beaumont A, Vagnozzi R. N-Acetylaspartate reduction as a measure of injury severity and mitochondrial dysfunction following diffuse traumatic brain injury. J Neurotrauma. 2001; 18: 977–991

[118] Brenner RE, Munro PM, Williams SC et al. The proton NMR spectrum in acute EAE: the significance of the change in the Cho:Cr ratio. Magn Reson Med. 1993; 29: 737–745

[119] Holshouser BA, Tong KA, Ashwal S. Proton MR spectroscopic imaging depicts diffuse axonal injury in children with traumatic brain injury. AJNR Am J Neuroradiol. 2005; 26: 1276–1285

[120] Bitsch A, Bruhn H, Vougioukas V et al. Inflammatory CNS demyelination: histopathologic correlation with in vivo quantitative proton MR spectroscopy. AJNR Am J Neuroradiol 1999; 20: 1619–1627

[121] Anderson ML, Smith DS, Nioka S et al. Experimental brain ischaemia: assessment of injury by magnetic resonance spectroscopy and histology. Neurol Res. 1990; 12: 195–204

[122] Go KG, Kamman RL, Mooyaart EL et al. Localised proton spectroscopy and spectroscopic imaging in cerebral gliomas, with comparison to positron emission tomography. Neuroradiology. 1995; 37: 198–206

[123] Shutter L, Tong KA, Holshouser BA. Proton MRS in acute traumatic brain injury: role for glutamate/glutamine and choline for outcome prediction. J Neurotrauma 2004; 21: 1693–1705

[124] Garnett MR, Corkill RG, Blamire AM et al. Altered cellular metabolism following traumatic brain injury: a magnetic resonance spectroscopy study. J Neurotrauma. 2001; 18: 231–240

[125] Garnett MR, Blamire AM, Corkill RG, Cadoux-Hudson TA, Rajagopalan B, Styles P. Early proton magnetic resonance spectroscopy in normal-appearing brain correlates with outcome in patients following traumatic brain injury. Brain. 2000; 123: 2046–2054

[126] Signoretti S, Marmarou A, Fatouros P et al. Application of chemical shift imaging for measurement of NAA in head injured patients. Acta Neurochir Suppl (Wien). 2002; 81: 373–375

[127] Brooks WM, Stidley CA, Petropoulos H et al. Metabolic and cognitive response to human traumatic brain injury: a quantitative proton magnetic resonance study. J Neurotrauma. 2000; 17: 629–640

[128] Friedman SD, Brooks WM, Jung RE et al. Quantitative proton MRS predicts outcome after traumatic brain injury. Neurology. 1999; 52: 1384–1391

[129] Ross BD, Ernst T, Kreis R et al. 1 H MRS in acute traumatic brain injury. J Magn Reson Imaging 1998; 8: 829–840

[130] Vagnozzi R, Signoretti S, Tavazzi B et al. Temporal window of metabolic brain vulnerability to concussion: a pilot 1H-magnetic resonance spectroscopic study in concussed athletes—part III. Neurosurgery. 2008; 62: 1286–1296

[131] Yeo RA, Gasparovic C, Merideth F, Ruhl D, Doezema D, Mayer AR. A longitudinal proton magnetic resonance spectroscopy study of mild traumatic brain injury. J Neurotrauma. 2011; 28: 1–11

[132] Henry LC, Tremblay S, Leclerc S et al. Metabolic changes in concussed American football players during the acute and chronic post-injury phases. BMC Neurol. 2011; 11: 105.

[133] Maugans TA, Farley C, Altaye M, Leach J, Cecil KM. Pediatric sports-related concussion produces cerebral blood flow alterations. Pediatrics 2012; 129: 28–37

[134] Cecil KM, Hills EC, Sandel ME et al. Proton magnetic resonance spectroscopy for detection of axonal injury in the splenium of the corpus callosum of brain-injured patients. J Neurosurg 1998; 88: 795–801

[135] Cimatti M. Assessment of metabolic cerebral damage using proton magnetic resonance spectroscopy in mild traumatic brain injury. J Neurosurg Sci 2006; 50: 83–88

[136] Kirov I, Fleysher L, Babb JS, Silver JM, Grossman RI, Gonen O. Characterizing 'mild' in traumatic brain injury with proton MR spectroscopy in the thalamus: Initial findings. Brain Inj. 2007; 21: 1147–1154

[137] Cohen BA, Inglese M, Rusinek H, Babb JS, Grossman RI, Gonen O. Proton MR spectroscopy and MRI-volumetry in mild traumatic brain injury. AJNR Am J Neuroradiol 2007; 28: 907–913

[138] Kraus MF, Susmaras T, Caughlin BP, Walker CJ, Sweeney JA, Little DM. White matter integrity and cognition in chronic traumatic brain injury: a diffusion tensor imaging study. Brain 2007; 130: 2508–2519

[139] Ashwal S, Holshouser B, Tong K et al. Proton spectroscopy detected myoinositol in children with traumatic brain injury. Pediatr Res. 2004; 56: 630–638

[140] Govindaraju V, Gauger GE, Manley GT, Ebel A, Meeker M, Maudsley AA. Volumetric proton spectroscopic imaging of mild traumatic brain injury. AJNR Am J Neuroradiol. 2004; 25: 730–737

[141] Son BC, Park CK, Choi BG et al. Metabolic changes in pericontusional oedematous areas in mild head injury evaluated by 1 H MRS. Acta Neurochir Suppl (Wien). 2000; 76: 13–16

[142] Garnett MR, Blamire AM, Rajagopalan B, Styles P, Cadoux-Hudson TA. Evidence for cellular damage in normal-appearing white matter correlates with injury severity in patients following traumatic brain injury: a magnetic resonance spectroscopy study. Brain. 2000; 123: 1403–1409

[143] Bayly PV, Cohen TS, Leister EP, Ajo D, Leuthardt EC, Genin GM. Deformation of the human brain induced by mild acceleration. J Neurotrauma 2005; 22: 845–856

[144] Viano DC, Casson IR, Pellman EJ, Zhang L, King AI, Yang KH. Concussion in professional football: brain responses by finite element analysis: part 9. Neurosurgery. 2005; 57: 891–916

Index